Person-Centered Planning

Person-Centered Planning

*Research, Practice,
and Future Directions*

edited by

Steve Holburn, Ph.D.

and

Peter M. Vietze, Ph.D.

New York State Institute for
Basic Research in Developmental Disabilities
Staten Island

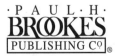

·P·A·U·L·H·
BROOKES
PUBLISHING CO. ®

Baltimore • London • Sydney

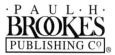

Paul H. Brookes Publishing Co.
Post Office Box 10624
Baltimore, Maryland 21285-0624

www.brookespublishing.com

Typeset by Auburn Associates, Inc., Baltimore, Maryland.
Manufactured in the United States of America by
Versa Press, Inc., East Peoria, Illinois.

Permission to reprint the following is gratefully acknowledged:

Excerpt on p. 399 from "Numbers and Faces," copyright 1951 by W.H. Auden, from W.H. AUDEN: THE COLLECTED POEMS by W.H. Auden. Used by permission of Random House, Inc.

Excerpt on p. xxi from Eliade, M. (1985). *Symbolism, the sacred, and the arts.* New York: The Crossroad Publishing Company; reprinted by permission.

The stories in this book are based on the authors' experiences. In some cases, individuals' names and other identifying information have been changed to protect their identities. Other vignettes are composite accounts that do not represent the lives or experiences of specific individuals, and no implications should be inferred.

Library of Congress Cataloging-in-Publication Data

Person-centered planning : research, practice, and future directions /
edited by Steve Holburn and Peter M. Vietze.
    p.   cm.
  Includes bibliographical references and index.
  ISBN 1-55766-590-7
  I. Holburn, Steve. II. Vietze, Peter, 1944–
HV1570 .P47 2002
362.1'968—dc21

2002022759

British Library Cataloguing in Publication data are available from the British
Library.

Contents

Self determinatia

About the Editors

Steve Holburn, Ph.D., Research Scientist, New York State Institute for Basic Research in Developmental Disabilities, 1050 Forest Hill Road, Staten Island, NY 10314. Dr. Holburn's career has focused on research and treatment of people with developmental disabilities and challenging behavior. He is best known for his work in the areas of clinical interventions for self-injurious air swallowing, reducing residential overregulation, and the effects of person-centered planning on problem behavior.

After receiving a master's degree in clinical psychology at Ball State University in 1973, Dr. Holburn worked in a large residential setting until receiving his doctoral degree in special education from the University of New Mexico in 1984. His residential research included the areas of employee job satisfaction, evaluating the impact of standards for intermediate care facilities for people with mental retardation, and applied behavior analysis of self-injury. In 1993, Dr. Holburn assumed his position at the New York State Institute for Basic Research in Developmental Disabilities, where he has continued his interests in residential issues and is conducting research and treatment in the areas of person-centered planning, assistive technology, health promotion, and parents with cognitive disabilities. He is an active member of the American Association on Mental Retardation and the Association for Behavior Analysis as well as a consulting editor for *Mental Retardation.*

Peter M. Vietze, Ph.D., Deputy Director, Chairman of the Department of Infant Development, New York State Institute for Basic Research in Developmental Disabilities, 1050 Forest Hill Road, Staten Island, NY 10314. Dr. Vietze is a developmental psychologist and educator who received his doctoral degree from Wayne State University in 1969. After completing a postdoctoral fellowship at University of California, Berkeley, he joined the faculty of George Peabody College for Teachers in Nashville. There he conducted research on early learning, perception, and socialization in human infants. In 1976, he moved to the National Institute for Child Health and Human Development (NICHD), where he conducted research on infant motivation and social development. Dr. Vietze became the Head of the NICHD Mental Retardation Research Centers Program in 1980 and remained there until 1987, when he moved to his present position in New York. He is also a Professor at the City University of New York.

Dr. Vietze has published more than 95 research articles, chapters, and reviews and is co-author or co-editor of seven books on infant development and developmental disabilities. He is known for developing new techniques for studying infants and for his work on the causes of child maltreatment. Most recently, Dr. Vietze has been involved in projects concerned with person-centered planning, parents with learning problems, and assistive technology.

About the Contributors

Brian Abery, Ph.D., Project Director, Institute on Community Integration, University of Minnesota, 150 Pillsbury Drive Southeast, 107 Pattee Hall, Minneapolis, MN 55455. Dr. Abery is Coordinator of School-Age Services at the University of Minnesota's Institute on Community Integration, Research Associate in the Rehabilitation Research and Training Center on Community Living, and an adjunct faculty member within the university's school psychology program. He has been a principal investigator and director of numerous federal projects funded through the Office of Special Education and Rehabilitative Services, the National Institute on Disability and Rehabilitation Research, and private foundations designed to promote person-centered planning, self-determination, and the social inclusion of people with disabilities. Dr. Abery has published journal articles and technical reports and has developed products on the topics of person-centered planning, self-determination, and residential services. He has also presented at numerous national and international conferences. Dr. Abery is co-editor of the book *Challenges for a Service System in Transition: Ensuring Quality Community Experiences for Persons with Developmental Disabilities* (1994, Paul H. Brookes Publishing Co.), which speaks to the challenges that professionals face in providing supports to people with developmental disabilities.

Angela Novak Amado, Ph.D., Executive Director of the Human Services Research and Development Center, 1195 Juno Avenue, St. Paul, MN 55116; Research Associate, Institute on Community Integration, Research and Training Center on Community Living, University of Minnesota, Minneapolis, MN 55455. For more than 25 years, Dr. Amado has worked with people with developmental disabilities in a variety of capacities, including national research, state government, direct support, and university teaching. Her books, manuals, articles, and training in person-centered planning and promoting friendships between people with and without disabilities is internationally recognized. She has traveled throughout the United States, Canada, and other countries, providing training and consultation on community bridge-building.

Heather Becker, Ph.D., Research Scientist, Lecturer, School of Nursing, The University of Texas at Austin, 1700 Red River, Austin, TX 78701. Dr. Becker holds a doctoral degree in educational psychology from The University of Texas at Austin, with a concentration in program evaluation. Since the early 1980s, she has conducted applied research projects and program evaluations for various human services programs, primarily in the areas of education, health, and disability services. She is a co-developer of the Functional Skills Screening Inventory, an assessment of functional skills in people with developmental disabilities that is used in schools and rehabilitation facilities throughout the United States. Dr. Becker is past chairperson for the Health Evaluation Topical

Interest Group of the American Evaluation Association and was appointed to the evaluation review panel of the U.S. Department of Health and Human Services. She has taught graduate courses and made community presentations on research design, measurement issues, and program evaluation. She assesses evaluation activities for the Texas Center for Disability Studies. Dr. Becker has authored or co-authored more than 40 publications, including *Making Evaluation Work for You: A Guidebook for Programs that Serve Persons with Developmental Disabilities* (1992, Texas Consortium for Developmental Disabilities).

Stan Butkus, Ph.D., Director, South Carolina Department of Disabilities and Special Needs, 3440 Harden Street Extension, Post Office Box 4706, Columbia, SC 29240. Dr. Butkus has extensive experience in the field of developmental disabilities at the local, regional, and state levels in roles ranging from live-in community group-home coordination to local/regional service development and management. He has directed Virginia's state office of mental retardation, served as Chief Executive Officer of a large institution, and served as an associate commissioner for community and facility services. In his work in South Carolina, Dr. Butkus has established policies and practices to increase self-determination for people with disabilities, to simplify funding and equalize service resources through a capitated funding model, and to implement outcome evaluation methodologies for services. His academic training includes graduate degrees in social work, public administration, and special education and a doctoral degree in social welfare.

Paula Davis, Ph.D., Professor, Rehabilitation Institute, Southern Illinois University, Carbondale, IL, 62901. Dr. Davis has a master's degree in behavior analysis and therapy and a doctoral degree in special education. She is the coordinator of the undergraduate program in Rehabilitation Services at Southern Illinois University at Carbondale. Her areas of interest include self-determination and choice for people with disabilities. Previously, Dr. Davis was the co-director of an interdisciplinary program to prepare special educators and rehabilitation professionals to work with students with disabilities as they leave high school. She has presented and published on the topic of community living skills and supported living.

Denise De La Garza, Ph.D., CRC, LPC, Director of Distance Learning, Texas Center for Disability Studies, A University Center for Excellence in Disability Education, Research, and Service, The University of Texas at Austin, 4030 West Braker Lane, Building 1, Suite 180, Mail Code L4000, Austin, TX 78759. Dr. De La Garza received a master's degree in social and psychological services and holds a doctoral degree in special education, with a specialization in rehabilitation counselor education. She taught for more than 10 years in a rehabilitation counselor education program. Dr. De La Garza also worked at both the Texas School for the Blind and Visually Impaired and the Texas Commission for the Blind. She is a licensed psychotherapist and maintains a part-time private practice. Dr. De La Garza's research interests and publications focus on disability-related cultural and gender issues.

Shelley Dumas, Ph.D., Director of Community Education, Texas Center for Disability Studies, A University Center for Excellence in Disability Education, Research, and Service, The University of Texas at Austin, 4030 West Braker Lane, Building 1, Suite 180, Mail Code L4000, Austin, TX 78759. Since the late 1980s, Dr. Dumas has worked on program development and evaluation and training and technical assistance in the areas of self-determination, person-centered planning, and inclusive community and education practices for people with developmental disabilities and their families. Dr. Dumas has conducted this work with individuals and families as well as with national, state, and local agencies and organizations. She is the parent of a young adult with developmental disabilities.

Sarah Elkin, M.A., Doctoral Candidate, Department of Educational Psychology, University of Minnesota, Minneapolis; School Psychologist Intern, Stillwater Area High School, Stillwater, Minnesota. Ms. Elkin has a bachelor of arts degree in psychology from Trinity University in San Antonio, Texas, and a master of arts degree in educational psychology from the University of Minnesota. She worked for 4 years as a research assistant at the University of Minnesota's Institute on Community Integration, studying the self-determination of adults with developmental disabilities. Ms. Elkin is co-author of two articles on self-determination. She has also helped develop training curricula for residential service staff about supporting the self-determination of the people whom they serve. In addition, as part of the sibling support programs of The Arc of Hennepin and Carver Counties (Minnesota), Ms. Elkin has written curricula for children who have siblings with developmental disabilities.

Gerald Faw, M.S., Behavior Analyst, Center for Comprehensive Services, Post Office Box 2825, Carbondale, IL 62902. Mr. Faw has a master's degree in behavior analysis and therapy. With more than 25 years of experience working with people with a variety disabilities—including mental retardation, dual diagnoses, and traumatic brain injury—his areas of interest include the development of behavioral systems for assessing a person's lifestyle satisfaction and functional analysis of the environmental factors affecting mood.

David Felce, Ph.D., Research Professor, Director, Welsh Centre for Learning Disabilities Applied Research Unit, University of Wales College of Medicine, Meridian Court, North Road, Cardiff, CF14 3BG, Wales. Dr. Felce's first research post (1973–1986) was at the University of Southampton, where he conducted research on the quality of residential services for people with severe or profound mental retardation. After 3 years as the Director of the British Institute of Mental Handicap, Dr. Felce was appointed to his current post. His research interests include the measurement of quality of life, the determinants of quality in community housing services, the analysis and amelioration of challenging behavior, and general service development in intellectual disabilities. He is co-editor of the *Journal of Applied Research in Intellectual Disabilities* and serves on the editorial board of seven other mental retardation journals. He is a fellow and President-Elect of the International Association for the Scientific Study of Intellectual Disabilities.

Lise Fox, Ph.D., Associate Professor, Department of Child and Family Studies, Louis de la Parte Florida Mental Health Institute, University of South Florida, 13301 Bruce B. Downs Boulevard, Tampa, FL 33612. In addition to her work at the Department of Child and Family Studies, Dr. Fox's publications and research interests include supporting children with disabilities and challenging behavior in developmentally appropriate environments, positive behavior support, and family support.

Carolyn W. Green, Ed.D., School Administrator, Rosewood Resource Center, Western Carolina Center, 300 Enola Road, Morganton, NC 28655. Dr. Green has more than 25 years of experience designing, implementing, and supervising education and residential services for people diagnosed with severe and profound multiple disabilities. She has co-authored more than 30 refereed journal articles and book chapters on program development and evaluation. Dr. Green has received recognition from the readership of the *Journal of The Association for Persons with Severe Handicaps* for providing the most useful information for effective classroom services for students with profound multiple disabilities. Most recently, Dr. Green received the North Carolina Eugene A. Hargrove Mental Health Research Award for practical application of research focusing on service delivery systems for people with significant disabilities.

Edwin Jones, Ph.D., Senior Research Fellow, Welsh Centre for Learning Disabilities Applied Research Unit, University of Wales College of Medicine, Meridian Court, North Road, Cardiff, CF14 3BG, Wales. For several years, Dr. Jones was a senior manager of community-based supported housing services for people with learning disabilities. He provides training in Active Support to enable staff teams to adopt a more structured approach to supporting clients to participate in a wide range of typical activities. His main research interest concerns the impact of training staff in Active Support and the extent of tenant participation in supported housing for people with learning disabilities. Dr. Jones also teaches postgraduate courses concerning challenging behavior and the management of supported housing services. He maintains an interest in rights-based approaches, is involved with self-advocacy groups, and has previously worked with homeless people and on housing rights in Wales.

Diane Bannerman Juracek, Ph.D., Senior Administrator, Community Living Opportunities, 2113 Delaware Street, Lawrence, KS 66046. Dr. Juracek has been working in the field of developmental disabilities for 20 years, specializing in self-determination and effective teaching techniques. In addition to her work at Community Living Opportunities, a not-for-profit organization providing supports to children and adults with severe developmental disabilities, Dr. Juracek is an adjunct faculty member in the Department of Human Development and Family Life at The University of Kansas and is a Board Certified Behavior Analyst.

Don Kincaid, Ed.D., Associate Professor, Department of Child and Family Studies, Louis de la Parte Florida Mental Health Institute, University of South Florida, 13301 Bruce B. Downs Boulevard, Tampa, FL 33612. Dr. Kincaid directs the Center for Autism and Related Disabilities and Florida's Positive Behavior Support Project at the University of South Florida. His professional interests include person-centered planning, positive behavior support, disabilities, and school and systems change.

Kevin P. Klatt, Ph.D., Assistant Professor, Psychology Department, University of Wisconsin, Eau Claire, WI 54702. Dr. Klatt has a master's degree in behavior analysis from Southern Illinois University and a doctoral degree in developmental and child psychology from The University of Kansas. Dr. Klatt is a Board Certified Behavior Analyst whose primary interests include using applied behavior analysis in community settings for people diagnosed with developmental disabilities, autism, and attention-deficit/hyperactivity disorder. His research includes investigating contextual variables and identifying conditions that promote active engagement. Dr. Klatt teaches courses and conducts research in the new emphasis in behavior analysis at the University of Wisconsin–Eau Claire.

Kathi Kelly Lacy, Ph.D., Director, Office of Policy and Division of Mental Retardation, South Carolina Department of Disabilities and Special Needs, 3440 Harden Street Extension, Post Office Box 4706, Columbia, SC 29240. Dr. Lacy is responsible for policy analysis and development of all services and supports to people with mental retardation and related disabilities in South Carolina. She has been influential in the statewide development and implementation of person-centered planning for people with lifelong disabilities.

K. Charlie Lakin, Ph.D., Director, Rehabilitation Research and Training Center on Community Living, 150 Pillsbury Drive Southeast, 214 Pattee Hall, University of Minnesota, Minneapolis, MN 55455. Dr. Lakin has 30 years of experience in services to individuals with developmental disabilities as a teacher, researcher, trainer, consultant, and advocate. He has authored or co-authored 200 books, monographs, journal articles, book chapters, and published technical reports. Dr. Lakin has been a frequent consultant to federal and state agencies in matters of policy, research, and evaluation, and he actively works with numerous state and local government agencies and with academic and private research organizations. Dr. Lakin has been an officer or director of numerous professional, advocacy, and service organizations at local, state, and national levels. He is Associate Editor of *Mental Retardation* and serves as an editorial board member of the *Journal of The Association for Persons with Severe Handicaps, Journal of Intellectual and Developmental Disability,* and the *Journal of Social Science and Disability.* Recognition afforded to Dr. Lakin includes the Dybwad Humanitarian Award of the American Association on Mental Retardation, appointments by former President Clinton to the President's Committee on Mental Retardation, and the University of Minnesota's Outstanding Community Service Award.

Kathy Lowe, Ph.D., Senior Research Fellow, Welsh Centre for Learning Disabilities, Department of Psychological Medicine, University of Wales College of Medicine, Meridian Court, North Road, Cardiff, CF14 3BG, Wales. Dr. Lowe has

25 years of experience of education and research in learning disabilities. In the 1980s, she worked on the development and longitudinal evaluation of NIM-ROD, a keynote government-funded feasibility project in community-based services. Dr. Lowe has since undertaken research in a variety of areas, including specialist community intervention in challenging behavior, quality and costs of residential services, staff training and selection, and primary health care. She has published widely in these areas. In addition, she directs two postgraduate courses on staffed housing and challenging behavior for senior service personnel, supervises master's and doctoral students, and trains direct care staff in Active Support. She is also the book review editor for the *Journal of Intellectual Disability Research*; is an external consultant with the Community Care Development Centre, King's College in London; and retains an active role in several local voluntary sector agencies.

Darlene Magito-McLaughlin, Ph.D., Clinical Psychologist, Co-founder of Positive Behavior Support Consulting, 68 Oakdale Road, Centerport, NY 11721. Dr. Magito-McLaughlin is an independent consultant who works directly with families who are pursuing person-centered approaches through self-determination or waiver services. She also serves as Lecturer and Testing Supervisor at the State University of New York at Stony Brook, and she works as a consultant for school districts in the area of transition planning for adolescents. Previously, Dr. Magito-McLaughlin served as the Clinical Director at Developmental Disabilities Institute in New York state. She has been working in the field of disabilities for more than 15 years, and her credits include numerous publications and presentations.

Paul H. Malette, Ph.D., Director, CBI Consultants, 6862 Copper Cove Road, West Vancouver, British Columbia, V7W 2K5, Canada. Since 1990, Dr. Malette has been one of the directors of CBI Consultants. He has more than 20 years of experience working with children and adults with autism and cognitive disabilities who engage in challenging behavior and require extensive supports to learn new skills. In 1992, he and his colleagues co-authored a paper describing the Lifestyle Development Process (LDP) that was published in the *Journal of The Association for Persons with Severe Handicaps*. Dr. Malette and his colleagues at CBI Consultants have used the LDP to create a person-centered consulting and training framework. Dr. Malette continues to focus his research and training on positive, person-centered supports that are designed to improve the quality of life of the focus person and his or her family.

Michael D. Marsalis, B.A., Program Manager/Coordinator, Developmental Disabilities Institute, 19 Bond Lane, Nesconset, NY 11767. Mr. Marsalis has more than 5 years of experience in the human services field. He is a human services initiator and is employed by the Developmental Disabilities Institute at Bond Lane, where he is responsible for the community inclusion of individuals with autism and mental retardation. Mr. Marsalis and his staff include and assess the consumers whom they serve and handle all facets of everyday life in a 24-hour residential facility. He is a trained counselor for parent and government intervention and is pursuing a master's of science degree in special education, with a specialization in early childhood intervention, at Hofstra University in Hempstead, New York.

Carolyn Martin, M.S.W., Program Director, Parsons State Hospital and Training Center, 2601 Gabriel, Parsons, KS 67357. Ms. Martin is a credentialed Essential Lifestyle Planner. In addition to her social work background, she has clinical and research experience in parent training, adult education, and applied behavior analysis, as well as in assessment and treatment of aggression, self-injury, and deviant sexual behavior in people with developmental disabilities.

David B. McAdam, Ph.D., Behavioral Psychologist, The Lindens Neurobehavioral Stabilization Program, Bancroft NeuroHealth, Hopkins Lane, Post Office Box 20, Haddonfield, NJ 08033. Dr. McAdam received his doctoral degree in developmental and child psychology from The University of Kansas. His research interests include behavioral analysis in developmental disabilities.

Marijo W. McBride, M.Ed., Institute on Community Integration, College of Education and Human Development, University of Minnesota, 150 Pillsbury Drive Southeast, 103 Pattee Hall, Minneapolis, MN 55455. On a personal and professional level, Ms. McBride has been involved in disability issues for more than 30 years. She coordinates a number of activities at the Institute on Community Integration, including person-centered planning outreach and training, the Certificate on Disability Policy and Services program, and the community component of the developmental disabilities rotation for pediatricians. Ms. McBride has developed and delivered innumerable workshops for parents, consumers, and professionals in the areas of self-determination, self-advocacy, empowerment, and person-centered planning, and she has worked as a consultant on these topics for state and national agencies. Her credits include numerous presentations and publications.

K. Renee Norman, M.A., Behavioral Dimensions, 415 Blank Road North, Hopkins, MN 55343. Ms. Norman received a master's degree in behavior analysis and early childhood education from The University of Kansas. Ms. Norman is a Board Certified Associate Behavior Analyst who has worked in the field of human services and applied behavior analysis for more than 14 years. She works as a consultant for children with autism and their families.

Connie Lyle O'Brien and **John O'Brien,** Responsive Systems Associates, 58 Willowick Drive, Lithonia, GA 30038. The O'Briens work in partnership to learn about building more just and inclusive communities for people with disabilities, their families, and their allies. They use what they learn to advise people with disabilities and their families, advocacy groups, service providers, and governments and to spread the news among people interested in change by writing and through workshops. They are affiliated with the Center on Human Policy at Syracuse University and the Centre for Integrated Education and Community in Toronto, Ontario, Canada.

Jerry A. Rea, Ph.D., Assistant Research Professor, Schiefelbusch Institute for Life Span Studies, The University of Kansas; Program Director, Parsons State Hospital and Training Center; 2601 Gabriel, Parsons, KS 67357. Dr. Rea has a background in applied behavior analysis. His clinical research experience has involved the assessment and treatment of clinically significant behaviors such as cigarette smoking cessation, deviant sexual behavior, self-injury, and aggression in individuals with developmental disabilities. He is also a credentialed Essential Lifestyle Planner.

Dennis H. Reid, Ph.D., Director, Carolina Behavior Analysis and Support Center, Post Office Box 425, Morganton, NC 28680. In addition to his work at the Carolina Behavior Analysis and Support Center, Dr. Reid serves in a part-time capacity as Co-director of the Leadership and Management Training Project of the Louisiana State University Health Sciences Center. Dr. Reid has more than 25 years of experience as a practitioner in settings providing supports for people with severe disabilities, and he has contributed more than 100 applied research articles to the published literature. He serves on the editorial boards of numerous journals, including the *Journal of Applied Behavior Analysis* and the *Journal of The Association for Persons with Severe Handicaps.*

David A. Rotholz, Ph.D., Clinical Associate Professor and Project Director, Center for Disability Resources, Department of Pediatrics, University of South Carolina School of Medicine, Columbia, SC 29208. Dr. Rotholz has more than 20 years of experience working with adults, children, and youth with developmental disabilities. His work during the past several years includes statewide systems change in positive behavior support and evaluation and planning activities in person-centered planning. His previous positions include Director of Evaluation and Clinical Studies for the South Carolina Department of Disabilities and Special Needs; Clinical Director, Director of Behavioral Services, and Training Director at the New England Center for Autism; and Psychology Director at Whitten Center in South Carolina. He has also worked as a senior clinical/ research staff member at the University of Minnesota's Institute for Disabilities Studies and as a learning specialist and teacher at the May Institute. Dr. Rotholz has published works on positive behavior support, ecobehavioral analysis, augmentative and alternative communication, and national trends in residential setting use. His other professional efforts include leadership positions with national, state, and local disability organizations and consultation/training work in the areas of positive behavior support, teaching methods, and system enhancement for people with developmental disabilities.

Helen Sanderson, Ph.D., Advisor, North West Training and Development Team, 34 Broomfield Road, Heaton Moor, Stockport, Cheshire, SK4 4ND, England. Dr. Sanderson has a master's degree in quality assurance in health and social care and a doctoral degree in person-centered planning and organizational change. She is the primary author of *People, Plans and Possibilities: Exploring Person Centred Planning* (1997, SHS Ltd.), a book on person-centered planning that emerged from 3 years of research and was supported by the Joseph Rowntree Foundation.

In addition, with Martin Routledge, Dr. Sanderson has written guidance on person-centered planning for England's Department of Health.

Penny Seay, Ph.D., Executive Director, Texas Center for Disability Studies, College of Education, A University Center for Excellence in Disability Education, Research, and Service, The University of Texas at Austin, 4030 West Braker Lane, Building 1, Suite 180, Mail Code L4000, Austin, TX 78759. Dr. Seay holds a doctoral degree in special education from The University of Texas at Austin, with a concentration in severe disabilities. Dr. Seay has worked in the disability advocacy field for more than 25 years, particularly in promoting the full inclusion of people with disabilities through public policy and person-centered community supports. Her interests include developing individual supports and strategies to facilitate community inclusion for people with disabilities, inclusion of students with disabilities in general education classrooms, research related to service system inequities, and assistive technology. In addition, Dr. Seay has extensive experience in researching and writing grant proposals. She is the past president of the Association of University Centers on Disabilities (formerly the American Association of University Affiliated Programs) and served 6 years on the association's board of directors. She teaches graduate and undergraduate courses and gives community presentations on topics related to the inclusion of people with disabilities in schools and community life.

Jan Bowen Sheldon, Ph.D., J.D., Professor, Department of Human Development and Family Life, School of Law, Director, Edna A. Hill Child Development Center, The University of Kansas, 4001 Dole Center, Lawrence, KS 66045. Dr. Sheldon has a doctorate degree in developmental and child psychology and a juris doctorate degree. She is a consultant for and member of the board of directors for Community Living Opportunities, a community-based program serving children and adults with severe and profound developmental disabilities. Dr. Sheldon has conducted research and published numerous articles on intervention programs for people with disabilities, children and youth, and families. She has also written extensively on the legal rights of and ethical issues involved with dependent populations. She is a fellow of the American Psychological Association and a licensed attorney.

James A. Sherman, Ph.D., Professor, Department of Human Development and Family Life, The University of Kansas, 4001 Dole Center, Lawrence, KS 66045. Dr. Sherman has conducted research in and published on the social skill development of children and adults, the evaluation of methods to teach language to children with developmental disabilities, and the evaluation of community intervention programs for adults with developmental disabilities. He has also participated extensively in the development of community programs serving children with autism and adults with developmental disabilities. Previously, he served as Chair of the Department of Human Development and Family Life at The University of Kansas for 25 years. Dr. Sherman is a fellow of the American Psychological Association.

Michael Smull, Director, Support Development Associates, 3245 Harness Creek Road, Annapolis, MD 21403. Mr. Smull has been working with people with disabilities since 1973. He has had extensive experience in nearly all aspects of developing community services. He founded two community agencies; helped a number of agencies convert from programs to supports; and helped states, regions, and counties change their structures to support self-determination. He has also worked to help people leave institutions and, most recently, was a consultant in the closure of Fairview Training Center in Oregon. He has written extensively on issues related to supporting people with challenging behaviors, person-centered planning, and the challenge of changing the system to support self-determination. From 1982 through 1997 he was affiliated with the University of Maryland. By 1997, he was Research Assistant Professor with the Department of Counseling and Personnel Services at the university's College Park campus and Clinical Assistant Professor with the Department of Pediatrics at the University of Maryland School of Medicine in Baltimore. Mr. Smull is a consultant who helps agencies, regions, and states learn how to conduct person-centered planning, implement the developed plans, and make the organizational changes needed for successful implementation. He recently developed a manual and process for families and individuals to develop their own person-centered plans without relying on people in the system to do it for them. Mr. Smull is the co-developer of Essential Lifestyle Planning and has worked in 47 states, Canada, and the United Kingdom.

Thomas R. Spinosa, M.A., P.D., Lead Teacher/Supervisor, Applied Behavior Analysis Programs, TheraCare: Medical, Educational, and Evaluation Services, 97–45 Queens Boulevard, Rego Park, NY 11374. Mr. Spinosa has a master's degree in special education and a professional diploma in educational administration and supervision. He has more than 25 years of experience in working with children and adults with autism. Mr. Spinosa has served as a classroom teacher, home-based itinerant teacher, parent trainer, and teacher trainer. In addition, he has directed various programs for individuals with autism including respite care; education; and adult residential, adult day, and vocational programs. Mr. Spinosa has participated in extensive programmatic and research efforts, including the provision of community-based support utilizing positive behavior support strategies and person-centered planning for individuals with autism and severe problem behavior. (The author can be reached at rochsroom@cs.com.)

Gregory A. Wagner, Ph.D., Senior Psychologist, California Department of Developmental Services, 1600 9th Street, Room 340 (MS 3-15), Sacramento, CA 95814. Dr. Wagner received his doctoral degree from The University of Kansas and was a fellow at the Kennedy Krieger Institute, an affiliate of The Johns Hopkins University School of Medicine. For more than 25 years, he has worked in several states in a variety of settings and roles in the field of developmental disabilities. For 10 years, Dr. Wagner has provided statewide consultation and oversight regarding behavioral and psychological services for people with developmental disabilities in California. He is President of the California Association for Behavior Analysis.

Michael L. Wehmeyer, Ph.D., Associate Professor, Department of Special Education, School of Education, Associate Director, Beach Center on Disability, The University of Kansas, Haworth Hall, 1200 Sunnyside Avenue, Room 3136, Lawrence, KS 66045. Dr. Wehmeyer is engaged in teacher personnel preparation in the area of severe multiple disabilities. He also directs multiple federally funded projects to conduct research in and develop methods and materials to promote the causal agency and self-determination of children, youth, and adults with cognitive and developmental disabilities. He is the author of more than 80 articles or book chapters on self-determination, student involvement, transition, and assistive technology; has authored, co-authored, or co-edited 10 books on topics including self-determination, student involvement, gender equity, and mental retardation; and is a frequent conference speaker. Dr. Wehmeyer holds undergraduate and master's degrees in special education from The University of Tulsa and a master's degree in experimental psychology from the University of Sussex in Brighton, England. He earned his doctoral degree in human development and communication sciences from The University of Texas at Dallas.

Kasey Wright, Client Training Specialist, Parsons State Hospital and Training Center, 2601 Gabriel, Parson, KS 67357. Ms. Wright has been a client training specialist for 8 years. Her duties are to assist in the development and implementation of research programs at Parsons State Hospital and Training Center. Ms. Wright has co-authored research in the areas of assessment and treatment of deviant sexual arousal, assessment and treatment of chronic aberrant behavior, and smoking cessation in individuals with developmental disabilities.

Foreword

It is good to find that, in these times, there are those who meet to
exchange their ideas concerning the ultimate goals of existence.
What could be more moving in our community here on earth than to
listen closely to a human heart, to hear in it the throbbings of
a world, its sighs and its dreams?
—*Marc Chagall, 1963*

The essence of person-centered planning is to listen closely to the
hearts of people with disabilities and to imagine with them a better
world in which they can be valued members, contribute, and belong.
This quest involves building a more compassionate, cooperative community in which people with disabilities can take their rightful place as
respected citizens. The task requires all of us in human services to radically reexamine our assumptions, commitments, and investments, then
change the way that we relate to people with disabilities, each other,
and the organizations through which we work. Individually, in our
own small ways, if we are involved in person-centered work, we are
remaking the world. Collectively, this is a big job.

In these times of deep searching, it is important to exchange ideas
about these ultimate goals, to find new ways to understand the scope of
our work together, and to see if we are doing the right things on behalf
of people with disabilities. *Person-Centered Planning: Research, Practice,
and Future Directions* makes an important contribution to this exploration. It helps us see the big picture, validate our experience, build
knowledge and understanding, and stay committed to the struggle. As
human services providers, we need to seek and comprehend many perspectives, which include the viewpoints of people with disabilities and
their loved ones, activists, direct support staff, artists, philosophers, scientists, academics, innovators, teachers, and policy makers.

Person-centered planning is both a philosophy and a set of related
activities that leads to simultaneous multilevel change. From its beginnings, person-centered work has been a complex, interactive, dynamic,
long-term process of personal, organizational, and social change—a
process that can never authentically be reduced to or measured by its
smallest parts. Artists, scientists, and policy makers each face the limits
of their media, their inability to capture and present the total reality of
this comprehensive change. Each selects an angle on reality that will
contribute to transforming the whole. As we work on behalf of people

with disabilities toward social change, families, storytellers, and artists are challenged to represent their truths through honest and inspiring stories and images. Academic researchers are challenged to find new ways to measure the causes and effects of multidimensional change. Policy makers confront the awesome task of translating powerful platforms for change into the real world of more and more people with disabilities. Multiple and diverse perspectives enable all of us to validate whether we are doing the right thing, then commit ourselves to the hard work of doing more of it.

This book's contributors assume that person-centered planning is a valid investment. The researchers among them use their preferred perspectives and tools of inquiry to examine part of the big picture—and, thus, identify conditions under which person-centered planning works or does not work—to make worthwhile changes. Taken together, their findings contribute to a greater understanding of the complexity of person-centered planning, and they add to the growing body of knowledge and experience that causes us to reflect on what we are doing and whether we are truly making a difference. Each perspective represented in this book points to bodies of theory and practice that enrich the practice of person-centered planning and extend our collective ability to do the right thing. It facilitates conversation among practitioners of positive behavior support, self-efficacy theorists, advocates for self-determination, and agents of organizational and systemic change. Every reader is likely to encounter new ideas and new ways to understand how people with disabilities want to live as full citizens and, therefore, act to realize that understanding.

Taken together, these studies confirm my 20 years of experience with person-centered planning. The most significant changes happen in people's lives when person-centered planning catalyzes the commitment of a small group of people who work toward many levels of change, which usually lead to small, individualized service environments that are focused on a positive vision for a particular person. When concentrated, committed listening to people incites the activism necessary to invent individualized supports. Then, the preferences of people are most likely to be respected, and responses are more likely to lead to daring and imaginative connections to community life. When person-centered planning is implemented without fundamentally changing traditional service settings, it may lead to some interesting programmatic tweaking, but positive outcomes are less impressive and often impossible to sustain over time.

Person-centered work awakens our connection to the basic experience of the lives of people with disabilities, and it renews our desire to build a better world with and for them. This involves us in a journey with people through their lives. We make our way by learning to listen more closely and compassionately to the many ways through which people communicate their despair and desires, by working together to build community, and by going together to whatever rivers of hope keep the work alive. *Person-Centered Planning: Research, Practice, and Future Directions* will increase our understanding of the many elements of the journey.

Beth Mount, Ph.D.
Graphic Futures
New York, NY

Preface

In the space of just one decade, person-centered planning has risen from a little-known way of helping disenfranchised people to a popular philosophy and approach in the field of developmental disabilities. Unlike other practices common to the field, such as special education and applied behavior analysis, person-centered planning did not evolve gradually from professional practice and research. To the contrary, this method differs from traditional professional practice, and it is a challenge to traditional research methods. Nonetheless, person-centered planning *is* widely practiced and it *does* have a methodology. Thus, it has become clear that it is possible to conduct a systematic investigation of person-centered planning. The field now needs information to guide the further planning and development of this popular method. In *Person-Centered Planning: Research, Practice, and Future Directions,* we hope to supply that information and to signify that the research exists.

One might speculate about why a service system would adopt an approach that is antithetical to system-centered service provision (Mount, 1992; O'Brien, & Lovett, 1992). We are more interested in speculating about why there has been almost no published research on how that might be accomplished. From our vantage point, there are many aspects of the process that, until recently, have discouraged investigators from tackling questions such as "Does person-centered planning really work?" and "How can we best adopt person-centered planning to maximize its effectiveness?" In short, there has been a dearth of research investigating this important area because those who conduct applied research have faced difficulties in implementing person-centered planning and assessing its effects.

We have learned firsthand that the process itself is not easy—it can be very complex, it takes longer to complete than other interventions, and its success often hinges on the cooperation of interlocking organizational systems. Person-centered planning asks for nurturance, even if resources are already stretched to the limit. It requires agencies to reach beyond the usual procedural boundaries and assist people in ways that, in the past, were considered unwarranted or superfluous. Perhaps the most challenging hurdle in researching person-centered planning is that in its mission to achieve individualized outcomes, person-centered planning resists standardization of procedures. These challenges present significant complications for researchers who are trying to evaluate person-centered planning in a faithful manner. In the realm of intervention research, close adherence to the process is important not only to ensure that the researcher reports findings about a given method (and not something else), but also because the process requires replication to form a body of evidence about the effectiveness of the procedure under investigation.

In addition to the challenges of faithful and replicable intervention, investigators must also grapple with the problem of reliable assessment of person-centered planning outcomes. In 2002, it is common to promote goals such as personal autonomy and meaningful relationships for people with developmental disabilities, but it is not so common for *researchers* to venture into these territories. Axiomatic to applied research, including person-centered planning investigations, is that long-term, multifaceted interventions that target broad, life-defining outcomes are the least amenable to a scientific analysis.

It is encouraging that researchers have begun to clearly define and measure quality-of-life goals, which heretofore have remained elusive to investigators and, therefore, not within their purview. Even so, improvements in quality of life are not as tangible as dollars earned or number of words spelled correctly, nor are they easily represented on a graph. For example, a two-fold increase in a variable called "life satisfaction" is harder to conceptualize, and perhaps less believable, than a doubling in the percentage of housing costs. Thus, even when investigators are able to implement person-centered planning in a faithful manner, they still face the problems of measuring, displaying, and interpreting its outcomes. Because of these challenges, we believe that person-centered planning is the most difficult approach to research that the field of developmental disabilities has confronted. Fortunately, in the scientific search for invention and discovery, the most difficult challenges often lead to the most important findings.

We know that there is a need to provide an outlet for person-centered planning research, but we also know that it is important for the research to be of high quality. Accordingly, all original research chapters in this book were peer reviewed by researchers who understand the challenges in implementing the components of person-centered planning and measuring its outcomes. Yet, the reviewers also held the investigators to a standard of proof that reflected an acceptable level of believability. Conceptual and practice-oriented chapters were reviewed by experts who understand that advances in the effectiveness of person-centered planning will be informed by variations of the process and frank discussion of the surrounding issues.

In addressing the challenges of implementing and evaluating person-centered planning, the book's authors present creative solutions to these obstacles. They have made some interesting discoveries that will no doubt affect ways in which service providers will apply current person-centered planning principles. Through the successes and failures described in *Person-Centered Planning: Research, Practice, and Future Directions,* the authors have demonstrated conditions under which person-centered planning does and does not work, and they have provided the field with information about how individuals and agencies can best adopt person-centered planning to maximize its effectiveness. We hope that this book will serve as an important reference for applying the principles of person-centered planning in today's service systems and for disseminating effective person-centered practices.

REFERENCES

Mount, B. (1992). *Person-centered planning: Finding directions for change. A sourcebook of values, ideals, and methods to encourage person-centered development.* New York: Graphic Futures.

O'Brien, J., & Lovett, H. (1992). *Finding a way toward everyday lives: The contribution of person centered planning.* Harrisburg: Pennsylvania Office of Mental Retardation.

Acknowledgments

We thank the following people for their careful and repeated reviews of chapter manuscripts: Angela Novak Amado, John Butterworth, Robert Davies, Jane Everson, Patricia Fratangelo, Randy Fulton, Carolyn W. Green, Susan Havercamp, Mary Jo Hebert, Martin Ivancic, John Jacobson, Connie Lyle O'Brien, Darlene Magito-McLaughlin, Paul H. Malette, Dong Nguyen, Greg Olley, Al Pfadt, Bertram Ploog, Laura Quinn, Rodney Realon, Dennis H. Reid, Sherry Rose, David A. Rotholz, Helen Sanderson, Maureen Schepis, Chris teKampe, Gregory A. Wagner, David Wetherow, and Philip Wilson.

*To Wolf Wolfensberger, whose life's work set the stage
for the emergence of person-centered planning*

*To Tommy, who died in an institution without
having the benefit of person-centered planning*

and

*To applied researchers and advocates for social change,
whose alliances are fostering the discovery
of better ways to help people with disabilities*

I

Person-Centered
Planning in Context

1

The Origins of Person-Centered Planning

A Community of Practice Perspective

Connie Lyle O'Brien and John O'Brien

To aid those who use person-centered planning to improve life conditions for people with disabilities, this chapter offers one account of how the family of approaches to person-centered planning developed. It describes the context shared by the first four methods to emerge (Twenty-Four Hour Planning, Personal Futures Planning, Individual Design Sessions, and Getting to Know You) and indicates some of their formative influences.

This account is recent history as viewed by insiders (i.e., those whom we interviewed as well as ourselves). We view person-centered planning as a systematic way to understand a person with a developmental disability as a contributing community member. Thus, this chapter identifies 12 distinct but related approaches to person-centered planning that developed during its formative period (1979–1992). To prepare, we interviewed originators of each approach, as well as col-

More detailed information is available from the Center on Human Policy's web site at http://soeweb.syr.edu/thechp.

Thanks to the people who participated in interviews or reviewed this chapter: Brian Abery, Marcie Brost, Emilee Curtis, Marsha Forest, Charles Galloway, Susan Burke Harrison, Terri Johnson, Susannah Joyce, Jo Krippenstaple, Sandra Landis, Marijo McBride, Karen Green McGowan, Beth Mount, Jack Pealer, Cyndi Pitonyak, David Pitonyak, Michael Smull, Steve Taylor, Alan Tyne, Ann P. Turnbull, John VanDenBerg, Terri Vandercook, John Winnenberg, Wolf Wolfensberger, and Jack Yates.

Preparation of this chapter was partially supported through a subcontract to Responsive Systems Associates from the Center on Human Policy, Syracuse University, for the Research and Training Center on Community Living. The Research and Training Center on Community Living is supported through a cooperative agreement (Grant No. H133B980047) between the National Institute on Disability and Rehabilitation Research (NIDRR) and the University of Minnesota Institute on Community Integration. Members of the Research and Training Center on Community Living are encouraged to express their opinions; these do not necessarily represent the official position of NIDRR.

lected and read training materials, reports, manuals, and accounts of person-centered planning that were published before 1992.

COMMUNITIES OF PRACTICE

It is reasonable to look at person-centered planning as a collection of techniques, each of which has particular defining features and a distinct history associated with particular leaders. However, this discussion explores the emergence of person-centered planning from the point of view of communities of practice. This approach puts learning in the context of social engagement by providing an understanding of how knowledge and skill are created and shared (Wenger, 1998). Wenger and Snyder defined *communities of practice* as "groups of people informally bound together by shared expertise and a passion for a joint enterprise" (2000, p. 139). People place themselves in communities of practice because of their personal interest in building and exchanging knowledge with others who share their commitment to an issue or a task. Communities of practice develop knowledge and invent necessary skills by allowing people to build a shared context— that is, a set of common meanings and stories that allow them to understand and effectively change a social world that matters to them.

In adopting this point of view, we want to promote an agenda. Agencies that seek to benefit from person-centered planning often act as if it is a toolbox of techniques that can be taught in staff training workshops by studying protocols, hearing about ideas, and perhaps trying out a technique or two for homework. Such context-free training no doubt teaches something, but it deprives learners of the kinds of social supports for inventive action that were available to the people who developed the first approaches to person-centered planning. This absence of a community of practice prescribes an easy system fix that is destined to fail in its purpose of promoting better lives.

The community of practice that shaped all of the earliest approaches to person-centered planning functioned between 1973 and 1986. It existed among people across North America who shared a passion for understanding and teaching how the principle of normalization might be applied to improve the quality of services to people with developmental disabilities. As the work spread to Britain in 1979, this community of practice became transatlantic, generating cross-national exchanges that extended available perspectives and skills and offered a ready channel for sharing and refining approaches. (For an account of person-centered planning in Britain, see Sanderson, Kennedy, & Ritchie, 1997.) This community of practice provided the originators of person-centered planning with the following: 1) a laboratory for closely observing how services affect people's lives, 2) a forum for discussing the difficult questions that arise in providing services and formulating ideas grounded in their experience, 3) a workshop for inventing new ways to explore the experience of people with developmental disabilities, and 4) a medium for communicating new ideas and techniques.

In describing the community of practice from which these first approaches emerged, we are not yearning for the good old days. However, proficient person-centered planning requires investment in the kind of long-term, regular, and face-to-face sharing (of activities, stories, and questions) that builds communities of practice that are able to create knowledge and skills relevant to today's opportunities and challenges. We believe that such conditions are necessary for real changes in the lives of people with disabilities. We also hope that describing some of the beliefs and assumptions that shaped the emergence of person-centered planning helps those who were not involved then to make sense of what has since developed.

A FAMILY OF APPROACHES

In 1979, Karen Green and Mary Kovaks began a series of workshops on Twenty-Four Hour Planning for people with severe disabilities sponsored by the Canadian National Institute on Mental Retardation (NIMR). By 1980, Beth Mount was training her Georgia colleagues in Personal Futures Planning, and Jack Yates was leading people in Southeastern Massachusetts in Individual Design Sessions for people moving out of Dever State School. Marcie Brost, Terri Johnson, and their co-workers in Wisconsin were using Getting to Know You to plan with people from three county service boards to define the necessary capacities for delivering individualized services. These distinct efforts grew from common roots in a network of normalization teachers.

By 1988, person-centered planning had grown well beyond the immediate reach of the people who developed the first approaches. More and more people were spreading the techniques, which they learned in workshops or by reading about them, into new settings for new purposes. A few regional and state administrators were considering how to make person-centered planning routinely available on a large scale. Over the 4 following years, interest continued to grow. In June 1992, the Pennsylvania Office of Mental Retardation sponsored a conference that included people involved in various approaches to person-centered planning to inform the implementation of the state's strategic plan (O'Brien & Lovett, 1992). We have chosen this event, with its debate about the costs and safeguards for mandating person-centered planning as a matter of state policy, to mark the close of person-centered planning's formative period.

The family tree depicted in Figure 1.1 identifies 12 approaches to person-centered planning that developed between 1979 and 1992 and suggests generational influences among them. (Brief references to approaches other than the first four are discussed in the last section of this chapter.)

Since 1992, a growing number of practitioners and agencies have developed their own variations. Some approaches, such as Essential Lifestyle Planning, are widely practiced in 2002 and continue to spread. Others, such as Individual Design Sessions, continue to develop in the niche where they were born. Still others, such as Getting to Know You, have nearly dropped from use.

The general term *person-centered planning* became common by 1985. It expresses the family resemblance among these different methods and suggests that they share common genes. This heritage includes the following characteristics: 1) see individuals as people first rather than use diagnostic labels; 2) use ordinary language and images rather than professional jargon; 3) actively search for a person's gifts and capacities in the context of community life; and 4) strengthen the voices of the person and of those who know the person best in accounting for his or her history, evaluating his or her present conditions in terms of

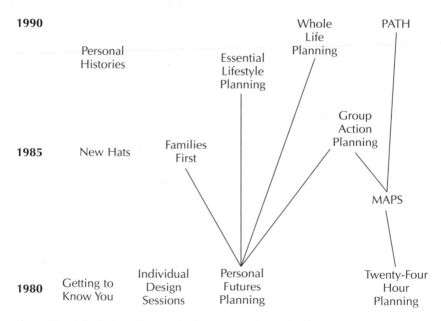

Figure 1.1. A family tree of approaches to person-centered planning.

valued experiences, and defining desirable changes in his or her life (Mount, 1992).

Person-centered planning did not emerge full blown. Scores of people worked out its methods in a common attempt to support people with disabilities to compose their lives. People did not begin to apply these approaches systematically to individual planning until about 1979. Nonetheless, the four at the base of the family tree have common roots in the community of practice that promoted adopting the principle of normalization between 1973 and 1986.

Comprehending the origins of person-centered planning requires a broad sense of how trends shape disability services. It also requires a more particular sense of how understanding and practice evolved among the people who were interested in teaching and applying the principle of normalization in the development of community services.

DEVELOPMENTS IN THE NORMALIZATION TEACHING COMMUNITY OF PRACTICE

From 1973 to approximately 1986, certain forces shaped the context in which the normalization teaching community of practice emerged (see Figure 1.2). The leading influence was the articulation of the principle of normalization in the second and third editions of the Program Analysis of Service Systems (PASS; Wolfensberger & Glenn, 1972, 1975), a systematic way of operationalizing the principle to assess human service programs. This community of practice provided the people who originated the first approaches to person-centered planning with a laboratory, a forum, a workshop, and a medium for communication. Each function played a direct role in shaping the early years of person-centered planning.

This community of practice grew up among people who believed that PASS was a powerful way to understand the relationship among disability, service policy and practice, and community life. PASS was designed primarily as an instrument for quantitative program evaluation across all of the human services and is still presented in that way by Wolfensberger and his associates (see Flynn, 1999). It was designed secondarily as a way to teach the normalization principle. Yet, many teachers found PASS to be most beneficial as a way of learning about the relationship between service programs and people with disabilities from the perspective of the principle of normalization. PASS workshops were intensive, taking 5 demanding days and involving 60–70 participants. The participants worked as a large group to learn the conceptual foundation and in teams of 10–12 to practice the process of looking at services from the perspective of the principle of normaliza-

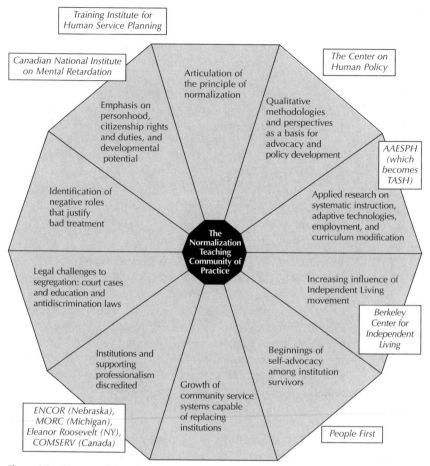

Figure 1.2. Forces and organizations shaping the context of the normalization teaching community of practice (1973–1986). (*Key:* AAESPH = American Association for the Education of the Severely and Profoundly Handicapped, ENCOR = Eastern Nebraska Community Office of Retardation, MORC = McComb Oakland Regional Center.)

tion. Team practice, which was guided by an experienced team leader and usually an assistant team leader, included at least one practicum visit to assess a service program. Practica included observation and extensive discussion of program quality from the following perspectives: 1) the 34 dimensions of the normalization principle as defined by PASS and 2) 16 dimensions of program quality relating to administrative effectiveness.

A PASS workshop typically required 10 to 14 teachers. By the late 1970s, there were as many as 40 workshops per year in North America and Britain. Some workshop sponsors made a practice of inviting teachers from other states and countries to join in building up their local cadre. Many strong relationships were built through the hard work of offering training on a controversial way to understand services. Nonetheless, for many reasons PASS did not catch on widely as an official evaluation tool, and, except in a few regions, PASS training was not funded well or systematically (Thomas, 1999).

As noted previously, this community of practice provided its originators with a laboratory, a forum, a workshop, and a medium for communication. The following subsections describe each facet in detail.

Laboratory

Members of the normalization teaching community of practice created various activities that provided a laboratory for close observation of service program functioning. Although practitioners of either qualitative or quantitative research could find much to criticize in the process, PASS encouraged looking carefully at a program from the point of view of the people whom the program served. Observation and evaluative discussion were based on a set of questions and criteria, which were derived from the principle of normalization. The practice of seeking a consensus among team members on conclusions about each dimension of service quality stimulated extensive discussion that often surfaced different understandings, values, and mindsets. Feelings often ran high in these discussions as participants struggled to digest the implications of what they had observed. Writing reports on consultation assessments demanded deeper thinking and offered a vehicle for disseminating ideas.

Members of the community of practice had repeated chances to look at the same world in which they functioned every day from a different position—that of outsiders whose charge was to identify with the people whom programs served and to think about those people's experiences. The discipline of asking team members to explore what they observed rather than explaining why it had to be that way built awareness of the potential damage that human services can unknowingly inflict. Many participants changed their own practices based on what they learned by assessing another program.

Through the lenses provided by PASS, the originators of person-centered planning learned difficult lessons. First, opportunities for improvement that were evident to people with disabilities and those who care about them were often obscured, ignored, or dismissed by powerful professionals and managers as being "impossible" or "unrealistic"—based solely on the untested assumptions of the powerful people. Second, it was difficult to consistently and intensively provide people assistance that was truly relevant to their development. Even individual plans that specified relevant assistance typically did not predict what people did day to day with the staff who were available to them. Third, people's social worlds were typically very constricted, even when services were provided in ordinary-looking buildings on ordinary, local streets. Fourth, alternatives to controlling and disciplining people with disabilities in stigmatized groups were rare and raised significant dilemmas. Fifth, a disconnection between a program's stated aims and its daily activities could be expected, and only a few service organizations had any way to discuss and work toward closing this gap. Finally, meeting ordinary security needs for the security of a comfortable home, people to love and care for, and good work was typically beyond the reach of a human service program that did not consciously and systematically commit to developing its own organizational capacity.

Despite the hard lessons, there was good news. Many network members avidly collected examples of good practice. Stories about and data on people with disabilities who were pioneers in employment, supported living, and community membership traveled quickly and widely to an audience that was sensitized to appreciate their importance.

A few projects were funded to apply what community of practice members had learned in new contexts. Two that were widely discussed among the network focused on linking individual plans to individualized budgets. One of these two projects assessed the capacity of three Wisconsin county service boards based on plans and individual budgets that were developed with 92 people and their families. As noted by Brost and Hallgren-Ferris, this study pursued a two-part question:

> What specific goods, services, and other supports does each individual need in order to be a respected, participating member of his/her community *and* what needs to happen for these services and other supports to be made available by the right people in the right place at the right time? (1981, p. 1)

The second of the two projects focused on a single individual, in response to a judge's order to develop effective community supports for a young woman who was institutionalized (Galloway, 1981). In framing Sharron Tapia's move from the institution as a "passage to community participation," this detailed plan evidenced imaginative use of the PASS teaching notion of designing services that were based on culturally valued analogues. This means asking, "What does this service compare to in the world of valued citizens and what would it take to offer the same kind and variety of opportunities to people who rely on services?" Figure 1.3 illustrates the pursuit of this question and the view of the ensuing work as assisting someone to journey safely

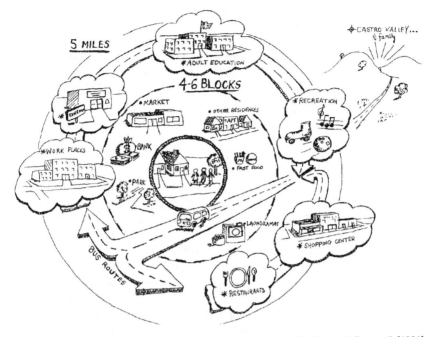

Figure 1.3. Graphic summary of Sharron Tapia's desired community. (From Galloway, C. [1981]. *Passage to community participation: A plan for Sharron Tapia and those who follow* [p. 16]. Sacramento, CA: Author; reprinted by permission.)

from surviving in the culture of an institution to moving competently in the unfamiliar culture of community. These factors defined a setting for Sharron and her two "teaching companions" that was far from the specialized group home design anticipated by the service system. The figure represents where Sharron would be spending her time rather than in human service settings. The house in the middle of the graphic is where she might live and is surrounded by the places within four to six blocks that Sharron could possibly seek membership in or use.

Those who shaped the first approaches to person-centered planning knew from their time in this laboratory that mission statements—as well as regulations, inspections, policies, and individual plans—on paper are useless unless people act out of commitment to each other. They knew the hellish difficulty of overcoming isolation from community life and escaping reproduction of the web of control that surrounds most people with developmental disabilities. They knew that with disciplined effort and careful listening, it is possible to learn a little bit about a person's perspective on his or her life and what the person thinks would improve it. They knew from experience that attending closely, openly, and thoughtfully to a person with a disability even for a little while can draw one into caring about that person's life.

Forum

Every careful look at a service program raised additional, deeper questions about the relationship among disability, organized services, and community. Looking closely at and thinking carefully about brief snapshots of people's experiences troubled the understanding of each term (i.e., disability, organized services, and community).

For example, the struggle to realize the value of social integration—understood as the active opportunity to grow in a variety of good relationships with others, including people without disabilities—made the shared understanding of community deeply problematic. Members of the community of practice knew that such relationships were possible. Indeed, all of the originators of the various approaches to person-centered planning had (and have) such relationships themselves. Yet, they learned that services seldom do well in facilitating such relationships outside their own boundaries.

In the forum created by ongoing teaching, members explored both the meaning of social integration and the means of building good relationships. This made news from citizen advocacy initiatives (local organizations that match and support people in a variety of one-to-one relationships) and in the growing number of Circles of Support relevant to the development of Personal Futures Planning (Mount, 1984; Mount, Beeman, & Ducharme, 1988).

The continued forum for refining and developing new ways to understand and explain the relationship among disability, community, and organized services led some to explore alternative ways of framing the search for service quality. The most elaborate understanding found expression at approximately the same time that the first approaches to person-centered planning emerged. Interest in the work of Thomas Gilbert (1978) led Charles Galloway and John O'Brien to rethink service effectiveness in terms of accomplishments (Galloway, 1978; O'Brien, Poole, & Galloway, 1981). The idea of accomplishments provided part of the conceptual structure for Getting to Know You, Personal Futures Planning, and Twenty-Four Hour Planning. The number of and labels for the accomplishments bounced around for a time before settling on five dimensions of experience in which service practice can make a significant difference in the lives of people with disabilities: community presence, choice, respect, competence, and community participation (O'Brien, 1987).

Workshop

Members of the network of normalization teachers regularly faced groups of people with different outlooks, values, and styles of learning.

Normalization teaching provided a workshop for inventing and testing new ways to facilitate learning about the effects of services on the quality of people's daily experiences and their connections to community life. Three innovations in the process of normalization teaching were of particular importance in the development of person-centered planning.

First, as experience grew, it became clear that PASS teams benefited from spending time in thoughtful discussion of the overall situations of the people who rely on the service whose quality the team is assessing before jumping into a discussion of service particulars. Two simple questions guided these discussions, which often moved the group to surface and to work through significant differences among themselves: "Who are the people being served?" and "What are their most important human needs?" These discussions proved most fruitful when team members used ordinary language rather than professional jargon to describe people's needs and the consequences of their impairments.

By adding one more question—"What would have to happen to meet these needs?"—Jack Yates (1980) developed a format for engaging staff in reviewing their own program, which he called Individual Design Sessions. When Bertha Young, the director of a community service agency and an active member of the normalization teaching community of practice, asked Jack Yates, "Why not work through these questions around one person instead of a group of people?" the format for Individual Service Design emerged. Because these questions are so simple, facilitating a discussion that moves below superficial comments and clichéd understanding requires great mastery on the part of the group leader. Repeated practice in teaching PASS helped a number of community of practice members develop such mastery, though such experience was not the only source of the necessary skill, as demonstrated by Herb Lovett's long and creative use of Individual Design Sessions.

Second, the power in striving to look at a service program from the point of view of the people who rely on the program led a number of teachers to shift the service assessment's perspective. Teachers learned simple, effective ways of pairing team members with particular people whom a program served to encourage professionals to view the program from those people's place within it. For example, team members observed what happens for a person who needs assistance during meals or training sessions. As team members considered their observations, they asked, "What are the likely consequences for the people we met if current practice does not change?" (Note that the focus is on noticing what happens; team members were not asked to pretend to understand the other person's inner experience.) This activity gave the originators of person-centered planning a good deal of practice in facil-

itating group thinking from a person's point of view. Twenty-Four
Hour Planning makes explicit use of this kind of predictive question,
asking, "What is this person at greatest risk for, if we do not change his
or her life?" (Green & Kovaks, 1984).

Third, Graphic Facilitation (Sibbet, 1977) introduced a way of
guiding discussion and gathering information by combining words
and simple graphics. It also stimulated the creation of graphic templates and tasks to structure the collection and display of information.
For several years, the growing number of these templates circulated as
hand-to-hand photocopies until they were collected in a handbook
(O'Brien, 1981). Some graphic facilitation found application in Twenty-
Four Hour Planning and Individual Design Sessions, and it became a
hallmark of Personal Futures Planning.

Medium of Communication

The normalization teaching community of practice grew yearly. It
engaged most person-centered planning originators with one another
and with a growing number of people who shared the demanding and
exciting experience of teaching people about normalization through
PASS. As person-centered planning took shape, some members of this
growing network would become early adopters of an approach, others
would collaborate in developing the approach, others would sponsor
projects that refined and extended the reach of the approach, and still
others would become its critics.

People in the community of practice could count on each other to
facilitate and usefully record discussions about the tough questions
and interesting possibilities found at the intersection of people's lives
and the daily reality of services. They also spoke a common language.
When Jack Yates (1980) wrote about his preference for using "wallpaper" at meetings, he knew that his readers would picture writing on
big sheets of paper that were taped to the wall. When he referred to
"age-appropriateness," he knew that most of his readers would grasp
the issue's nuances. A common language and skill set made it reasonably easy for people across the community of practice to try out different person-centered planning approaches. These factors also provided
originators with fast feedback on results and news about variations that
they had invented to address particular problems arising in practice.

A COMMON AGENDA

A typical way to communicate the goals of person-centered planning
was to draw a strong contrast between usual practices and beliefs and
person-centered practices and beliefs. The first approaches to person-

centered planning shared a common agenda which reflected their originators' involvement in the normalization teaching community of practice. This agenda was expressed in themes that each approach to person-
centered planning followed in its own distinct way:

- Increase choice
- Avoid depersonalizing labels and stigmatizing procedures
- Honor the voices of the person and those who know the person best
- Build relationships
- Individualize supports based on high expectations for the person's development
- Demand that agencies adopt new forms of service and organization to provide newly conceived supports

Perhaps the most powerful idea underlying person-centered planning is that the way a person who receives services is seen and understood by those who deliver that service generates a powerful internal
consistency in the ways that the person is served. Altering procedures
or settings offers far less leverage for changing services than shifting
the understanding of a person. Table 1.1 expresses this contrast. The
table deconstructs the logic of the activity center that currently serves
George and outlines a common-sense response to him as a person,
which is masked by the internal consistency of the program.

The person-centered planning process makes three important conceptual moves. First, it reframes differences in performance that justify
diagnostic labels as differences in life experience. As Table 1.1 shows,
George acts age-inappropriately, in part, because those close to him
treat him as a child. He needs more people in his life who treat him as
an adult and facilitate his participation in the adult world of work and
community. Second, it directs attention outside the orbit of service programs. George is poor and has missed many typical experiences. He
needs the sort of job that is only available in the real world, not at his
group's table in the activity center. Third, it brings George's capacities
to the foreground. George is a delightful man to those who know him.
He needs more people to enjoy him. Those who use the logic of congregate services will experience dissonance if they make these three
moves. This dissonance can motivate change but, paradoxically, it can
also stimulate a recommitment to the familiar logic of congregation. To
support this retreat, people recast person-centered planning in terms
that make it consistent with service-as-usual. Managing this paradox in
ways that preserve person-centered planning's leverage for systems
change continues to trouble its originators (Lyle O'Brien, O'Brien, &
Mount, 1997).

Table 1.1. Programmatic consequences of contrasting ways of understanding a person

Congregate service perspective		Connections perspective	
Who is George?	What does he need?	Who is George?	What does he need?
A person with a mental age of 4 years, 3 months	A program for children	A 40-year-old man who has missed most typical experiences and has never had a real job	A lot of experiences
A person with IQ < 30	To be protected from the world		A real job
A person who is severely mentally retarded	To learn very simple tasks	A person with no income who is poor	An income
A person who has "an indication of organicity, including difficulty with angles, closure, retrogression, oversimplification, and an inability to improve poorly executed drawings"	To learn these skills separately from non-disabled people because he is so different from them	A person who has been isolated all his life	To be included and present in the community
		A person who has no contacts or connections to the wider community	Relationships to other people, connections to community
	Highly specialized staff who can address issues of retrogression, closure, etc.		Friends
		A person who has little control over the direction of his life	Vision for the future and support in getting there
	An environment where his temper can be controlled	A person who has more difficulty learning new skills than most people	Someone who can speak out on his behalf
A person with acute temper flare-ups directed at staff	To be repaired and sent back to the real world when he is better controlled	A person who is treated as a child by his mother	A lot of support for learning
			More people who see and treat him as an adult
		A delightful man who makes a difference in the lives of those who care about him	People who can enjoy him

From Mount, B. (1984). *Creating futures together: A workbook for people interested in creating desirable futures for people with handicaps* (p. 11). Atlanta: Georgia Advocacy Office; adapted by permission.

Typical individual service planning occurs within the logic of the sponsoring service program. The way that individual planning is conducted reflects and reinforces the assumptions underlying the program. Person-centered planning confronts these assumptions explicitly and seeks to build its practice on a different logic.

DISTINCTIVE METHODS

Because people can belong to and be influenced by more than one community of practice at a time, and because over time people can move from one community of practice to another, the community of practice idea helps explain how approaches with common roots and common agendas differentiated from each other. Differences grew because practitioners engaged distinct issues and settings, drew on different theories and tools to shape their processes, and formed new communities of practice around each approach.

The First Four Approaches

As Figure 1.4 suggests, person-centered planning developed at the points of overlapping membership between the normalization teaching community of practice and other communities of practice that were active in reforming services. These communities of practice were concerned with directly improving life for people with developmental disabilities in school, in the transition to adult life, in employment, and in the move from institution to community—especially when difficult behavior or severe disability threatened to leave people no alternative to institutionalization.

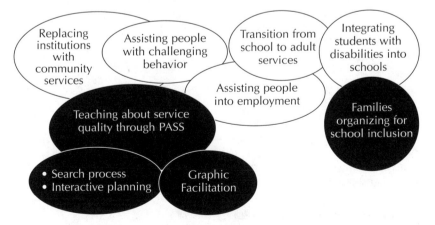

Figure 1.4. Communities of practice whose overlapping memberships differentiated approaches to person-centered planning.

Twenty-Four Hour Planning   The Twenty-Four Hour Planning approach grew from a concern for people whose chances for effective community services were significantly reduced by the complexity
of their disabilities. Karen Green and Mary Kovaks drew on their own
successful work in creating effective services for people with profound,
multiple disabilities to develop training and consultation. This training
and consultation focused service development on careful individual
plans that specified the exact settings and supports that a person would
need to engage in functional and meaningful activity. Jerry, a 20-year-
old man identified as "the most medically fragile" person in a 1,200-
person institution, and his family developed such a plan. Those in the
service system perceived Jerry as having a devastating disability and
needing institutional services for survival. Thus, a plan that called for
Jerry to live in his own place—with peers who did not have disabilities—and to make choices among community activities profoundly
challenged the imagination and skill of those responsible for Jerry's
services (Green & Kovaks, 1984). In formulating these goals, Jerry and
his family presumed that the institution could not offer Jerry what he
needed to grow and develop (see Figure 1.5). As might be imagined, the
plan became the locus of controversy between advocates for institutional improvement and advocates for institution closure—a controversy in which Jerry's family and advocates prevailed.

Balancing participation to ensure that professional voices did not
drown out the contributions of those who knew and loved a person
deeply concerned the originators of Twenty-Four Hour Planning. They

---

From: living in a ward with 60 persons labeled "medically fragile" in an institution of 1,200; being worked with by nurses and
aides who bathe, feed, dress, change, and give medication; getting one hour of "music therapy" a week, staying in bed when
he had seizures

↓

To: living in the home with at least one non-handicapped age peer and no
others with handicaps; being worked with by his peer on experiencing five
other environments per week (i.e., leisure time, basic necessity,
watching/helpful with real work); being allowed individualized recovery
time after seizures

Figure 1.5.   Jerry's goal for community presence. (From Green, K., & Kovaks, M. [1984]. Twenty-
four hour planning for persons with complex needs. *The Canadian Journal on Mental
Retardation, 34*[1], 3–11; reprinted by permission.)

adopted nominal group process techniques (Delbecq, Van de Ven, & Gustafson, 1975) as a way to ensure equality of involvement and a balance of influence on the group's results.

This style of planning blended a deep understanding of how to assist people with significant disabilities in very practical and detailed ways with the task of forming an appreciation of the unique identity of each person. It gave people who knew and loved a person with profound disabilities a privileged voice in formulating a sense of the person's individuality and worth as a community member, as well as in defining what mattered in that person's life. It gave people with specialist knowledge and skills the chance to define how these things that mattered could be supported and to specify the exact conditions of service under which professionals could most effectively practice. Accordingly, Twenty-Four Hour Plans were more technically specific and detailed across people's weekdays, evenings, nights, and weekends than the other three approaches, and they particularly appealed to people with specialist training. The plans became a gathering point for nurses and occupational, physical, and speech-language therapists who were committed to creating powerful supports for people with complex physical needs.

Personal Futures Planning   Personal Futures Planning intersected several communities of practice. Beth Mount's work took her from helping people move into employment from a work activity center in a rural South Georgia county to helping people move from institutions into community living settings in northeast Georgia. Then, she did her doctoral research with young African American adults and their families who were completing special education in areas with limited service funding and went on to work with people who were identified as having the most severe behavior problems in Connecticut's institutions. At each step, new issues and problems tested, refined, and extended the approach as new colleagues brought new skills and knowledge. Mount's involvement with Citizen Advocacy (a program that makes and supports one-to-one relationships between people with disabilities and other citizens) and with Circles of Support (a way of organizing a person's allies around shared concerns) oriented Personal Futures Planning toward organizing and extending a person's social supports (Mount et al., 1988).

Personal Futures Planning incorporated more extensive exploration of planning ideas than other early approaches to person-centered planning. Some of these ideas came from Mount's doctoral work in public administration. This study brought her into contact with research on people-centered development efforts in Asia (Korten, 1981) and with the life/work planning processes that were created to assist former clergy and displaced engineers in discovering new career paths (Crystal & Bolles, 1974). Some ideas came from her shared reading and discussion with a subgroup of the normalization training community of practice, which was interested in applying the insights of feminist thinkers to disability practice (e.g., see French, 1985). Other ideas came from her engagement with a community of practice concerned with service planning that intersected the normalization teaching community of practice.

Individual Design Sessions Individual Design Sessions (Yates, 1980) stayed close to its roots in PASS teaching. The process guided service workers to a deeper understanding of a person's experience and, thus, to increased empathy for the people they assist. This approach considered a person's identity by

- Carefully reviewing personal history
- Thoughtfully drawing out connections between the individual's experience and the processes of social devaluation that shaped institutional living
- Comparing and contrasting the life experiences of the focus person and other members of the group

By imaginatively pursuing a search for socially valued analogues—which were defined by asking "How does this ordinarily happen for valued citizens?"—the originators constructed a test for its own practice. If the focus person lived in a group home, for example, the question, "What is 'home' like for the rest of us here?" would be followed by the questions, "In what ways is this group home similar to and different from what the rest of us consider 'home'?" and "What changes would offer this person more of the benefits of home?"

Getting to Know You Getting to Know You (Brost & Johnson, 1982) was designed to define the service system capacities required to provide individualized supports. It enlisted 92 people with disabilities and their families as collaborators in system evaluation and service development rather than as consumers of a planning process and available services. Getting to Know You blended the normalization teaching perspective on gathering information and understanding people's needs with an approach to human service needs assessment and case management. This blend constructed General Service Plans, which specified services that holistically met an individual's needs.

General Service Plans are precise about the assistance that people need but are far less detailed about how support must be delivered than those constructed in Twenty-Four Hour Plans. Many of the original participants and their families, who chose to test their county service system by clearly specifying their individual needs and the costs of meeting them, reported some benefit for themselves in making the plans; however, what they created also influenced the evolution of their county's and state's developmental disabilities services systems.

Incorporating Lessons from Service Planners

Disappointing experiences in implementing comprehensive plans for community-based service systems led to disillusionment with the kind of rational planning that assumed it was possible to systematically implement a fully designed system from the top down. It proved nearly impossible to gather sufficient political power to pull off a complete solution. Worse yet, the approximations of a comprehensive solution that did get implemented demonstrated that the prevailing idea of *system* was mechanistic and inflexible, at least from the point of view of the people and families that these systems served.

Disillusionment pushed Alan Roeher and John O'Brien to discover different ways to understand planning and systems in a collaboration with Eric Trist, a seminal thinker in understanding and designing adaptive social systems, and David Morley. Through this collaboration, the search conference process and the social systems theory behind it became available in the normalization teaching network. (For an overview of this process and theory, see Emery, 1999.) Further exploration brought engagement with complementary systems theories and planning practice that Russell Ackoff and his colleagues (1974) developed under the heading "Interactive Planning."

These links provided four key ideas. First, rapid and connected change means that people and their organizations live in a turbulent environment. In such an environment, people can steer but cannot sustain walls that permit successful control from the top. Self-organization leads to success. Second, the best way to understand situations is to look at them whole, in terms of interactions and purposes, rather than break them down into ever-smaller pieces. Third, there are benefits to gathering people with diverse and conflicting interests to discuss the trends and forces shaping their shared environment, to assess the consequences of not changing, and to create vivid images that communicate shared possibilities for desirable change. Fourth, a shared vision of a desirable future provides a far more robust mechanism for coordinating action in a rapidly changing world than any bureaucratic blueprint for command and control. These insights powerfully influenced Personal Futures Planning and, later, MAPS and PATH.

Two Approaches with Distinct Roots

Two early streams of person-centered planning began apart from the community of practice concerned about normalization teaching. These approaches, New Hats and MAPS, are discussed in detail next.

New Hats

Emily Curtis worked in an activity center with people who had developmental disabilities. New Hats (Curtis & Dezelsky, 1996) grew from her recognition that many of these people had potential and dreams that were easily overlooked. Indeed, she concluded that service workers frequently tried to extinguish people's dreams. Encouraging people to communicate their dreams led her to develop a variety of aids to thinking, deciding, and communicating—for example, a deck of cards presenting an array of possible activities that people can use to identify, communicate about, and perhaps extend their interests. Links to other approaches with person-centered planning emerged later as Curtis connected with other practitioners and incorporated some of their ideas into her unique formats.

MAPS

MAPS (Making Action Plans, formerly known as the McGill Action Planning System; Forest, & Lusthaus, 1989) was developed from the Twenty-Four Hour Planning approach. Marsha Forest was led to learn about Twenty-Four Hour Planning out of her concern for including children with profound disabilities into a neighborhood school. A growing community of practice, driven by the desire of Ontario parents to open neighborhood schools and classrooms to students with disabilities, reshaped the Twenty-Four Hour Planning format into MAPS. The following questions provided the context for MAPS development: How might a school welcome and support a student with disabilities whose adaptation needs challenge typical classroom practice? How might a student whose place in school is threatened get the support to belong and learn in a classroom (O'Brien & Forest, 1989)? Two Ontario Separate (Roman Catholic) School Boards—in Hamilton-Wentworth and Kitchener-Waterloo—committed themselves to full inclusion, and their schools were visited by educators and families from around the world. Visitors learned what it takes for all children to be welcomed as active learners, including the usefulness of MAPS. Efforts to promote inclusion in schools across Canada convened a 10-year series of summer institutes at NIMR and McGill University. The institutes gathered parents, people with disabilities, teachers, and administrators to teach them—among other things—how to use MAPS as a foundation for inclusion (Forest & Lusthaus, 1989). Collaboration with Judith Snow, who lives with the support of a circle and has a deep and powerful interest in assisting people to guide their lives by listening to their dreams (Snow, 1992), extended the MAPS process and built strong bridges among MAPS, Circles of Support, and Personal Futures Planning.

Continued Development

By 1992, six other person-centered approaches were developed, bringing the total to 12. Explanations of these additional approaches follow.

Personal Histories The Personal Histories approach was initially incorporated into the work of Residential, Inc, a pioneer supported living agency in New Lexington, Ohio. It was part of the consultation Sandra Landis and Jack Pealer offered until about 1990 with agencies in Ohio. Personal Histories drew directly from the normalization teaching community of practice: It encouraged those who acted as planning assistants to invest time and imagination in helping people with developmental disabilities to construct and communicate their life stories (Landis & Pealer, 1990).

Families First Leah Holden (1990) developed Families First in Ohio. It was a way to teach the parents of children and young people how to use an adaptation of Personal Futures Planning to strengthen their advocacy for family support services and inclusive education.

Whole Life Planning With his colleagues in Connecticut, John Butterworth (1993) developed Whole Life Planning. This approach matched planning procedures to the individual preferences of people with developmental disabilities who were seeking employment.

Group Action Planning Ann and Rud Turnbull adopted ideas from Personal Futures Planning and MAPS to create Group Action Planning. The purpose of the approach was to empower parents in building brighter futures for their young and school-age children by linking family-controlled individual planning with organization for the needed local and state system changes to align education and human services with visions shared among families (Turnbull & Turnbull, 1996, 1999).

PATH In 1993, Jack Pearpoint, John O'Brien, and Marsha Forest developed PATH (Planning Alternative Tomorrows with Hope). PATH's purpose was to support individuals and groups in charting strategies for achieving valued futures when sustained and coordinated action is required.

Essential Lifestyle Planning After exploring Personal Futures Planning, Michael Smull and Susan Burke Harrison (1992) responded to the opportunity to specify what community services would provide for people who were so profoundly isolated and deprived by their years of institutionalization that they could not articulate a dream for themselves and lacked anyone to join a support circle who knew them beyond their reputation for challenging behavior. Essential Lifestyle Planning (ELP) aimed to discover and gain service provider agreements that addressed the simple but important issues for each person that if ignored lead to mistrust, unhappiness, and power struggles. A growing community of practice around ELP has generated an array of tools for discovering what matters to people by

- Building a finely grained understanding of the rituals and routines that allow people to express their uniqueness
- Reviewing quality of plans
- Incorporating the perspective of skilled service providers
- Dealing with conflicts
- Supporting necessary organizational changes
- Bridging to other person-centered approaches as a person's dreams grow bigger and stronger and a person's relationships with potential allies grow wider and deeper

CONCLUSION:
KEEPING PERSON-CENTERED PLANNING ALIVE

Person-centered planning grew out of a passionate concern to support people with developmental disabilities in discovering and contributing their gifts. This concern brought people together to form communities of practice. The skills and knowledge that these communities of practice created moved their members into alliances with people with developmental disabilities, as well as their families and friends. These alliances put person-centered planners' knowledge to work in supporting one person at a time, adding their talent to the task of shaping more just and more inclusive communities. This bold vision melded personal and social change. Discovering and realizing ways for people who have been marginalized to claim opportunities and contribute to community life serves justice in both small and significant ways.

Person-centered approaches that lose touch with this almost presumptuous vision will drown in a swamp of bureaucratic requirements. Practitioners without lifelines to a community of practice that renews and refines their energy—by firing imagination and creating knowledge—will wither into servants of rules and regulations. The meaning in person-centered planning today lies where it has since its beginnings. Meaning lies in serving people as they move from being segregated and controlled toward participation in and origination of lives that matter. Meaning lies in belonging to a community of practice that over months and years shares stories, lessons, and support.

REFERENCES

Ackoff, R. (1974). *Redesigning the future: A systems approach to societal problems.* New York: John Wiley.

Brost, M., & Hallgren-Ferris, B. (1981). *Getting there: Developing individualized service options.* Madison, WI: Bureau of Developmental Disabilities.

Brost, M., & Johnson, T. (1982). *Getting to know you: One approach to service assessment and planning for individuals with disabilities.* Madison: Wisconsin Coalition for Advocacy.

Butterworth, J. (1993). *Whole life planning: A guide for organizers and facilitators.* Cambridge, MA: Institute for Community Integration.

Crystal, J., & Bolles, R. (1974). *Where do I go from here with my life?* Berkeley, CA: Ten Speed Press.

Curtis, E., & Dezelsky, M. (1996). *My life planner series.* Salt Lake City, UT: New Hats.

Delbecq, A., Van de Ven, A., & Gustafson, D. (1975). *Group techniques for program planning: A guide to nominal group and Delphi processes.* Glenview, IL: Scott Foresman.

Emery, M. (1999). *Searching: The theory and practice of making cultural change.* Philadelphia: John Benjamins Publishing Co.

Flynn, R. (1999). A comprehensive review of research conducted with the program evaluation instruments PASS and PASSING. In R. Flynn & R. Lemay (Eds.), *A quarter century of normalization and social role valorization: Evolution and impact* (pp. 317–349). Ottawa, Ontario, Canada: University of Ottawa Press.

Forest, M., & Lusthaus, E. (1989). Promoting educational equality for all students: Circles and Maps. In S. Stainback, W. Stainback, & M. Forest (Eds.), *Educating all students in the mainstream of regular education* (pp. 43–57). Baltimore: Paul H. Brookes Publishing Co.

French, M. (1985). *Beyond power: Women, men, and morals.* New York: Simon & Schuster.

Galloway, C. (1978). *Conversion to a policy of community presence and participation.* Presentation to The 1978 Regional Institutes in Law and Mental Health, University of Southern California Schools of Medicine and Public Administration, Los Angeles.

Galloway, C. (1981). *Passage to community participation: A plan for Sharron Tapia and those who follow.* Sacramento, CA: Author.

Gilbert, T. (1978). *Human competence: Engineering worthy performance.* New York: McGraw-Hill.

Green, K., & Kovaks, M. (1984). Twenty-four hour planning for persons with complex needs. *The Canadian Journal on Mental Retardation, 34*(1), 3–11.

Holden, L. (1990). *Building brighter futures for our children.* Columbus, OH: Association for Retarded Citizens–Ohio.

Korten, D. (1981). Community organization and rural development: A learning process approach. *Public Administration Review, 41*(6), 480–510.

Landis, S., & Pealer, J. (1990). *Personal histories.* Chillicothe: Ohio Safeguards.

Lyle O'Brien, C., O'Brien, J., & Mount, B. (1997). Person-centered planning has arrived . . . or has it? *Mental Retardation, 35,* 480–484.

Mount, B. (1984). *Creating futures together: A workbook for people interested in creating desirable futures for people with handicaps.* Atlanta: Georgia Advocacy Office.

Mount, B. (1992). *Person-centered planning: A sourcebook of values, ideas, and methods to encourage person-centered development.* New York: Graphic Futures.

Mount, B., Beeman, P., & Ducharme, G. (1988). *What are we learning about circles of support?* Manchester, CT: Communitas Communications.

O'Brien, J. (1981). *Normalization training through PASS: Team leader manual* (version 1.0). Decatur, GA: Responsive Systems Associates.

O'Brien, J. (1987). A guide to life-style planning: Using The Activities Catalog to integrate services and natural support systems. In B. Wilcox & G.T. Bellamy, *A comprehensive guide to The Activities Catalog: An alternative curriculum for youth and adults with severe disabilities* (pp. 175–189). Baltimore: Paul H. Brookes Publishing Co.

O'Brien, J., & Forest, M. (1989). *Action for inclusion.* Toronto: Inclusion Press.

O'Brien, J., & Lovett, H. (1992). *Finding a way toward everyday lives: The contribution of person centered planning.* Harrisburg: Pennsylvania Office of Mental Retardation.

O'Brien, J., Poole, C., & Galloway, C. (1981). *Accomplishments in residential services: Improving the effectiveness of residential service workers in Washington's developmental services system.* Olympia, WA: Governor's Council on Developmental Disabilities.

Pearpoint, J., O'Brien, J., & Forest, M. (1993). *PATH (Planning Alternative Tomorrows with Hope): A workbook for planning positive futures.* Toronto: Inclusion Press.

Sanderson, H., Kennedy, J., & Ritchie, P. (1997). *People, plans, and possibilities: Exploring person-centered planning.* Edinburgh, Scotland: SHS Ltd.

Sibbet, D. (1977). *"I see what you mean!" A guide to group graphics.* San Francisco: Author.

Smull, M., & Burke Harrison, S. (1992). *Supporting people with severe reputations in the community.* Alexandria, VA: National Association of State Mental Retardation Program Directors.

Snow, J. (1992). *What's really worth doing and how to do it: A book for people who love someone labeled disabled (possibly yourself).* Toronto: Inclusion Press.

Thomas, S. (1999). Historical background and evolution of normalization-related and social role valorization related training. In R. Flynn & R. Lemay (Eds.), *A quarter century of normalization and social role valorization: Evolution and impact* (pp. 353–374). Ottawa, Ontario, Canada: University of Ottawa Press.

Turnbull, A.P., & Turnbull, H.R. (1996). Group Action Planning as a strategy for providing comprehensive family support. In L.K. Koegel, R.L. Koegel, & G. Dunlap (Eds.), *Positive behavioral support: Including people with difficult behavior in the community* (pp. 99–114). Baltimore: Paul H. Brookes Publishing Co.

Turnbull, A.P., & Turnbull, H.R. (1999). Comprehensive lifestyle support for adults with challenging behavior: From rhetoric to reality. *Education and Training in Mental Retardation and Developmental Disabilities, 34*(4), 373–394.

Wenger, E. (1998). *Communities of practice: Learning, meaning, and identity.* Cambridge, UK: Cambridge University Press.

Wenger, E., & Snyder, W. (January–February 2000). Communities of practice: The organizational frontier. *Harvard Business Review,* 139–145.

Wolfensberger, W., & Glenn, L. (1972). *Program Analysis of Service Systems (PASS) (2nd ed.)*. Toronto: National Institute on Mental Retardation.

Wolfensberger, W., & Glenn, L. (1975). *Program Analysis of Service Systems (PASS) (3rd ed.)*. Toronto: National Institute on Mental Retardation.

Yates, J. (1980). *Program design sessions: OOP (optional operating procedure)*. Carver, MA: Author.

2

Person-Centered Planning and Positive Behavior Support

Don Kincaid and Lise Fox

In recent years, there has been significant change in society's understanding and support of individuals with disabilities. The 1990s were characterized by a developing understanding that individuals with disabilities can and should have an active leadership role in determining why and how supports can be provided in their homes, schools, and communities. In fact, individuals with disabilities and their families have come to expect supports that are positive, person- and family-centered, effective, collaborative, and comprehensive.

These expectations were reinforced by two parallel approaches to supporting individuals with disabilities that experienced tremendous growth in use and allegiance during this decade: person-centered planning and positive behavior support (PBS). Perhaps no approaches in this 10-year time period redefined and shaped the values, philosophies, and supports that are provided for individuals with disabilities more than person-centered planning and PBS. However, few professionals, families, and individuals with disabilities are aware of how these two approaches share common values; philosophies; and, in some cases, techniques for supporting individuals with disabilities to live in typical home, school, and community settings.

The purpose of this chapter is to share some of our experiences in melding person-centered planning and PBS approaches to provide a values-driven, person-centered, and comprehensive support approach for individuals with disabilities who also have challenging behavior. This chapter explores some of the more common person-centered planning processes, as well as some of the themes and characteristics that person-centered planning and PBS share. The chapter also discusses outcomes of person-centered planning and PBS that extend beyond the focus individual to affect team participants, agencies, and systems. Then, the chapter examines how person-centered planning and PBS are able to enhance each other in process and practice. Finally, the chapter points to future directions for research and practice in PBS and person-centered planning.

PERSON-CENTERED PLANNING

Person-centered planning is a process for learning how a person wants to live and then describing what needs to be done to help that person move toward that life (Smull & Burke Harrison, 1992). Person-centered planning is rooted in the values, goals, and outcomes that are important to the person, but it also takes into account other critical factors that have an impact on the individual's life, including family and agency views, funding issues, and the person's disability and community (Lyle O'Brien, O'Brien, & Mount, 1997). In general, person-centered planning processes use 1) group graphics and facilitation techniques to assist a person in describing the kind of life that he or she wants to live and 2) a committed team of family members, friends, community members, and agency staff to identify the supports that will allow the person to develop this life. Person-centered planning processes also provide an opportunity—sometimes for the first time—for individual team members to understand the life that the person has experienced to this point, to understand more clearly the life that he or she is experiencing now, and to envision the kind of life that he or she wants to pursue and experience in the future.

Well-Known Person-Centered Planning Processes

Under the umbrella of person-centered planning, a variety of processes have been developed and expanded since the late 1980s. In addition, a variety of processes have begun to emerge for application at a local or agency level. These local processes are frequently patterned after some of the more well-known person-centered planning processes, such as Personal Profiling (O'Brien, 1987; O'Brien & Lyle, 1987; O'Brien, Mount, & Lyle O'Brien, 1990), Personal Futures Planning (Mount, 1987; Mount & Zwernik, 1988), MAPS (Making Action Plans, formerly known as the McGill Action Planning System; Forest & Lusthaus, 1989; Vandercook, York, & Forest, 1989), PATH (Planning Alternative Tomorrows with Hope; Pearpoint, O'Brien, & Forest, 1993), and Essential Lifestyle Planning (ELP; Smull & Burke Harrison, 1992). These well-known person-centered planning processes share underlying values and similarities but may differ in their application.

Personal Profiling   Personal Profiling (O'Brien et al., 1990) uses group graphics techniques to help a team reach a better understanding of an individual's identity and experiences. Team members are facilitated through the development of a series of frames, and the focus person takes an active role in this process. These frames identify critical areas for the team to address in the future and may depict

1. Important people in an individual's life
2. Community places in which the person spends time
3. Critical events in the person's history
4. An overview of the person's health issues
5. Which choices the individual does and does not make in his or her daily life
6. Ways in which the individual may gain or lose respect
7. Strategies that work or do not work for supporting the person
8. The individual's and the team's hopes and fears
9. Barriers to and opportunities for the team's continued support of the individual in a positive and possible future

Because frames reflect critical areas in the focus person's life, they may vary from person to person. These frames allow the team to uncover critical themes that may be further addressed in a futures planning process.

    Personal Futures Planning Personal Futures Planning focuses on what the team can do to address the themes or issues identified within a personal profile or other person-centered process (Mount, 1987; Mount & Zwernik, 1988). In Personal Futures Planning, the team identifies an appropriate time frame for achieving a futures plan that specifically addresses themes and issues in five areas (home, work or school, community, choices and preferences, and relationships). The identified themes or issues are interwoven into these critical areas. In conjunction with a personal profile process, Personal Futures Planning may take several hours or longer to complete. Personal Futures Planning can be extremely effective, even when some of the team members do not know the focus person well, because it gives the team a comprehensive understanding of many important areas of the individual's life.

    MAPS MAPS is a person-centered planning process that may assist a team in identifying a "roadmap" for working toward and achieving goals for the focus person (Forest & Lusthaus, 1989; Vandercook et al., 1989). MAPS identifies where the person currently is, what his or her goal is, and how a team will assist the individual in reaching the goal. Similar to the Personal Profiling, MAPS has an established framework that addresses the individual's history, identity, dreams, nightmares, strengths, and gifts. The person's needs and action steps for the team are also identified. The MAPS process may require as little as 1–2 hours to complete and is most effective when the focus person identifies some well-formed goals for the team to address.

PATH PATH may take a team 2 or more hours to complete (Pearpoint et al., 1993). It is an effective process for bringing together a team that may already know an individual well and has already shown commitment to supporting that individual in the future. PATH is ideal for addressing long- and short-term planning and for clearly identifying the focus person's dreams and desires. One of PATH's strengths is that it provides clear time lines for achieving goals and breaks those goals into measurable and achievable steps. It also identifies individuals who are responsible for completing each action step. PATH uses group graphics techniques and, like other person-centered planning processes, encourages and supports the individual in identifying dreams and goals while respecting the person's perceptions and concerns.

Essential Lifestyle Planning ELP is also a facilitated group meeting that uses "wallpaper" and may include group graphics techniques (Smull & Burke Harrison, 1992). ELP makes a significant commitment of time to ascertaining the individual's likes and dislikes. In fact, the ELP process is built on the concept of supporting the individual's expression of choices that are "non-negotiable," "strong preferences," and "highly desirable." These preferences lay the foundation on which a positive view of the individual is formed. Then, the team discusses the individual's history of challenging behavior, presents critical issues to success, and identifies action steps.

Similar Goals of Person-Centered Planning Approaches

Although these person-centered processes differ in terms of graphics approaches, facilitation, and the structure of the process and other features, most person-centered planning processes also share many similarities (Kincaid, 1996). For the most part, person-centered planning processes have similar valued accomplishments for an individual's life. The following subsections detail these goals.

Be Part of and Participate in Community Life This accomplishment stresses that the person should be part of the same community that is available to all other citizens. Furthermore, the person should be a full and active participant in that community to the degree that he or she wishes to participate.

Gain and Maintain Satisfying Relationships The individual with disabilities is supported in pursuing and maintaining satisfying relationships, including family, friend, community, and romantic relationships. In addition, person-centered planning identifies methods to support the individual in achieving healthy interactions with friends and family, who can provide the person with opportunities to give and receive love and affection.

Express Preferences and Make Choices in Everyday Life Person-centered planning operates on the expressed preferences of individuals with disabilities. These individuals indicate how they would like to live and how they would like to be supported in that life. Person-centered planning approaches pursue ways to support the individual to make choices in small and big life decisions.

Have Opportunities to Fulfill Respected Roles and to Live with Dignity Person-centered planning supports the person with disabilities in making community contributions and being valued as a person. This includes the individual's learning to behave with dignity and being treated with respect by others. Person-centered planning is built on the premise of respecting the individual for his or her achievements and identity. Yet, it also supports the individual to grow and fulfill even more respected roles in family, school or work, and community settings.

Continue to Develop Personal Competencies Person-centered planning provides opportunities and support for an individual to develop personal competencies. Through person-centered planning, the focus individual identifies areas for growth and development and is supported by the team to take advantage of life's opportunities and to control his or her own life and future. This includes making contributions to the community, learning new skills, and succeeding in tasks and activities with minimum assistance.

Shared Characteristics of Person-Centered Planning Approaches

In addition to having common goals, the different person-centered planning processes also have some common characteristics. These shared characteristics are discussed next.

Make Systems More Person Centered Person-centered planning, by its philosophy and values, centers on the person and the family. Yet, this focus requires more than an assertion that it is necessary to include the person and the family in the process. Significant systems issues often need to be addressed, including changes in how teams are formed, how individuals are supported, and how the planning process is conducted to better meet the needs of the individual and family members.

Develop Respect and Understanding Person-centered planning teaches and promotes respect for the individual, the family, and all team members. First and foremost, person-centered planning respects the information, perceptions, goals, and visions for the future of the person with the disability. However, person-centered planning also respects the visions, input, and experiences of family members and team members as they collaborate to provide support for the individual to succeed.

Give Priority to Preferences and Choices   Person-centered planning gives priority to the expressed choices and preferences of the individual and his or her family, depending on the individual's age. This characteristic of person-centered planning indicates not only that the individual has the opportunity to express choices and preferences, but also that team members listen and respond appropriately to those expressions.

Emphasize a Positive View   Person-centered planning approaches take a positive view of the individual and his or her dreams and plans for the future. As a result, person-centered planning differs from many traditional planning processes that emphasize deficits, disabilities, and problems. Rather, person-centered planning emphasizes strengths, abilities, and capacities. This positive view of an individual builds on the characteristic of respecting the individual and the life choices that he or she has made and wishes to make.

Develop a Unique and Creative Process   Person-centered planning is a creative process that does not accept the status quo. Each individual's view of his or her positive and possible future is unique. As a result, the supports and solutions to identified problems need to be diverse and creative. Person-centered planning should not be seen as a process to fit an individual into a predefined array of residential, employment, or educational settings. Rather, it should be viewed as an opportunity to explore and consider an expanded view of how an individual wishes to live and how to support him or her in that life.

Pursue Ideals   Person-centered planning seeks the ideal life for an individual. The process prompts and supports a team to consider what is possible and positive, and it often asks team members, "What can we do if everyone tries his or her best to help achieve this dream for the future?" This question often requires the team to consider options other than those present in the environment, as well as what is possible and ideal to support the individual in the future.

Gain Access to Typical Community Resources   Given the previously discussed characteristics of person-centered planning, it is not surprising that agencies are often concerned about the financial costs of such an approach. However, person-centered planning is not built on the idea of developing new programs or services but, rather, on gaining access to community resources that are available to all citizens. Gaining access to natural communities of support means that individuals may be supported in ways that are less affected by agency and funding systems changes. Person-centered planning may actually result in reduced financial supports for individuals as they begin to achieve the employment outcomes and community supports that they desire.

Support Learning and Growth Person-centered planning also creates an environment in which everyone is a learner. Person-centered planning is not built on a typical professional–expert model. Instead, it identifies and capitalizes on the expertise of each team member, particularly the individuals who know the person well. Thus, all team members learn from each other and learn new ways of thinking and acting as they help an individual to pursue and achieve his or her goals.

Empower Participants Person-centered planning also empowers the person, family, and team to explore options and consider futures that may differ from those previously considered. Person-centered planning is an essential component of self-direction and self-determination for individuals with disabilities. Individuals learn how to express their preferences about their futures, as well as how to collaborate with other people and to assume a leadership role in fostering a positive and possible future.

Outcomes of Person-Centered Planning

Person-centered planning has the potential to produce radical, long-term changes in the quality of life of individuals with disabilities. Person-centered planning has the capacity to change where people live, what they do, and who they do it with, as well as their satisfaction with their lifestyle (Lyle O'Brien et al., 1997). Professionals who use person-centered planning approaches to identify and develop the supports that they provide to individuals with disabilities have recognized its potential to produce significant, lasting, and comprehensive changes in a person's life.

In addition, person-centered planning has a positive and significant impact on team members and agencies (Lyle O'Brien et al., 1997). Through participation in person-centered planning, team members may also experience changed perceptions about and responses to fellow team members and the focus person. Person-centered planning teams often are not initially united and cohesive in their understanding and perceptions of the focus person and his or her life. However, person-centered planning can build a powerful team that shares a common vision and commitment.

Because person-centered planning can be an effective planning and team-building process, it also has the potential to motivate all of the team members, including the focus person. Often, teams are pulled together for a person-centered planning process because they do not know what else to do. Team members are burned out and having a difficult time identifying with and being motivated to pursue necessary supports for the focus person. A positive person-centered planning process can be an invigorating and exciting process for team participants (Lyle O'Brien et al., 1997). At its best, person-centered planning produces a team that cannot wait to start helping the focus person to achieve his or her dream for the future.

Person-centered planning can also be considered an important assessment process. It assesses the focus person's history, current environment, and dreams for the future. Person-centered planning does not produce supports that address a particular need in isolation from the person's entire life. Instead, it scans his or her entire environment to gather critical information that allows a team to more effectively fit supports with the context of the individual's life (Albin, Lucyshyn, Horner, & Flannery, 1996). For individuals who exhibit challenging behaviors, team members come to understand the individual beyond his or her behavior; they learn what is important to the person and the context in which challenging behaviors occur (Kincaid, 1996). As a result, behavioral supports that are developed are positive, respectful, and appropriate for the individual.

Finally, person-centered planning clearly lays the foundation on which effective supports and interventions can be built. Person-centered planning often points to areas of need within a person's life that are giving rise to challenging behaviors or other significant issues. A team planning process that identifies comprehensive, long-term needs for an individual can also identify positive, effective, comprehensive, and long-term supports for the individual.

POSITIVE BEHAVIOR SUPPORT

Positive behavior support is an applied science that uses educational and systems change methods to redesign an individual's living environment to achieve an enhanced quality of life and to minimize challenging behavior (Carr et al., 1999; Koegel, Koegel, & Dunlap, 1996). The primary goal of PBS is to affect an individual's lifestyle so that all of the relevant stakeholders—including teachers, employers, parents, and friends—perceive an improved quality of life for themselves and the individual with challenging behavior. While focusing on achieving broader lifestyle changes, PBS also seeks to make challenging behavior "irrelevant, inefficient, and ineffective" by teaching, strengthening, and expanding positive behavior (O'Neill et al., 1997).

PBS has emerged from three major sources: 1) the science of applied behavior analysis, 2) the principles of normalization, and 3) person-centered values (Carr et al., 2002). PBS owes much to applied behavior analysis and normalization. Early in its development as a science, however, PBS clearly shared a values base with person-centered planning. Those in the field of PBS also understood the benefits that this approach and its values could provide for individuals with disabilities and challenging behavior. Carr and colleagues (2002) indicated that science describes how one can change things, but values indicate what is worth changing. Science can answer the question of "How?" but values can answer the question of "Why?" Thus, PBS combines the values and technologies to produce strategies that are effective but that also enhance personal dignity and opportunities for choice. Due to this shared philosophy, person-centered planning is valuable for assisting teams in developing behavior support plans that emphasize the goals of the person-centered planning processes: community participation, meaningful social relationships, enhanced opportunities for choice, respected roles for the individual, and opportunities to develop personal competencies.

PBS is enhanced by person-centered planning in multiple ways. Person-centered planning provides a unique process for developing the behavior support team, understanding the distinct circumstances of the individual with challenging behavior, and creating a vision for an optimal lifestyle (Kincaid, 1996). Many professionals regard person-centered planning as the essential first step in the functional assessment process, as well as a useful mechanism for creating optimal supports and monitoring outcomes as required by PBS (Dunlap et al., 2000; Fox, Dunlap, & Buschbacher, 2000; Kincaid, 1996). In the process of PBS, person-centered planning may be used to bring together all of the people who care about the individual to create the circle of support or a team that will develop and implement the behavior support plan. The first task of the circle of support is to gain a deeper understanding of the individual, the individual's lifestyle, and his or her desires for the future. Through that discussion, the team can identify situations that may require a functional assessment, environments that may need to be changed or enriched, and the meaningful outcomes that will be used to evaluate the effectiveness of behavioral support efforts. Once a behavior support plan is constructed, person-centered planning meetings offer a forum for discussing implementation issues, the individual's progress, problem-solving strategies, and the achievement of meaningful outcomes.

Distinguishing Features of Positive Behavior Support in Relation to Person-Centered Planning

PBS has clear features that distinguish it from other contemporary approaches to addressing challenging behavior (Carr et al., 2002). These distinguishing features also share many underlying values, techniques, and pursued outcomes with person-centered planning. These factors are explored in the following subsections.

Comprehensive Lifestyle Change and Quality of Life Outcomes   Although decreasing challenging behaviors is still of central importance, PBS also goes beyond this change to look at lifestyle changes that reflect the broad emphasis of both PBS and person-centered planning (Carr et al., 1999; Dunlap, Fox, Vaughn, Bucy, & Clarke, 1997; Meyer & Evans, 1993). Of primary importance in PBS is an emphasis on quality of life outcomes that may or may not directly relate to changing challenging behavior, including developing relationships, obtaining employment, and having more daily control and choice.

The goal of person-centered planning is to support an individual with disabilities in identifying and achieving his or her vision for a desired lifestyle. It is critically important that meaningful outcomes are referenced to the dreams and desires of the focus individual, rather than to the expectations and perspectives of people who support the individual. Person-centered planning ensures that the voice of the focus individual is always heard or represented when the behavior support team discusses meaningful outcomes.

Life-Span Perspectives   PBS does not emphasize the provision of short-term intervention or support to decrease challenging behaviors (Carr et al., 1999). Instead, PBS emphasizes pursuing a life-span perspective that results in the maintenance of durable change and lifestyle outcomes for the individual. Although PBS may produce quick solutions to challenging behaviors, the production and maintenance of comprehensive lifestyle change may require months or years of continued team support.

This emphasis on a life-span perspective is also fundamental to person-centered planning. Time lines for achieving positive quality of life outcomes with the focus individual may be as short as 6 months or as long as 5 or more years. In both person-centered planning and PBS, the individual's circle of support focuses on identifying events and circumstances in the past, present, and future environments that are relevant to the vision for the individual.

Ecological Validity   Ecological validity refers to whether support activities and interventions can readily be applied to real-life settings such as homes, schools, workplaces, and communities. A distinguishing feature of PBS is that the methods of gathering information about the individual and the resulting supports and interventions can be applied by parents, teachers, school personnel, and agency staff in typical environments (e.g., homes, schools, communities). This distinguishes the approach from those that only involve individuals who have been highly trained in advanced behavioral techniques (i.e., masters- and doctoral-level practitioners) and that typically occur in inpatient or outpatient clinic settings.

The use of person-centered planning as the framework for identifying the appropriate environments and for the behavior support plan development and implementation safeguards ecological validity. The structure and process of person-centered planning explicitly guarantee that the context of a person's life is always considered first and that professional perspectives are only as important as they are pragmatic for supporting the individual (Lyle O'Brien et al., 1997). In person-centered planning, support strategies are developed by the individuals with the most knowledge about the focus person and his or her daily issues or challenges. As a consequence, when strategies and supports are developed, they are far more likely to be ecologically relevant.

Stakeholder Participation Participation by stakeholders is critical to a PBS approach. *Stakeholders* are individuals who know the person well and have a stake in his or her success. The stakeholders may include parents, friends, neighbors, community members, teachers, administrators, agency support staff, and, of course, the focus person. PBS is built on the concept of developing effective, collaborative relationships among stakeholder participants. As a result, team building and team process activities are critical to PBS.

Therefore, PBS cannot be conceptualized as an "expert" model for addressing challenging behaviors. Individual PBS practitioners do not necessarily take the leadership role with an individual's team but, rather, collaborate to facilitate team processes that result in gathering information, developing a behavior support plan, and implementing the behavior support plan for the individual with challenging behaviors (Dunlap et al., 2000). Thus, although the PBS practitioner may be identified as being an expert on facilitating effective team processes, understanding behavior, and developing behavioral interventions, he or she also understands the necessity of involving stakeholders in the process. PBS practitioners have a responsibility not only to provide needed knowledge to the team, but also to ensure a framework for arriving at consensus regarding why the challenging behaviors occur and which supports may be necessary. As a result of this collaborative model, the team can be more responsive to the individual's expressed choices and preferences.

The PBS team members also assume a variety of roles that go beyond simply providing information. Stakeholders on the team become active participants in gathering necessary information; exploring community options; addressing physical, social, and environmental issues; and implementing the identified supports within typical environments.

The circle of support or person-centered team is often the basis for the stakeholder group that will develop and implement a PBS plan. In person-centered planning, the members in a circle of support gather because of their shared commitment to support an individual with disabilities through creative problem solving. As the circle of support members work together, their struggles and accomplishments further strengthen their relationships to each other and their commitment to the focus individual (Lyle O'Brien et al., 1997). The strength of these relationships and this commitment is instrumental to using PBS to address challenging behavior.

Social Validity   *Social validity* refers to various characteristics and outcomes that are consistent with PBS approaches and is defined as the social importance and practicality of behavioral interventions (Baer, Wolf, & Risley, 1968; Wolf, 1978). In particular, social validity addresses the following items noted by Carr and colleagues (2002):

- The desirability of the interventions (e.g., Do typical support people believe that the interventions are worthy of implementation?)
- The goodness of fit of the interventions (e.g., Do stakeholders agree that the strategies are appropriate for the specific context in which they are implemented?)
- The subjective effectiveness of the interventions with respect to challenging behavior and quality of life (e.g., Do stakeholders perceive that challenging behaviors have been reduced to an acceptable level and that the implemented strategies are making meaningful differences for the individual in typical community settings?)
- The practicality of the interventions (e.g., Can typical support people carry out the strategy?)

Thus, concern with social validity reflects a PBS emphasis on issues beyond simple behavior change, including critical issues that may be neglected in traditional efforts at decreasing challenging behavior. For instance, in a PBS approach, it is not sufficient to produce decreases in challenging behavior without planning to produce comprehensive lifestyle and quality of life changes. In other words, an individual's challenging behavior may decrease significantly, but PBS practitioners are still concerned about whether

- Such a change can be practically maintained within typical environments
- Stakeholders are comfortable with the procedures and will likely continue using them in the future
- Interventions match the individual's values and the variety of contexts within his or her life

• Team members believe that there has been or will be sufficient change in challenging behavior and quality of life outcomes

The nature of person-centered planning is to continually ask, "Are we making a difference?" Pursuing outcomes that are socially valid to stakeholders and the individual is central both to person-centered planning and to PBS. Therefore, the effectiveness of PBS is not measured solely by assessed changes in behavior, but also in terms of individual or family comments such as, "Life is more fun," and family or support provider statements such as, "He is happy," or "She's doing what she likes." These changes are consistent with valued outcomes in a person-centered planning approach. They are obtained in both person-centered planning and PBS approaches because the voice of the individual with a disability is amplified and the presumptive expertise of professionals is attenuated when discussing lifestyle issues.

Systems Change in Multicomponent Intervention PBS is based on the understanding that supporting individuals to improve their challenging behavior and quality of life must move from an emphasis on "fixing" the individual to fixing his or her environments. Because this broader emphasis moves beyond a focus on discrete behavior change, PBS must look at larger systems that affect the individual's behavior and lifestyle. For instance, within an educational context, the PBS approach would likely examine the classroom environment, instructional strategies, functions of an individual's challenging behavior, social relationships, and other issues. However, PBS would also consider larger systems-level issues such as overall classroom management strategies, schoolwide support strategies, district- and state-level policies and procedures, and funding sources that may influence the individual's ability to participate in an inclusive educational setting and achieve academic success. This broadening of attention to include systems issues points to the complexity of achieving and maintaining changes in behavior and quality of life. Multicomponent interventions are directed not only at an individual's challenging behaviors and the immediate environment, but also at the systems of support that need to change to better meet the individual's current and future needs.

Systems change is a logical process and an outcome of person-centered planning (Holburn & Vietze, 1998, 1999). As members in the circle of support begin to think outside the box and to develop creative solutions to persistent problems, the need for changes in systems is inevitable. Those changes may be simple (e.g., scheduling meals so that the individual can eat when hungry or after a favorite television show) or they may be significant (e.g., providing a companion for supported living instead of asking the individual to live in a home with two roommates who have disabilities). It is the nature of person-centered planning to tackle whatever may affect the individual's pursuit of his or her vision for a desirable life.

Emphasis on Prevention   PBS emphasizes skill building and environmental design as primary procedures for producing desirable change in behavior and the environment. In fact, preventive strategies for supporting one individual with challenging behavior may produce systemic change that has a broader impact on all children or adults who are supported by the system. Systemwide applications of PBS focus on creating flexible environments that promote appropriate behavior and provide preventive support for others who are at risk of developing challenging behavior and not achieving successful quality of life outcomes (Sugai et al., 2000).

Person-centered planning provides the framework for identifying prevention strategies. A primary goal of the person-centered planning process is to assist the individual in achieving his or her desired lifestyle. As a consequence, it is expected that the focus individual will be happier and feel more supported and will use challenging behavior less frequently to express his or her needs or wants. The changes in environments, activities, and structure that are developed through person-centered planning are likely to be very similar to the prevention strategies that would be identified through a behavior support process.

Flexibility with Respect to Scientific Practices   The science and technology of behavior change, or applied behavior analysis, are the foundation of PBS. In addition, person-centered philosophy and practicality are essential to the PBS approach to behavior change. As such, PBS continues to expand the assessment and evaluation of behavior change and quality of life. This move beyond direct observation (which is standard practice in science) incorporates the use of various assessment and evaluation approaches, including interviews, rating scales, team discussions, naturalistic observations, logs, and self-reports. This expansion of data collection approaches is consistent with PBS's 1) expanding valued outcomes from discrete behavior change to the individual's quality of life and 2) assessing the process of implementing behavioral support and its impact on the team and the system. Such processes may not be amenable to traditional scientific analyses and require an array of new approaches and tools.

Person-centered planning processes are deliberately more humanistic than scientific. However, this emphasis does not diminish the value or credibility of the impressions presented by the circle of support members as they discuss the individual's life and desired outcomes. Planning meetings offer a forum in which rich qualitative data can be collected for understanding challenging behavior, developing interventions, and assessing meaningful outcomes. Person-centered planning provides the depth of information about the individual's life contexts that is critical to developing an effective PBS plan.

Multiple Theoretical Perspectives Although a functional assessment of an individual's challenging behavior is important in PBS, a greater emphasis is placed on broad-level analyses (Carr et al., 2002). As the emphasis expands from an individual's behavior, to the environment, to team behavior, and to the behavior of systems, PBS continues to evolve in its assessment practices and to incorporate relevant practical and theoretical perspectives.

Person-centered planning offers a mechanism for understanding diverse perspectives from key individuals. Questions of interest often include the impact of intervention on the individual, the resulting changes in systems (e.g., the family system, the support system, the work culture), and changes that have occurred in service policy and provision as a result of person-centered planning. Thus, person-centered planning offers exemplary qualitative assessment practices, which mesh well with PBS approaches that begin to identify and address issues at the molecular level (behavior) and expand to the molar level (systems and policies).

Intervention Strategies The intervention strategies that have been and will continue to be used within a PBS approach are consistent with its life-span perspective, commitment to ecological and social validity, and stakeholder involvement. Intervention strategies will continue to be provided in typical community settings such as homes, schools, workplaces, and communities. As a result, intervention agents may not be highly credentialed experts in the field but, rather, parents, friends, community members, teachers, and other typical support agents who are already available in the community of support. Because supports are provided by typical people in typical environments, the implementors also must consider that support strategies and interventions developed must also be acceptable in those environments. Behavior support strategies continue to reflect appropriate practices in the field but acknowledge the fact that best practices consist of support strategies that are understandable, applicable by diverse support personnel, and acceptable to the community and support providers. For instance, support approaches within a classroom that are both effective and practical include environmental changes, curriculum modifications, instructional presentation changes, and other typical classroom and teaching approaches. PBS interventions generally do not include rigorous scientific methodologies and complex interventions that cannot be implemented within typical environments and routines by teachers or other school personnel.

When PBS is integrated with person-centered planning, the efficacy of the behavior support strategies and their fit within the individual's routines and lifestyle are discussed by the person-centered planning team. For example, members of the circle of support might say that the behavior support plan is cumbersome and difficult to implement. Thus, person-centered planning not only lays the foundation for identifying effective behavior support interventions but also, as an ongoing process, is an ideal vehicle for evaluating and modifying PBS interventions.

CONCLUSION: FUTURE DIRECTIONS

It has been our experience that embedding the process of PBS into person-centered planning enhances the quality and effectiveness of behavioral support. As indicated in the previous section, person-centered planning offers a framework for achieving the essential elements of PBS. Although it is certainly possible to form a distinct team for the development and implementation of PBS, the process is deeply enriched by the structure, commitment, and creativity of established person-centered planning teams.

In many ways, we are advocating for the marriage of PBS methods and person-centered planning. Although it will always be possible to conduct person-centered planning without integrating PBS (i.e., when the individual does not have challenging behavior), we believe that PBS is always enhanced by person-centered planning. Person-centered planning ensures that the individual's desires are always represented, that behavior support efforts consider the diverse perspectives of the focus person and others who are closest to the person, and that intervention strategies result in meaningful lifestyle outcomes.

Implications for Research

Our call for a more clear and widespread marriage of person-centered planning and PBS approaches provides numerous opportunities for future research. Because person-centered planning and PBS both emphasize broad lifestyle outcomes, it follows that research on more effective approaches to measuring those outcomes is essential. In their review of PBS for people with developmental disabilities, Carr and colleagues (1999) found that lifestyle change was a stated goal for only slightly more than 10% of participants in published studies, and only 2.6% of the studies (involving a total of six participants) measured changes in lifestyle. Lifestyle changes were documented anecdotally for four of the six participants; quantitative data were provided to document the lifestyle changes for two participants. If PBS supporters continue to advocate for using person-centered planning to address broader lifestyle issues, then innovative research practices that are aimed at quantifying those outcomes will be necessary.

Although initial behavior change and some lifestyle outcomes can be measured in the early stages of PBS and person-centered planning processes, only longitudinal studies of outcomes are likely to address the maintenance and generalization of behavior change as well as long-term quality of life changes. Thus, research evaluating the effectiveness of PBS and person-centered planning must consider outcomes that may not be obtained for months or years, even after person-centered planning and PBS are complete. Longitudinal research is also necessary to identify the factors that are critical to the success and failure of person-centered planning and PBS.

As person-centered planning processes grow in number and use, there is also a need for research that addresses the development of person-centered planning processes that are uniquely matched to the needs and characteristics of the individual and the systems of support. Most practitioners who utilize PBS within a person-centered planning framework realize that different situations may be more amenable to one person-centered planning approach than to others. Indeed, practitioners who are competent in person-centered planning also realize that its techniques can and should be adapted to every situation. However, research and practice offer little guidance about the essential features of person-centered planning that actually promote the changes and outcomes discussed in this chapter. In other words, what makes person-centered planning work and how can it be made more effective?

Implications for Professional Practice

The marriage of PBS and person-centered planning has important implications for practitioners in the field. Relatively few professionals have been exposed to person-centered planning and even fewer are able to initiate and facilitate a person-centered planning process. Although person-centered planning is becoming increasingly visible in the literature, few personnel preparation programs include the ability to facilitate person-centered planning as a professional competency.

A related concern pertains to the ability of professionals to implement the process of PBS as it has been described in the literature (Dunlap et al., 2000; Schwartz, 1997; Singer, 2000; Snell, 1997). The 1997 amendments to the Individuals with Disabilities Education Act (IDEA; PL 105-17) mandate the use of PBS components such as functional behavioral assessment and positive behavior interventions. This mandate has led to efforts to offer training in PBS, but the number of professionals who are fluent in PBS remains limited.

As training programs begin to examine how to prepare professionals in person-centered planning and PBS, program developers must use caution. Person-centered planning and PBS were developed as nontraditional efforts to assist individuals with disabilities to achieve a quality lifestyle and meaningful outcomes (Horner et al., 1990; Lyle O'Brien et al., 1997). These processes could be compromised if participants come to the table to fulfill a mandated obligation rather than to think creatively and to problem-solve in support of the individual with challenging behavior. The values base of both person-centered planning and PBS must be respected because it is paramount to the success of each approach (Dunlap et al., 2000; Lyle O'Brien et al., 1997).

In addition to concerns related to training and personnel preparation, there are also serious implications for service systems that seek to adopt person-centered planning and PBS approaches. The issue of most importance is the tendency for any service system to compromise person-centered planning and PBS due to an inability to adopt the philosophies and to allocate adequate resources for true implementation of either or both approaches (Holburn & Vietze, 1998, 1999).

Person-centered planning and PBS require changes in how individual professionals and entire systems think and act. This process of change is difficult for any structured and bureaucratic support system and is also difficult for the professionals who comprise such a system. Both person-centered planning and PBS require significant changes in the functioning of teams and their individual members (Holburn & Pfadt, 1998). In particular, the roles of professionals who have significant input into behavioral concerns (i.e., psychologists, behavior analysts) may change significantly. These professionals may find themselves as change agents or facilitators of the person-centered planning and PBS processes. This change necessitates expanded areas of expertise for the "behavior expert," from only addressing behavioral concerns to also addressing broader quality of life issues and the entire team process. However, such a role expansion may actually produce better practice outcomes for the behavior expert: He or she may be better able to address the broad environmental factors that affect the individual's behavior and the systems and interpersonal factors that affect the team's functioning.

Although professionals, consumers, and agencies may become excited by the potential positive outcomes that person-centered planning and PBS can produce, a final concern that affects professional practice must be mentioned. The values underlying both approaches may have an impact on all children and adults supported by service systems. For instance, choice, positive approaches to addressing behavior, self-determination, and other values inherent in person-centered planning and PBS may have far-reaching effects on the services, supports, and funding provided to individuals, families, and agencies. Thus, it may seem that PBS and person-centered planning should be provided to all individuals who have support needs. However, the enthusiasm that accompanies these approaches must be tempered with the realities of scarce resources (Holburn & Vietze, 1999). Not all individuals need or desire their own person-centered plan or PBS process, and no system can be expected to authentically implement these processes for each consumer given the available time, personnel, and fiscal resources. System administrators must be very thoughtful about how to expand the underlying values of person-centered planning and PBS to all consumers while still preserving the integrity of true, individualized person-centered planning and PBS for those consumers who can benefit most from these positive and effective processes.

REFERENCES

Albin, R.W., Lucyshyn, J.M., Horner, R.H., & Flannery, K.B. (1996). Contextual fit for behavior support plans: A model for "goodness of fit." In L.K. Koegel, R.L. Koegel, & G. Dunlap (Eds.), *Positive behavioral support: Including people with difficult behavior in the community* (pp. 81–98). Baltimore: Paul H. Brookes Publishing Co.

Baer, D.M., Wolf, M.M., & Risley, T.R. (1968). Some current dimensions of applied behavior analysis. *Journal of Applied Behavior Analysis, 1*, 91–97.

Carr, E.G., Dunlap, G., Horner, R.H., Koegel, R.L., Turnbull, A.P., Sailor, W., Anderson, J.L., Albin, R.W., Koegel, L.K., & Fox, L. (2002). Positive behavior support: Evolution of an applied science. *Journal of Positive Behavior Interventions, 4*, 4–16, 20.

Carr, E.G., Horner, R.H., Turnbull, A.P., Marquis, J., Magito-McLaughlin, D., McAtee, M.L., Smith, C.E., Anderson-Ryan, K., Ruef, M.B., & Doolabh, A. (1999). Positive behavior support for people with developmental disabilities: A research synthesis. *Monographs of the American Association on Mental Retardation.*

Dunlap, G., Fox, L., Vaughn, B.J., Bucy, M., & Clarke, S. (1997). In quest of meaningful perspectives and outcomes: A response to five commentaries. *Journal of The Association for Persons with Severe Handicaps, 22*, 221–223.

Dunlap, G., Hieneman, M., Knoster, T., Fox, L., Anderson, J., & Albin, R. (2000). Essential elements of inservice training in positive behavior support. *Journal of Positive Behavior Interventions, 2*, 22–32.

Forest, M., & Lusthaus, E. (1989). Promoting educational equality for all students: Circles and Maps. In S. Stainback, W. Stainback, & M. Forest (Eds.), *Educating all students in the mainstream of regular education* (pp. 43–57). Baltimore: Paul H. Brookes Publishing Co.

Fox, L., Dunlap, G., & Buschbacher, P. (2000). Understanding and intervening with children's challenging behavior: A comprehensive approach. In S.F.

Warren & J. Reichle (Series Eds.) & A.M. Wetherby & B.M. Prizant (Vol. Eds.), *Communication and language intervention series: Vol. 9. Autism spectrum disorders: A transactional developmental perspective* (pp. 307–332). Baltimore: Paul H. Brookes Publishing Co.

Holburn, S., & Pfadt, A (1998). Clinicians on person-centered planning teams: New roles, fidelity of planning and outcome assessment. *Mental Health Aspects of Developmental Disabilities, 1*(3), 82–86.

Holburn, S., & Vietze, P. (1998). Has person-centered planning become the alchemy of developmental disabilities? A response to O'Brien, O'Brien, and Mount. *Mental Retardation, 36*(1), 485–488.

Holburn, S., & Vietze, P. (1999). Acknowledging barriers in adopting person-centered planning. *Mental Retardation, 37*(2), 117–124.

Horner, R.H., Dunlap, G., Koegel, R.L., Carr, E.G., Sailor, W., Anderson, J., Albin, R.W., & O'Neill, R.E. (1990). Toward a technology of "nonaversive" behavioral support. *Journal of The Association for Persons with Severe Handicaps, 15,* 125–132.

Individuals with Disabilities Education Act Amendments of 1997, PL 105-17, 20 U.S.C. §§ 1400 *et seq.*

Kincaid, D. (1996). Person-centered planning. In L.K. Koegel, R.L. Koegel, & G. Dunlap (Eds.), *Positive behavioral support: Including people with difficult behavior in the community* (pp. 439–465). Baltimore: Paul H. Brookes Publishing Co.

Koegel, L.K., Koegel, R.L., & Dunlap, G. (Eds.). (1996). *Positive behavioral support: Including people with difficult behavior in the community.* Baltimore: Paul H. Brookes Publishing Co.

Lyle O'Brien, C., O'Brien, J., & Mount, B. (1997). Person-centered planning has arrived . . . or has it? *Mental Retardation, 35,* 480–484.

Meyer, L.H., & Evans, I.M. (1993). Science and practice in behavioral interventions: Meaningful outcomes, research validity, and usable knowledge. *Journal of The Association for Persons with Severe Handicaps, 18,* 224–234.

Mount, B. (1987). *Personal futures planning: Finding directions for change* (Doctoral dissertation, University of Georgia). Ann Arbor: University of Michigan Dissertation Information Service.

Mount, B., & Zwernik, K. (1988). *It's never too early, it's never too late: A booklet about personal futures planning* (Publication No. 421-88-109). St. Paul, MN: Metropolitan Council.

O'Brien, J. (1987). A guide to life-style planning: Using The Activities Catalog to integrate services and natural support systems. In B. Wilcox & G.T. Bellamy, *A comprehensive guide to The Activities Catalog: An alternative curriculum for youth and adults with severe disabilities* (pp. 175–189). Baltimore: Paul H. Brookes Publishing Co.

O'Brien, J., & Lyle, C. (1987). *Framework for accomplishment.* Lithonia, GA: Responsive Systems Associates.

O'Brien, J., Mount, B., & Lyle O'Brien, C. (1990). *The personal profile.* Lithonia, GA: Responsive Systems Associates.

O'Neill, R.E., Horner, R.H., Albin, R.W., Storey, K., Sprague, J.R., & Newton, J.S. (1997). *Functional assessment of problem behavior: A practical assessment guide.* Pacific Grove, CA: Brooks/Cole Thomson Learning.

Pearpoint, J., O'Brien, J., & Forest, M. (1993). *PATH (Planning Alternative Tomorrows with Hope): A workbook for planning positive futures.* Toronto: Inclusion Press.

Schwartz, I.S. (1997). It is just a matter of priorities: A response to Vaughn et al. and Fox et al. *The Journal of The Association for Persons with Severe Handicaps, 22,* 213–214.

Singer, G. (2000). Ecological validity. *Journal of Positive Behavior Interventions, 2,* 122–124.

Smull, M., & Burke Harrison, S. (1992). *Supporting people with severe reputations in the community.* Alexandria, VA: National Association of State Mental Retardation Program Directors.

Snell, M.E. (1997). Parent–professional partnerships, the critical ingredient: A response to Vaughn et al. and Fox et al. *The Journal of The Association for Persons with Severe Handicaps, 22,* 218–220.

Sugai, G., Horner, R.H., Dunlap, G., Hieneman, M., Lewis, J.L., Nelson, C.M., Scott, T., Liaupsin, C., Sailor, W., Turnbull, A.P., Turnbull, H.R., Wickham, D., Wilcox, B., & Ruef, M. (2000). Applying positive behavior support and functional behavioral assessment in schools. *Journal of Positive Behavior Interventions, 2*(3), 131–143.

Vandercook, T., York, J., & Forest, M. (1989). The McGill Action Planning System (MAPS): A strategy for building the vision. *Journal of The Association for Persons with Severe Handicaps, 14,* 205–215.

Wolf, M.M. (1978). Social validity: The case for subjective measurement or how applied behavior analysis is finding its heart. *Journal of Applied Behavior Analysis, 11,* 203–214.

3

The Confluence of Person-Centered Planning and Self-Determination

Michael L. Wehmeyer

Since the early 1990s, the self-determination construct has become a focal point for designing supports in disability services, from education to adult services provision. In fact, it is now possible to refer to the self-determination movement in the same historical sense as the independent living movement or the normalization movement. These movements represent efforts to operationalize and widely implement core values, beliefs, or philosophies that were, in essence, organizing principles on which to base service delivery. Such values have included the importance of independence, the opportunity to live in and experience one's community, and to experience the rich routine of daily life. The self-determination movement fundamentally involves efforts to operationalize the societal value for personal control.

This chapter provides an overview of self-determination's application in the lives of people with severe disabilities. It examines the ways in which planning to achieve self-determination has occurred and discusses issues in the relationship between person-centered planning and self-determination. The chapter title's image of a river's confluence is purposeful—not to suggest that person-centered planning and self-determination are two different rivers that need to join but, instead, to suggest directions for person-centered planning that expand it to promote and enhance self-determination. Other works have focused on incorporating the values and processes from person-centered planning into student-directed planning (Wehmeyer & Sands, 1998; Wehmeyer, Sands, Knowlton, & Kozleski, 2002), but this chapter primarily examines the implications for person-centered planning.

THE TRIBUTARIES OF SELF-DETERMINATION: AN HISTORICAL OVERVIEW

Several sources have reviewed the emergence of the focus on self-determination in disability services (Nerney & Shumway, 1996; Ward, 1996; Ward & Kohler, 1996; Wehmeyer, 1998). The focus on self-determination emerged from and, in fact, was predicated on changes in societal views of disability, the disability rights and independent living movements, and the application of the principle of normalization to adult services. Ward (1996) acknowledged the importance of the disability rights movement to the self-determination movement, noting that the emergence of the disability rights movement as what Driedger (1989) called the " 'last civil rights' " movement aligned the struggle of people with disabilities for equality and equal protections with previous civil rights movements in labor, for women's suffrage and gender equity, and for people of color—most notably the struggle of African Americans in the 1950s and 1960s. Ward noted that the "concepts of the right to integration and meaningful equality of opportunity stressed by other civil rights groups, as well as the methods and tactics utilized, were adopted by disability rights efforts" and that leaders in this movement, such as Ed Roberts, "emphasized the connection between the struggle of other minorities for equality and the marginal status of people with disabilities" (1996, p. 6).

These themes in turn led to the emphasis on self-help and group organizing, both key elements of the independent living movement and, more recently, the self-advocacy movement. That the focus on self-determination in disability services had its genesis in these movements is evidenced by the fact that the earliest call for self-determination as it applied to people with disabilities appeared in a chapter by Bengt Nirje in Wolf Wolfensberger's now-classic 1972 text on the principle of normalization. Nirje's chapter, "The Right to Self-Determination," began

> One major facet of the normalization principle is to create conditions through which a handicapped person experiences the normal respect to which any human being is entitled. Thus the choices, wishes, desires, and aspirations of a handicapped person have to be taken into consideration as much as possible in actions affecting him. To assert oneself with one's family, friends, neighbors, co-workers, other people, or vis-à-vis an agency is difficult for many persons. It is especially difficult for someone who has a disability or is otherwise perceived as devalued. But in the end, even the impaired person has to manage as a distinct individual, and thus has his identity defined to himself and to others through the circumstances and conditions of his existence. Thus, the road to self-determination is both difficult and all important for a person who is impaired. (1972, p. 177)

Despite outdated language, Nirje's chapter has a contemporary feel in its depiction of the core values and principles of self-determination. First, Nirje clearly articulated the importance of self-determination for *all* people, excluding neither people with mental retardation nor people with other disabilities. Nirje equated self-determination with the respect and dignity to which all people are entitled; moreover, he recognized that people define themselves, and others define them, by the circumstances and conditions of their existence. An analysis of Nirje's chapter to determine the actions, beliefs, and opportunities that describe *self-determination* reflects the same breadth and scope seen in the literature today. Nirje identified the salient features of self-determination to be making choices, asserting oneself, self-management, self-knowledge, decision making, self-advocacy, self-efficacy, self-regulation, autonomy, and independence, although he often did not use those terms. Nirje emphasized the importance and right of people with mental retardation having personal control in their lives. Although efforts to promote self-determination seem to have different focal points in the field today (e.g., changing funding streams and systems for managing money; teaching students with disabilities to become more effective problem solvers, decision makers, or goal setters), these efforts essentially attempt to ensure personal control.

At the same time that Nirje was discussing self-determination, Perske was calling for the opportunity for people with mental retardation to experience the "dignity of risk":

> The world in which we live is not always safe, secure and predictable. . . . Every day that we wake up and live in the hours of that day, there is a possibility of being thrown up against a situation where we may have to risk everything, even our lives. This is the way the real world is. We must work to develop every human resource within us in order to prepare for these days. To deny any person their fair share of risk experiences is to further cripple them for healthy living. (1972, p. 199)

These calls to action by Nirje and Perske emphasized the universal importance of control over decisions and choices that affect one's quality of life. Thus, one can identify the value of personal control as a recognition of human dignity and worth, as well as the importance of such efforts to ensure a better quality of life, as overarching themes or values inherent in efforts to promote and enhance self-determination. Furthermore, these themes resonate with and illustrate the connections between self-determination and empowerment, which constitute yet another value underlying the focus on self-determination. Appropriately, the term *empowerment* is usually associated with social movements and is typically used, as Rappaport stated, in reference to actions that "enhance the possibilities for people to control their lives" (1981, p. 15). Individuals with disabilities have unequivocally understood self-determination as a form of empowerment (Kennedy, 1996; Ward, 1996). In a speech at the National Conference on Self-Determination, an event organized in 1989 by the U.S. Department of Education's Office of Special Education Programs (Ward, 1996), Robert Williams effectively captured this link between self-determination and empowerment:

> But, without being afforded the right and opportunity to make choices in our lives, we will never obtain full, first class American citizenship. So we do not have to be told what self-determination means. We already know that it is just another word for freedom. We already know that self-determination is just another word for describing a life filled with rising expectations, dignity, responsibility, and opportunity. That it is just another word for having the chance to live the American Dream. (1989, p. 16)

These principles—the value for personal control, the emphasis on improving quality of life, and the emphasis on empowerment—underlie efforts to promote self-determination, either at the level of ensuring that children and youth with disabilities receive an educational program that enables them to become more self-determined or at the level of ensuring that adults with disabilities achieve greater personal control over resources, services, and supports. The means to achieve these outcomes has differed, mostly because of the nature of the tasks (education versus health/residential/employment services) and, of particular relevance to this chapter, because two planning processes have been employed to achieve these outcomes. Although adult services provision has incorporated person-centered planning as a key strategy to achieve the outcome that people control resources, education has implemented self-directed or student-directed planning as the process by which self-determination is promoted and enhanced.

Student-Directed Planning

Historically, the educational experiences of most students, particularly students with disabilities, have not reflected a value for self-determination (Wehmeyer, 1998). Students have been recipients of instructional programs that are almost uniformly teacher delivered and based on plans and decisions made by others, including teachers, parents, administrators, school board members, and state legislators. There is no doubt in the minds of most students who is in control when they are in school. Sarason described the typical classroom as such:

> Our usual imagery of the classroom contains an adult who is "in charge" and pupils who conform to the teacher's rules, regulations and standards.

> If students think and act in conformity to the teacher's wishes, they will learn what they are supposed to learn. (1990, p. 78)

In special education services and supports, this situation began to change with the passage of the Individuals with Disabilities Education Act (IDEA) of 1990 (PL 101-476), which required the individualized education program (IEP) to include transition services for all students age 16 and older who receive special education services. IDEA also mandated student involvement in transition planning, stating that needed transition services must be based on student preferences and interests. This emphasis on the primacy of student involvement in the transition planning process spurred an emphasis in educational services to promote the self-determination of students with disabilities. Although the IDEA mandates do not state as such, the clear intent of the student-involvement language in IDEA is to ensure that students with disabilities have a meaningful voice in the process that is used to make decisions about their future. Wehmeyer and Ward (1995) argued that the student-involvement language places IDEA's intent and spirit in line with consumer choice, participatory planning, and empowerment language in civil rights legislation (e.g., the Americans with Disabilities Act [ADA] of 1990, PL 101-336).

IDEA's student-involvement language has resulted in a growing number of processes and resources designed to promote active student involvement in education and transition planning (Wehmeyer & Sands, 1998). In fact, in many cases the involvement of students with disabilities in their educational planning and decision-making process has become the fulcrum for efforts to promote self-determination. For example, one of the earliest and most widely used curricular packages to promote self-determination was the ChoiceMaker program (overviewed in Martin & Marshall, 1996), which promotes self-determination through student self-management of the IEP process. The ChoiceMaker Self-Determination Transition Curriculum (Martin & Marshall, 1995) consists of three sections: 1) Choosing Goals, 2) Expressing Goals, and 3) Taking Action. Each section contains two to four teaching goals and numerous teaching objectives that address six transition areas. The package includes an assessment tool, lessons on choosing personally valued goals, lessons on taking action to achieve those goals, and a planning process titled the Self-Directed IEP. This component provides teacher and student materials that focus on enabling the student to chair his or her own IEP meeting. Through instruction and practice, students learn 11 steps for running their own IEP (see Table 3.1); then, they chair their own IEP meeting.

The ChoiceMaker materials, specifically The Self-Directed IEP, are examples of the emphases on planning in education to promote or

Table 3.1. Eleven steps for transition planning from the ChoiceMaker program

Step	Activity
1	Begin the meeting by stating the purpose.
2	Introduce everyone.
3	Review past goals and performance.
4	Ask for others' feedback.
5	State your school and transition goals.
6	Ask questions if you don't understand.
7	Deal with differences in opinion.
8	State the support you will need.
9	Summarize your goals.
10	Close meeting by thanking everyone.
11	Work on IEP goals all year.

From Martin, J.E., & Marshall, L.H. (1996). ChoiceMaker: Infusing self-determination instruction into the IEP and transition process. In D.J. Sands & M.L. Wehmeyer (Eds.), *Self-determination across the life span: Independence and choice for people with disabilities* (pp. 215–236). Baltimore: Paul H. Brookes Publishing Co.; adapted by permission.

enhance self-determination. Most such processes embody similar features. First, these efforts emphasize student control over the process itself, even to the extent of chairing the IEP meeting. Second, there is emphasis on preparing students to take an active role in setting goals that are included in the IEP, particularly as they pertain to transition-related outcomes. Third, these processes emphasize self-advocacy skills to employ in the course of the meeting. Finally, the processes emphasize ongoing student self-regulation and self-monitoring of progress on goals.

Self-Determination and Person-Centered Planning

Person-centered planning processes share common beliefs and attempt to put those shared beliefs into a planning framework. Schwartz, Jacobson, and Holburn (2000) used a consensus process to define *person-centeredness*. This effort provided a useful picture of the values underlying person-centered planning as it exists at the beginning of the 21st century. Specifically, Schwartz and colleagues identified eight "hallmarks" of a person-centered planning process:

1. The person's activities, services, and supports are based on his or her dreams, interests, preferences, strengths, and capacities.

2. The person and people important to him or her are included in lifestyle planning and have the opportunity to exercise control and make informed decisions.

3. The person has meaningful choices, with decisions based on his or her experiences.

4. The person uses, when possible, natural and community supports.

5. Activities, supports, and services foster skills to achieve personal relationships, community inclusion, dignity, and respect.

6. The person's opportunities and experiences are maximized, and flexibility is enhanced within existing regulatory and funding constraints.

7. Planning is collaborative and recurring and involves an ongoing commitment to the person.

8. The person is satisfied with his or her relationships, home, and daily routine.

There is no question that at this point in time, most practitioners view the promotion and enhancement of self-determination as both a core value of and an anticipated outcome from person-centered planning. Indeed, efforts to promote self-determination through adult services have identified as a key strategy the implementation of person-centered planning. Given the hallmarks of person-centered planning that Schwartz and colleagues identified, it is not hard to see why person-centered planning and self-determination are viewed as closely related, if not synonymous.

However, a side-by-side examination of person-centered planning processes and student-directed or self-directed planning processes suggests differences—not so much in the values evident in the process, as those are virtually identical, but in the priority assigned to those values. To some degree, the ingredients to these two processes are the same, but they are mixed differently, with varying proportions of each value reflected in each respective process. For example, person-centered planning has always emphasized the role of significant others in planning, whereas student-directed planning processes have emphasized building student capacity to set or track goals or to make decisions.

Although it is inaccurate to draw too stark a contrast between the two processes or to imply that every instance of person-centered planning differs from every instance of student-directed planning, there is evidence that the different values for various components of planning have differential effects on promoting self-determination. Cross, Cooke, Wood, and Test (1999) examined the effects of two planning processes on the self-determination of adolescents with disabilities: 1) a person-centered approach, MAPS (Making Action Plans, formerly known as the McGill Action Planning System; Pearpoint, Forest, &

O'Brien, 1996) and 2) the previously discussed ChoiceMaker process. Both processes resulted in enhanced self-determination (as measured by student-report and teacher-report indicators), but the ChoiceMaker process, which includes the Self-Directed IEP process, had a greater overall effect. The generalizability of the study's findings was limited by sample size (five students per group), and both processes were beneficial for students. However, because it focuses the student-directed process on capacity building, it appeared that ChoiceMaker is more beneficial in promoting self-determination.

A number of variables likely account for why the self-directed planning and person-centered planning processes emphasize different components. One variable is the individuals with whom these processes have been implemented. Person-centered planning emerged from efforts to plan for individuals with significant cognitive, developmental, or multiple disabilities who often lived in institutional environments. Most student-directed planning processes have focused on students with mild levels of impairment.

In using the metaphor of a confluence between person-centered planning and self-determination, I am not implying that person-centered planning does not already value self-determination or does not already promote or enhance self-determination. Because both person-centered and self-directed planning processes share the value of promoting self-determination, however, it may be useful to examine self-directed planning processes to see how person-centered planning might more effectively promote self-determination.

POINT OF CONFLUENCE: TOWARD PERSON-CENTERED, SELF-DIRECTED PLANNING

One of the key issues to consider is who is responsible for plan making. Who is or should be the plan maker in efforts to enhance self-determination? With certain caveats (see Wehmeyer, 1998), the person for whom the services and supports are being designed should ultimately be the plan maker. What does that mean for individuals who cannot engage in plan making because of age or limitations imposed by the severity of their disability? Does this mean that they cannot be "self"-determined and that others should plan for them? Clearly, the misinterpretation of *self-determination* as being synonymous with *doing it yourself* is a barrier for many people with more significant disabilities. In other words, some people believe that unless one can independently make complex decisions or solve difficult problems, one cannot be self-determined. However, Wehmeyer (1998) argued that the capacity to make complex decisions, solve complex problems, or engage in any of the skills and knowledge-based activities that enable one to better exert control over one's life is secondary in importance for self-determination to being the causal agent in one's life and making things happen in accordance with one's preferences, wants, needs, and interests. Rousso provided an excellent example of how exerting control in one's life and independent performance are often decoupled:

> I know a sculptor who is quadriplegic. She sculpts by giving precise instructions to her assistants, who serve as her hands. While it is tempting to think that her assistants are the true artists, she is, in fact, the sculptor in charge. When she has given the same directions to two assistants who have had no contact with each other, they both produce identical pieces of sculpture. Through the experience of disability, this woman has learned to articulate her vision and her needs in direct, specific ways—so much so, that she gets precisely the help she needs in forms that are replicable. (1997, p. 134)

Wehmeyer (1998) suggested that this is equally true for individuals with significant cognitive impairments. Such impairments limit the types and complexity of skills a person can perform. If the person remains at the center of the decision-making process (e.g., decisions are made based on the person's preferences and interests and the person has a voice in the decision-making process), however, he or she does not need to be able to independently make the decisions. Being self-determined does not mean that one does everything for oneself. For most adults, plan making takes into account the needs, interests, and preferences of many others (e.g., spouse, significant other, children, parents, friends, co-workers). In many such cases, decision making is a group process, whether making a decision as a family about what vacation to take or a work group making a decision about a specific work activity or objective. This fact is central in person-centered planning and at least implied in most self-directed planning processes. The emphasis is on interdependence, not independence, and planning activities encourage active involvement of key stakeholders. Indeed, many family-directed planning models embody the same intent. Levitz and Fowler described a family-directed process in which "both the student and parent(s) or guardian(s) are involved in the process" (2000, p. 7).

Nonetheless, this does not mitigate the need to do everything possible to ensure that it is the person, to the greatest extent feasible, who is the plan maker. Whether or not each of us typically includes others in our own plan-making process, we reserve the fundamental right to disregard that information if we want to pursue a highly preferred goal that others may not value. For example, adolescents often have to "rebel" against their parents to pursue their own dreams, sometimes successfully and sometimes not. A person-centered planning process centers on the person's dreams and visions, then the team carries out a plan to achieve those dreams and visions. The person's cognitive ability or other limitations may serve as barriers to that person's communicating those dreams or may limit the types and numbers of experiences enabling him or her to understand the scope and breadth of options available. In such cases, it becomes necessary to piece together that dream and vision with the input of individuals who are closest to the person.

Wehmeyer and colleagues (2002) suggested that this visioning process is one of two components of person-centered planning that should be incorporated into most student-directed or self-directed planning processes. (The other component is the meeting itself being informal and user-friendly.) Within the person-centered planning process, considerable value is given to identifying and documenting—often through elaborate (and creative!) formats—the individual's dream and vision, as well as those of his or her family members.

However, describing the dream or vision of another person, as is often necessary in planning for people with the most significant disabilities, introduces the possibility that the dream or vision represents the other person's dreams more than those of the person for whom planning is occurring. A similar concern exists in determining the preferences of people with significant cognitive disabilities. Interviewing significant others about their perceptions of the person's preferences is an important component in supporting choice making, but there is a need to go beyond that step by implementing additional ways to more objectively evaluate preferences through direct observations or systematic evaluations of preferences (see Wehmeyer, Agran, & Hughes, 1998, for examples from the literature). The point is not that parents, family members, or friends purposefully subjugate the individual's dreams with their own but that it can be very difficult to make an external determination of a person's dreams, however well one knows that person. As such, there is a need to consider what checks and balances can be put in place to provide a mechanism for ensuring that the person's dreams and visions drive the system.

Moreover, in most cases of person-centered planning, determining a person's dream or vision leads directly to designing a plan of action to achieve that dream or vision. That plan quite often consists of the provision of opportunities to achieve the vision (e.g., opportunities for inclusion, opportunities to exert greater control) as well as the design of supports needed to take advantage of those opportunities. Those supports often take the form of accommodations to mitigate the impact of the disabling condition on the person's capacity to take advantage of the opportunity. The 1992 American Association on Mental Retardation manual defined *supports* as

> Resources and strategies that promote the interests and causes of individuals with or without disabilities; that enable them to access resources, information and relationships inherent within integrated work and living environments; and that result in their enhanced interdependence, productivity, community integration, and satisfaction. (Luckasson et al., 1992, p. 101)

It is the case, then, that education and instruction in areas that enable people to become more self-determined—such as decision making or problem solving—are supports in that they enable people to gain access to resources, information, and relationships that enhance independence and integration. Although self-directed planning processes probably focus too much on teaching skills that are related to self-determination, person-centered planning processes may sometimes overlook the importance of teaching as a support. Providing opportunities to exert control are important but probably are not sufficient. If individuals are to actually achieve greater control over their lives, then it is important to provide 1) opportunities to exert control and make choices, 2) the supports and accommodations needed, and 3) the experiences to extend existing and learn new skills and knowledge that are related to exerting control. The fact that most student-directed or self-directed planning processes have this capacity-enhancement focus is not surprising, as these have emerged from educational efforts to promote self-determination, and education is a capacity-building enterprise. The mission of schools is to enhance knowledge and skills leading to effective citizenship, self-reliance, and self-sufficiency. Likewise, it is not surprising that person-centered planning processes emphasize opportunity enhancement and accommodations—many people working with individuals with significant disabilities are skeptical about adopting "flow-through" models of service delivery, in which individuals must achieve certain prerequisite skills before moving to the next level or step. Historically, the emphasis on skills attainment as a prerequisite for community inclusion has relegated people with the most significant disabilities to segregated settings (e.g., sheltered workshops, group homes) and limited their progression into more normative, community-based experiences.

However, legitimate concerns about creating a "flow-through" model of self-determination must be balanced with the seemingly self-evident fact that providing opportunities and supports alone is unlikely to enable people to become as self-determined as possible. Napoleon Bonaparte is credited with stating, "Ability is of little account without opportunity." However, it is also worth noting that in many circumstances, opportunity is of little account without ability. That is, if professionals and stakeholders do not do whatever they can to better prepare and enable people to exert control more effectively and to take more responsibility for plan making, then they limit the likelihood that people will succeed when opportunity comes knocking. This does not imply an emphasis on the ability to master certain skills as a prerequisite to taking more control; instead, it suggests that individuals are better able to control their own lives if they are provided both the opportunity to do so and the supports to improve their capacity to respond to that opportunity.

By focusing on building the capacity to self-determine (as well as providing opportunities and designing accommodations), professionals and stakeholders also address the previously identified concern about suppressing the person's dream by supplanting others' dreams for that person. A means is put into place to check the legitimacy of the visioning process by ensuring that part of the action plan emerging from person-centered planning is to promote skills and knowledge related to areas such as problem solving, decision making, goal setting, self-advocacy, self-regulation, self-management, and self-knowledge. More accurately, perhaps, a mechanism is put into place to better enable people, through successful experiences, to refine and individualize those visions and dreams and to make them known to others.

For better or worse, the focus on self-determination in education has been largely on developing curricular materials that address the needs of youth with less severe cognitive disabilities or other disabilities. The result has been that teachers who work with students with more significant cognitive or developmental disabilities tend not to see such activities as feasible for their students, and there are fewer strategies to promote skills related to self-determination for youth with more significant disabilities (Wehmeyer, Agran, & Hughes, 2000). However, there are numerous ways to promote the skills and abilities related to self-determination for individuals with more significant disabilities (see Wehmeyer et al., 1998, for a comprehensive overview). One can, for example, apply the principle of maximal participation to learning a complex process such as decision making, goal setting, or problem solving. Some individuals may not be able to be fully independent in any of these activities, but there are steps in each of these skills that people with significant disabilities can master and, as a result, exert greater control over the process.

PROCESSES THAT MERGE
PERSON-CENTERED, SELF-DIRECTED PLANNING

The remainder of the chapter highlights two processes that have been designed to merge person-centered planning and the self-directed planning processes seen in education settings. They are meant to illustrate possibilities. The two efforts also demonstrate the struggle of researchers at the Beach Center on Disability at The University of Kansas to incorporate principles of person-centered planning into student- and self-directed planning processes.

Group Action Planning

The Group Action Planning (GAP) process was developed by Turnbull, Blue-Banning, and colleagues (1996) to enable adolescents with severe cognitive and multiple disabilities to be more actively involved in transition planning and decision making. With funding from the U.S. Department of Education, these researchers set out to merge what was best practice in student-directed planning within a person-centered planning context. Their method focused on actively involving students to maximally participate in their transition program and planning process. Turnbull, Blue-Banning, and colleagues noted that although the focus of GAP was consistent with student-directed planning's emphasis on enabling young people to direct the process, it was accomplished within the following fundamental characteristics:

1. Actively invite people who can be helpful to participate in a reciprocal and interdependent manner.
2. Create a context of social connectedness and caring among all participants.
3. Foster dynamic and creative problem solving fueled by great expectations.
4. Continuously affirm and celebrate the progress that is being made.

One factor that distinguishes GAP from traditional person-centered planning processes is that students who are involved in the process are enrolled in a high school course in self-determination, through which they receive individualized instruction in areas such as decision making or self-advocacy. Moreover, an "action group" is formed for each student; this group enables the student to express, practice, and benefit from his or her newly developing self-determination related skills (Turnbull, Blue-Banning, et al., 1996, p. 240). This action group forms the planning and decision-making team that works with the student to plan for his or her future. The student's role in the process varies according to student preferences, but he or she is actively involved in developing goals for the action plan through the school course. Thus, the capacity-enhancement process is linked directly to planning activities. Like most person-centered planning processes, the action group assembled in the

GAP process meets frequently or as often as necessary; the meetings are convened in comfortable, nonthreatening environments and emphasize community inclusion and participation.

GAP has been implemented widely (see Turnbull & Turnbull, 2000, for an overview; see Turnbull, Turbiville, Schaffer, & Schaffer, 1996, and Turnbull & Turnbull, 1996, for more process detail). For example, Blue-Banning, Turnbull, and Pereira (2000) examined GAP's responsiveness to youth and young adults with disabilities from Hispanic backgrounds and their families.

It's My Future! Planning for What I Want in My Life

The GAP process, on the one hand, bears a family resemblance to person-centered planning processes while embodying some key aspects of student-directed planning. *It's My Future! Planning for What I Want in My Life* (Bolding & Wehmeyer, 1999), on the other hand, more closely resembles student- or self-directed processes with key components of person-centered planning incorporated. Briefly, *It's My Future!* is a self-directed planning process designed for use by adults with cognitive and developmental disabilities. The process provides opportunities for individuals to identify personal abilities and interests and acquire skills in decision making, goal setting and small-group communication so that they are better prepared to take an active, meaningful role in their habilitation planning process. The *It's My Future!* process is designed with the person with the disability as the intended end user. Support personnel are provided recommendations for enabling individuals to self-direct the process.

Many components of *It's My Future!* resemble the types of activities in student- or self-directed planning processes. For example, individuals working through the process are introduced to a five-step decision-making process called DO IT!, which they learn by making decisions about potential recreation and leisure goals that they might want to pursue. The steps to the DO IT! process are listed in Table 3.2.

Participants also learn more about the goal-setting process, their rights and responsibilities, leadership skills, effective communication skills, how to negotiate to achieve a desired outcome, and other skills and knowledge that are aimed at enhancing their capacity to direct both planning and implementation. However, *It's My Future!* differs from more traditional self-directed planning programs in that the process is based on the outcome of an exercise titled "What is my Dream?" The exercise begins by the person selecting the primary support person in the process, learning about who must be involved in the planning process, and identifying who else he or she wants involved. Like person-

Table 3.2. Steps in the DO IT! process

D	**D**efine your problem.
O	**O**utline your options.
I	**I**dentify the outcome of each option.
T	**T**ake action.
!	Get excited!

From Bolding, N.L., & Wehmeyer, M.L. (1999). *It's my future! Planning for what I want in my life.* Silver Spring, MD: The Arc of the United States; adapted by permission.

centered planning processes, *It's My Future!* emphasizes active and meaningful involvement of parents, family members, friends, and other key stakeholders. The dreaming or visioning process in *It's My Future!* centers around the development of a Life Visions Book.

As with person-centered planning, this planning process occurs over frequent meetings or sessions. In the *It's My Future!* process, however, those meetings are structured around the self-paced sessions, without an emphasis on having all team members present for every meeting. In fact, the person him- or herself determines who needs to be at which meeting or session. The Life Visions Book is constructed as the individual addresses questions about his or her life dreams, interests, abilities, and supports, as well as the resources that are available to him or her. The Life Visions Book is often graphically based and represents dreams about where to live and work; who to spend time with; what learning or educational activities to pursue; and subjects such as hobbies, pets, travel desires, and transportation needs. Moreover, the individual uses the decision-making and goal-setting processes to design action plans that achieve self-selected goals, which are also entered in the Life Visions Book, along with means to record progress toward those goals. The latter item reflects the emphasis in the process on self-monitoring.

It is anticipated that many people with mental retardation (for whom the process was developed) will need considerable support across all activities, and the goal of the process is not to become independent in goal setting or decision making. Instead, the goal is to provide a framework that is unambiguously person directed and places the individual in the driver's seat for planning, decision-making, and goal-attainment activities. Pilot testing of the process suggested that because the participants' reading skills varied considerably, facilitators (e.g., people supporting the participants in the planning process) often had to adapt the process, most commonly by condensing and consolidating some sessions to reduce repetition and hold the interest of the participants. Facilitators emphasized key concepts rather than a word-for-word reading of each entire session, and they simplified language to help increase participants' comprehension.

Interviews of support staff and participants during and after the process provide some examples of the value of including capacity enhancement in a context of person-centered planning and some pitfalls to be aware of as well. Support personnel at almost all pilot sites gave high marks to the Life Visions Book for capturing participants' interest and attention, being useful for participants to immediately record their interests and ideas, and giving participants a way to more easily communicate their interests and desires to those at their planning meeting, as well as to family, friends, and support staff.

One benefit communicated by support staff was that participants learned more about decision-making, problem-solving, and goal-setting skills than anticipated, and they were more capable of heading up their own planning meeting than expected. *It's My Future!* was developed as a self-directed process to give the individual control over planning; however, when capacity enhancement is introduced in the planning process, there is a need to ensure that support staff do not just assume the role of "teacher" and thus exert unwarranted power and control over the person's life.

When asked to share their insights and stories about the process, support staff placed a great deal of value on the Life Visions Book. One respondent stated, "What amazed me the most was that many of the participants who I have known for years had dreams and aspirations and interests that I had never been aware of." Another support person said, "Most of the consumers I spoke with said how good they felt when completing the program. They seemed more self-assured and confident." Support staff also commented on changes in the way in which participants perceived themselves and their ability to take more control. One staff person stated, "Some were surprised that they had the 'powers' or ability to say more or take more control of their staff meetings and could ask anyone they wanted to be there. I heard a lot of '. . . really?' "

An interesting finding was that when participants responded to queries about their satisfaction with the process, they tended to emphasize the value of setting their own goals and making their own decisions. Participants generally pointed to their Life Visions Book as an important outcome of the process, but they also usually articulated pride in their goal-setting achievements or in their capacity to "learn what I want to do," "lead my meeting," or "show people about my goals."

CONCLUSION

The examples in this chapter have illustrated attempts to merge person-centered planning with self-directed planning. My work has focused on getting those who plan the delivery of education services to incorporate characteristics of person-centered planning into student-directed planning. Yet, there is also benefit in enhancing person-centered planning by incorporating aspects of self-directed planning to better support and enhance self-determination. Given that promoting self-determination is a core value of person-centered planning, it seems worth the effort to examine the capacity-building aspects of self-directed planning processes to ensure that both opportunity and capacity are supported.

REFERENCES

Americans with Disabilities Act (ADA) of 1990, PL 101-336, 42 U.S.C. §§ 12101 *et seq.*

Blue-Banning, M.J., Turnbull, A.P., & Pereira, L. (2000). Group Action Planning as a support strategy for Hispanic families: Parent and professional perspectives. *Mental Retardation, 38,* 262–275.

Bolding, N.L., & Wehmeyer, M.L. (1999). *It's my future! Planning for what I want in my life.* Silver Spring, MD: The Arc of the United States.

Cross, T., Cooke, N.L., Wood, W.W., & Test, D.W. (1999). Comparison of the effects of MAPS and ChoiceMaker on student self-determination skills. *Education and Training in Mental Retardation and Developmental Disabilities, 34,* 499–510.

Driedger, D. (1989). *The last civil rights movement: Disabled Peoples' International.* New York: St. Martin's Press.

Individuals with Disabilities Education Act (IDEA) of 1990, PL 101-476, 20 U.S.C. §§ 1400 *et seq.*

Kennedy, M.J. (1996). Self-determination and trust: My experiences and thoughts. In D.J. Sands & M.L. Wehmeyer (Eds.), *Self-determination across the life span: Independence and choice for people with disabilities* (pp. 37–49). Baltimore: Paul H. Brookes Publishing Co.

Levitz, B.G., & Fowler, J.T. (2000). *Family-directed transition planning guide.* Westchester, NY: Westchester Institute for Human Development.

Luckasson, R., Coulter, D.L., Polloway, E.A., Reiss, S., Schalock, R.L., Snell, M.E., Spitalnick, D.M., & Stark, J.A. (1992). *Mental retardation: Definition, classification, and systems of supports.* Washington, DC: American Association on Mental Retardation.

Martin, J.E., & Marshall, L.H. (1995). ChoiceMaker: A comprehensive self-determination transition program. *Intervention in School and Clinic, 30,* 147–156.

Martin, J.E., & Marshall, L.H. (1996). ChoiceMaker: Infusing self-determination instruction into the IEP and transition process. In D.J. Sands & M.L.

Wehmeyer (Eds.), *Self-determination across the life span: Independence and choice for people with disabilities* (pp. 215–236). Baltimore: Paul H. Brookes Publishing Co.

Nerney, T., & Shumway, D. (1996). *Beyond managed care: Self-determination for people with disabilities.* Durham: University of New Hampshire.

Nirje, B. (1972). The right to self-determination. In W. Wolfensberger (Ed.), *Normalization: The principle of normalization* (pp. 176–200). Toronto: National Institute on Mental Retardation.

Pearpoint, J., Forest, M., & O'Brien, J. (1996). MAPS, Circles of Friends, and PATH: Powerful tools to help build caring communities. In S. Stainback & W. Stainback (Eds.), *Inclusion: A guide for educators* (pp. 67–86). Baltimore: Paul H. Brookes Publishing Co.

Perske, R. (1972). The dignity of risk. In W. Wolfensberger (Ed.), *Normalization: The principle of normalization in human services* (pp. 194–200). Toronto: National Institute on Mental Retardation.

Rappaport, J. (1981). In praise of a paradox: A social policy of empowerment over prevention. *American Journal of Community Psychology, 9,* 1–25.

Rousso, H. (1997). Seeing the world anew: Science and disability. In N. Kreinberg & E. Wahl (Eds.), *Thoughts and deeds: Equity in mathematics and science education* (pp. 131–134). Washington, DC: American Association for the Advancement of Science.

Sarason, S.B. (1990). *The predictable failure of educational reform: Can we change course before it's too late?* San Francisco: Jossey-Bass.

Schwartz, A.A., Jacobson, J.W., & Holburn, S. (2000). Defining person-centeredness: Results of two consensus methods. *Education and Training in Mental Retardation and Developmental Disabilities, 35,* 235–258.

Turnbull, A.P., Blue-Banning, M.J., Anderson, E.L., Turnbull, H.R., Seaton, K.A., & Dinas, P.A. (1996). Enhancing self-determination through Group Action Planning: A holistic emphasis. In D.J. Sands & M.L. Wehmeyer (Eds.), *Self-determination across the life span: Independence and choice for people with disabilities* (pp. 237–256). Baltimore: Paul H. Brookes Publishing Company.

Turnbull, A.P., Turbiville, V., Schaffer, R., & Schaffer, V. (1996). Getting a shot at life through Group Action Planning. *Zero to Three, 16*(6), 33–40.

Turnbull, A.P., & Turnbull, H.R. (1996). Group Action Planning as a strategy for providing comprehensive family support. In L.K. Koegel, R.L. Koegel, & G. Dunlap (Eds.), *Positive behavioral support: Including people with difficult behavior in the community* (pp. 99–114). Baltimore: Paul H. Brookes Publishing Co.

Turnbull, A.P., & Turnbull, H.R. (2000). *Families, professionals and exceptionality: Collaborating for empowerment.* Columbus, OH: Charles E. Merrill.

Ward, M.J. (1996). Coming of age in the age of self-determination: A historical and personal perspective. In D.J. Sands & M.L. Wehmeyer (Eds.), *Self-determination across the life span: Independence and choice for people with disabilities* (pp. 1–16). Baltimore: Paul H. Brookes Publishing Co.

Ward, M.J., & Kohler, P.D. (1996). Teaching self-determination: Content and process. In L.E. Powers, G.H.S. Singer, & J. Sowers (Eds.), *On the road to autonomy: Promoting self-competence in children and youth with disabilities* (pp. 275–290). Baltimore: Paul H. Brookes Publishing Co.

Wehmeyer, M.L. (1998). Self-determination and individuals with significant disabilities: Examining meanings and misinterpretations. *Journal of The Association for Persons with Severe Handicaps, 23,* 5–16.

Wehmeyer, M.L., Agran, M., & Hughes, C. (1998). *Teaching self-determination to students with disabilities: Basic skills for successful transition.* Baltimore: Paul H. Brookes Publishing Co.

Wehmeyer, M.L., Agran, M., & Hughes, C. (2000). A national survey of teachers' promotion of self-determination and student-directed learning. *Journal of Special Education, 34,* 58–68.

Wehmeyer, M.L., & Lawrence, M. (1995). Whose future is it anyway? Promoting student involvement in transition planning. *Career Development for Exceptional Individuals, 18,* 69–83.

Wehmeyer, M.L., & Sands, D.J. (Eds.). (1998). *Making it happen: Student involvement in education planning, decision making, and instruction.* Baltimore: Paul H. Brookes Publishing Co.

Wehmeyer, M.L., Sands, D.J., Knowlton, H.E., & Kozleski, E.B. (2002). *Teaching students with mental retardation: Providing access to the general curriculum.* Baltimore: Paul H. Brookes Publishing Co.

Wehmeyer, M.L., & Ward, M.J. (1995). The spirit of the IDEA mandate: Student involvement in transition planning. *Journal of the Association for Vocational Special Needs Education, 17,* 108–111.

Williams, R.R. (1989). Creating a new world of opportunity: Expanding choice and self-determination in lives of Americans with severe disability by 1992 and beyond. In R. Perske (Ed.), *Proceedings from the National Conference on Self-Determination* (pp. 16–17). Minneapolis: University of Minnesota, Institute on Community Integration.

II

Changes in Organizational Culture

4

Using Person-Centered Supports to Change the Culture of Large Intermediate Care Facilities

Jerry A. Rea, Carolyn Martin, and Kasey Wright

Parsons State Hospital and Training Center (PSH&TC) has moved from being a residential training center for children with epilepsy to a residential center for adults with mental retardation and severe behavior problems. In 2000, PSH&TC served 198 individuals with intellectual disabilities. There are 11 residential buildings, with 8–20 people residing in each living unit. Ninety percent of these individuals also have a mental illness (as defined by the *Diagnostic and Statistical Manual of Mental Disorders, Fourth Edition* [DSM-IV]; American Psychiatric Association, 1994). Almost one third of these individuals receive medication to control behaviors, and 10% are on restrictive behavior programs. People come to reside at PSH&TC when community agencies are unable to support them due to their challenging behaviors. The majority of the individuals admitted from 1989 to 1999 engaged in challenging behaviors.

Many changes have increased the quality of services for individuals who live at PSH&TC. The first efforts were aimed toward developing more humane treatment and were based on a psychiatric model (Bair, 1958). This model did not fully meet the educational and rehabilitation needs of children, but it was an improvement over the earlier conception of mental retardation as an incurable disease which required only custodial care. Later, attempts were made to change the culture by introducing programs based on operant principles (Girardeau & Spradlin, 1964; Lent, LeBlanc, & Spradlin, 1970).

The authors thank Gary Daniels, Superintendent of Parsons State Hospital and Training Center, for his leadership and vision during this transformation process. We acknowledge our appreciation and immense respect for all of the qualified mental retardation professionals and other support staff at Parsons State Hospital and Training Center who have made this change effort possible. Also, we thank Kathryn Saunders, Joseph Spradlin, and Pat White for their insightful comments and editorial assistance.

In the mid-1980s, the enforcement of Health Care Financing Administration (HCFA; now known as the Centers for Medicare & Medicaid Services) regulations of active treatment brought about major changes in institutional practices. Both operant and active treatment models were based on a philosophy of rehabilitation. Although each of these movements brought about various temporary (and some permanent) improvements in living conditions, neither resulted in a culture that focused on meeting the desires, values, and expectations of individuals.

This chapter presents a retrospective review of our attempts since 1989 to change the culture of PSH&TC to person-centered support services. The chapter presents data that demonstrate an increase in job choices and a reduction in the use of restrictive procedures. In addition, it describes the use of person-centered planning to eliminate a contingent electrical shock program and to reduce the use of restraints for a woman with challenging behaviors.

THE HABILITATION MODEL OF THE 1980s

In 1989, the facility served 266 individuals. Habilitation was the primary clinical model from the 1980s through early 1991. Mental retardation and associated disabilities were viewed as conditions to be remediated through programming. Program services were primarily facility based and prescribed by staff. A driving force for the habilitation model was the HCFA guidelines for active treatment standards in intermediate care facilities. Professional assessments identified the strengths and deficits of individuals, with deficits prioritized from least to most debilitating. Treatment efforts focused predominantly on altering the most debilitating deficits through behavioral teaching programs.

To remediate deficits, professional staff established schedules for each individual. Activities were planned throughout the day so staff could teach new skills or maintain existing skills that allowed an individual to move to a less restrictive environment. For instance, a treatment team might have required an individual to learn vocational skills in the wood shop with the belief that these skills would facilitate moving into the community. Teams seldom considered input from the person regarding preferences (e.g., whether he or she enjoys working with wood, hates noisy environments, prefers sedentary work). Teams seldom asked whether the job fit the person's values. Professional staff made decisions with little regard for the individual's desired lifestyle, leaving the person with little control over his or her life.

Individuals who did not want to participate in their scheduled activities often became noncompliant. Opposition to staff directives frequently included challenging behaviors such as aggression. Treatment teams often responded by writing behavior programs that specified reinforcement for compliance, concurrent with extinction procedures for noncompliance. If challenging behaviors, such as aggression, continued and placed the individual or others at risk for injury, then aversive behavior reduction strategies were implemented.

Motivation System and Compliance Objectives

One strategy used to encourage individuals to participate in their assigned activities was a facility-wide token economy. The Teaching Family Model (Phillips, Phillips, Fixsen, & Wolf, 1972) was used to teach prosocial behaviors to individuals with mild cognitive impairments. Staff delivered points when individuals displayed appropriate prosocial behaviors such as accepting critical feedback, following instructions, or being polite. Points were also given for participation in scheduled activities such as household chores or attending family conferences. Points were exchanged for preferred objects or activities (e.g., special outings, decreased supervision, favorite foods, a late bedtime on the weekend). Points and privileges were lost (response–cost) for displays of challenging behaviors or for not following the assigned schedule. To monitor the staff's program implementation, we collected quality assurance data on staff behaviors such as keeping groups on schedule, delivering clear teaching instructions, and reinforcing appropriate behaviors. These data indicated that for the most part, clients were engaged in scheduled activities and interactions were positive.

With the deficit model, individuals who showed resistance to staff directives were considered noncompliant. Staff frequently targeted compliance training objectives for individuals who resisted following staff instructions. The expectation for compliance was often specified as a prosocial training objective linked to the token economy motivation system.

Centralized Vocational, Dietary, Leisure, and Transportation Services

Services from the vocational, dietary, leisure, and transportation departments were centralized, and department heads administered clinical control. The vocational director created jobs without considering what was important to the individuals. Professional staff selected worksite assignments; most worksites grouped individuals who lived together. Vocational training objectives focused on reinforcing appropriate work behaviors (e.g., compliance, staying on task). If the person did not demonstrate acceptable work behaviors, then restrictive strategies targeting inappropriate behaviors were implemented. For example, suspension from work or the loss of privileges might be the consequence of noncompliance.

Meals were served in a large cafeteria at three fixed times each day. Menus were established without input from individuals or staff about food preferences. Cooking and meal preparation skills (e.g., cooking, grocery shopping, menu planning) were seldom taught in the living units.

Leisure services were administered by the directors of the art, music, and recreational therapy departments. Leisure staff were assigned to living units, and they implemented programs that were developed by their department supervisors. Participation in leisure "zones" (classes that taught leisure skills) was a major programming component for individuals with mild cognitive disabilities. Leisure staff determined zones with little input from these individuals.

Transportation services were centralized. All vehicles were maintained in a central parking lot. Requests for the use of vehicles required multiple levels of approval, with the final determination made by the director of transportation. Requests had to be submitted as much as a week in advance, even for local trips.

CHANGING THE APPROACH: PERSON-CENTERED SUPPORTS

People without disabilities have a great deal of control over what they do with their lives. People with disabilities often lack such control. In seeking to change this discrepancy, a number of consultants such as Michael Smull, Michael Mayer, and Thomas Coval helped us to rethink how we provide services. Our perspective has changed from prescribing professionally driven treatment programs to identifying and creating person-centered services. This change has involved decentralizing services to increase flexibility and individualization. The role of treatment teams has evolved from trying to "fix" the person to asking the individual and the people who know and care about that person how that individual wants to live his or her life. The following section describes changes in our program philosophy and service provision that began in late 1991 and have continued through 2002. These changes have occurred without staff or budget increases.

Decentralization of Vocational, Dietary, Leisure, and Transportation Services

We began identifying which aspects of work were important to individuals and consequently reallocated resources to fit those values. Instead of placing people in worksites, we developed work opportunities based on each person's preferences for type of work; work schedule (e.g., full or part time, morning or afternoon); work conditions (e.g., location, noise level, number of people); and characteristics of co-workers, supervisors, or staff. Individuals were encouraged to sample different jobs and were allowed to quit these jobs without consequences other than the natural consequence of monetary loss. Instead of acting out to get time off from work, an individual was encouraged to request a vacation. Direct support staff who knew the individuals well helped each person choose vocational options. This help was especially important for identifying and interpreting preferences for individuals with limited communication.

We gradually began cooking all meals in the living units and eliminated dining in the cafeteria. This transition took approximately 15 months. We wanted to create a more personalized environment, to better satisfy individual meal preference, and to create more teaching opportunities during cooking and mealtimes.

Leisure services were decentralized and staff were challenged with a new mission of moving from group-oriented leisure activities to individual leisure interests. Rather than using "programs" that were developed by department heads and implemented by living-unit leisure staff, the latter were now responsible for identifying each individual's leisure interests. Staff assessed whether the person preferred learning skills related to an activity or simply wanted to participate in it. For example, one individual may have wanted to learn bicycle road safety rules so she could ride her bike to the store. Another individual might have been interested in bike riding only as a form of exercise to lose weight, without a desire or need to learn the safety rules. Support for this second person would have included ensuring that staff were available as companions for daily bike rides. Yet another person may have required adaptive devices or staff assistance. For instance, one individual had a severe physical disability and was unable to operate a bike independently. Based on other activities that he enjoyed, however, his support team believed that he might enjoy the fresh air and movement of bicycle rides. The team decided to support his participation by adapting a bicycle to transport him as a passenger.

Previously, the centralized vehicle pool of the transportation department lacked flexibility to meet individual needs. These services were decentralized by assigning a vehicle to each living unit. This allowed greater flexibility to meet individual choices and respond to impromptu leisure opportunities.

Elimination of Compliance Objectives

Compliance objectives, which targeted a generalized compliance response to staff instructions, were eliminated. These programs were designed to eliminate noncompliance and other aberrant behaviors. Often the noncompliance was motivated by avoidance or escape. As a result, these programs required compliance responses with little utility for the individual because of the context in which the request was made. For example, interrupting someone during a pleasurable activity, such as watching a favorite TV show, and then requiring the person to comply with a staff directive, such as setting the table, is aversive. Thus, staff inadvertently created aversive conditions that people wanted to avoid or escape.

Rather than expecting individuals to comply with all staff directives, we began looking at the context in which instructions were delivered. As a first step, teams were asked to identify specific situations in which compliance was necessary, typically for health and safety reasons. These situations were considered nonnegotiable. For all other situations, when individuals resisted requests, the staff were asked to consider the context of the request to determine whether compliance was necessary (e.g., Why the person was resisting? Was health or safety in jeopardy if the person did not comply?). If staff determined that compliance was necessary, they were encouraged to work with the individual to develop methods that made completing these tasks more pleasant. For instance, a woman who once refused gynecological exams kept her appointments and allowed the exams to be conducted once she was allowed to select the person who accompanied her to the exams and was paid for completing them.

Advocacy

Attorney Thomas Coval[1] conducted a workshop for staff on the right to risk. His message was that too often people who live in an intermediate care facility are overprotected. He pointed out that in their everyday lives, people without disabilities often engage in activities that have some element of risk. In these situations most people consider the

[1]We gratefully acknowledge the expertise and training that Thomas Coval provided. Correspondence concerning the right to risk in human services should be addressed to Thomas Coval, 809 North Eastson Road, Willow Grove, PA 19090.

element of risk and what actions would minimize the risk. To do this at PSH&TC, we helped individuals consider the degree of risk associated with activities, then supported them through teaching the necessary skills and/or providing other supports to minimize risk.

One such example involved Pam, who had become prediabetic. Pam enjoyed vending machine food and soda, both of which have high sugar and fat contents. Her physician believed that Pam would become diabetic if she continued to eat and drink these items in such large quantities. Carrying her own money was also very important to Pam. Rather than restricting access to her money, Pam was involved in problem-solving discussions with her support team. Through these discussions, Pam learned how much she could spend on food and drinks and still maintain safe blood sugar levels. Pam, her doctor, and her support team agreed to check Pam's blood sugar on a monthly basis. During this time, Pam continued carrying her money. At her request, staff accompanied her when shopping and helped her learn to make better choices when buying from vending machines. Over the course of several months, Pam lowered her blood sugar and lost weight. Her support team took a risk, but a monitoring system enabled an evaluation of the effectiveness of their supports.

We also began asking staff to serve as "champions" or "buddies" (Mount, 1994). The champions served as advocates, speaking on behalf of individuals who were uncomfortable about or unable to speak or advocate for themselves. The champion attended meetings during which discussions about the person occurred, and they worked directly with the team to achieve the lifestyle and/or services that were compatible with the person's preferences. Not all champions were assigned by the staff. Some individuals selected a person who knew them well; others had people who volunteered to serve as a champion when the need arose.

In November 1994, Michael Mayer presented a workshop on the role of champions (Mayer, 1997). He stressed that the staff's responsibility was to do more than just protect individuals. Instead, they were to help people stay safe and healthy while the individuals learned to make informed choices by considering options and natural consequences. Champions took active roles in teaching choice-making skills through consideration of the risks, responsibilities, and options that were present during choice-making situations. Champions could also stage "safe" situations in which individuals could learn these abilities. Mayer suggested using "confederates" (staff whom the individual did not know) to minimize and monitor risks as part of the teaching process. For example, when a person began riding a bus independently, a confederate could be planted on the route to assist the person if necessary.

Modification of the Motivation System

With the exception of a few individuals, the token response–cost system was eliminated throughout the facility. Instead of attempting to control unwanted behaviors through a token response–cost system, staff were instructed to listen to individuals and attempt to meet requests through negotiation, rationale, and compromise. This shift was accomplished through in-service sessions and discussions with teams, staff, and individuals living at PSH&TC. Treatment teams continued to use token response–cost systems with a few individuals. In these instances, teams decided the procedures were warranted after balancing rights with safety concerns.

Focus discussions with residents and staff at PSH&TC were held to identify what would make the facility a better place to live. The members of these groups agreed on ways to try to meet resident requests while balancing staff obligations to keep the residents healthy and safe. During in-service sessions, we provided the conceptual framework to person-centered services and explained why we were eliminating the response–cost and token economy system. We also provided examples to foster collaboration and problem solving rather than to control behaviors through the loss of privileges and points.

Essential Lifestyle Planning

As part of the cultural change process, Michael Smull began training staff in Essential Lifestyle Planning (ELP; Smull & Burke Harrison, 1992). The ELP process promotes the view that individuals with disabilities do not need repair; instead, the systems in which they live need repair to meet lifestyle preferences. It is important to understand that an Essential Lifestyle Plan itself is not the important outcome; rather, it is listening to how the individual wants to live and then helping him or her achieve that lifestyle.

Even modest changes can enrich the quality of life for an individual. For example, through the ELP process, a team discovered the importance of cultural identity for an African American woman who was nonverbal and had a severe disability. Previously, staff kept her healthy and safe, but they did not place much emphasis on her cultural identity. This oversight was not discovered until the team used the ELP process as a tool to listen, observe, and interpret what she valued. The team noticed her enjoyment while watching the TV program *Thea* on the Black Entertainment Television cable network and her differential eye gazes at African American staff. Various things were encouraged to support the woman's cultural identity. She began attending an African American church, and staff volunteered to take her to a community-wide African

American celebration. Staff decorated her room with African American art, and they made sure that she had opportunities to watch *Thea* and had her African American doll with her at bedtime. They ensured that her relationship with preferred African American staff was maintained by organizing staff schedules to support her preferences.

Due to the complexity and the time involved in the ELP process, we prioritized the development of plans for individuals who were preparing to move out, complained verbally or through challenging behaviors, or had limited communication skills. These individuals were given priority because the changes in our service philosophy enabled most verbal individuals to meet their preferences through self-advocacy.

Essential Lifestyle Planning Credentialing Program and Peer Reviews

Smull developed a credentialing program for ELP facilitators. Trained facilitators taught and mentored new facilitators in developing Essential Lifestyle Plans. This process ensured that facilitators were able to 1) develop plans that reflected how individuals wanted to live; 2) create plans to support those preferences; 3) identify issues to be resolved, such as conflicts between preferred lifestyle choices and health and safety issues; and 4) build support strategies that reconciled differences between lifestyle choices and health and safety issues. An ELP peer review committee was formed as a strategy to maintain the integrity of the plans. This committee, composed of credentialed facilitators, reviewed the Essential Lifestyle Plans to ensure that facilitators identified and addressed their essential components.

Smull and Burke Harrison (1992) proposed that when individuals with disabilities engage in noncompliant or other challenging behaviors, they are telling others that something is wrong with the system (i.e., they are engaging in nonverbal complaining). Moreover, they contend that when systems do not support desired lifestyles, individuals learn to rely on extraordinary displays of challenging behaviors to be heard. When these "inappropriate" behaviors escalated at PSH&TC, a typical response was to develop more restrictive behavior control programs while drastically limiting lifestyle options. Smull and Burke Harrison (1992) proposed that rather than setting goals to control behavior, staff should listen and respond to individual lifestyle preferences, then work to accommodate choice while maintaining a safe and healthy environment. As we implemented these changes, the need for restrictive behavioral procedures (e.g., emergency physical restraints, restrictive behavior reduction programs) to maintain safe, healthy environments diminished.

JOB OPPORTUNITIES
AND RESTRICTIVE PROCEDURES

Having an enjoyable job is an important lifestyle preference for many individuals. We believed that if job opportunities were increased, the need for restrictive control procedures would decrease. Thus, we collected data in three particular areas.

Definitions

Data were collected on 1) jobs, 2) emergency physical restraints, and 3) restrictive behavior reduction procedures. Each item is defined next.

Jobs   A *job* was defined as a specific task that is completed for payment during a payroll period. Some jobs consisted of only a few hours of work per week; however, the majority of jobs consisted of 30–40 work hours per week. A few individuals were employed at more than one job during the year. The data were collected at the end of each year by counting the total number of jobs performed by all residents during the last payroll period of each year.

Emergency Physical Restraints   An *emergency physical restraint* was 1 second or more of limb immobilization to restrict an individual's movement. Staff could physically restrain a person who was attacking someone else or hurting him- or herself 1) when the person or others were in immediate danger or 2) as a last resort after other efforts were ineffective in stopping the behavior. For example, if an individual physically attacked another person and was unresponsive to verbal redirection by staff, then staff might have held the individual's arm or even held the individual on the floor until the individual was calm. Excluded from this definition were 1) physical prompts for a correct response during a teaching task (e.g., guiding a hand to pick up a glass) and 2) restraints that were implemented as part of an approved behavior reduction program (i.e., programmatic restraints). Restraint data were collected 24 hours per day, 7 days per week. Because PSH&TC census data decreased during the 1990s, data were calculated in percentages. A percentage measure was derived by taking the monthly count of the number of individuals who received an emergency physical restraint and dividing it by the average number of individuals at the facility for the month.

Restrictive Behavior Reduction Procedures   *Restrictive behavior reduction procedures* involved the application of an aversive stimulus or the removal of a reinforcer contingent on a target behavior. To ensure the individuals' safety and rights, PSH&TC policy required safeguards and supervision for programs that included these procedures.[2] Approved restrictive procedures had been demonstrated to be effective with a low probability of harm in published research (see Axelrod & Apsche, 1983) and were recognized as acceptable in the clinical community (e.g., response–cost, restitution, time-out, overcorrection, sensory reduction, aversive stimulation). As with emergency physical restraints, data were calculated in percentages. The percentage measure was derived by taking the number of individuals at the end of each year who were on a restrictive behavior reduction program and dividing it by the average number of individuals at the facility in December.

Review of Longitudinal Data

Figure 4.1 indicates the number of jobs performed during each year and the percentage of individuals who received an emergency physical restraint each month. Jobs and emergency physical restraints are depicted on the same graph to demonstrate the increase of choice opportunities through jobs and its relationship to reduced emergency physical restraints. During the multiyear baseline, the number of jobs performed was 14. The percentage of individuals who received an emergency physical restraint was variable and reached a peak of 31%. During this time, the mean percentage of individuals who received an emergency restraint was 25% (range 17%–31%).

When we began restructuring vocational services, the number of jobs performed increased to 27, almost a 100% increase from baseline. The percentage of individuals who received an emergency physical restraint began a downward trend during this period. The mean percentage of individuals who received a restraint during this phase was 17% (range 12%–23%), a 32% decrease from baseline.

In 1994, as we continued efforts to expand our vocational supports, we also began to revise the motivation system. The systemwide token economy system and response–cost components were replaced by helping individuals learn to make informed choices. When confronted with challenging behaviors, staff were encouraged to try to understand what the individual wanted to communicate. Staff were also encouraged to support individual preferences through negotiation and compromise when possible. As Figure 4.1 demonstrates, the num-

---

[2]The use of any of these strategies required a written individualized behavior program specifying use of the procedure. Approvals from the individual, his or her parent and/or guardian, his or her treatment team, and a facility behavior peer review committee were required before any of these restrictive strategies could be implemented. More restrictive strategies, as categorized within our defined hierarchy, required additional prior approval from Parsons State Hospital and Training Center's human rights review committee and the superintendent of the facility.

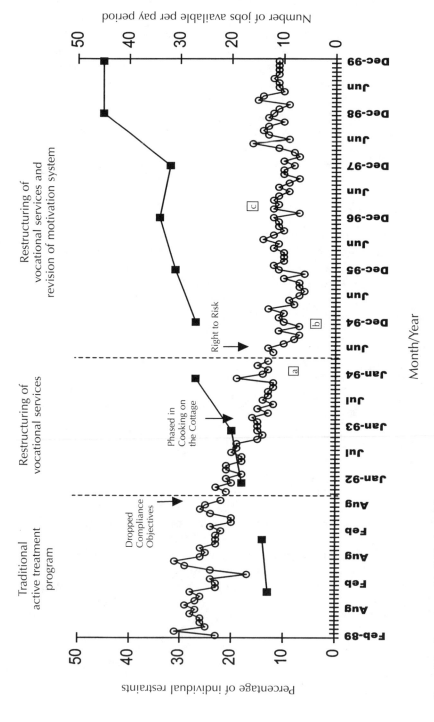

Figure 4.1. Percentage of individuals receiving an emergency physical restraint and the number of jobs performed. (*Key:* ○ = emergency restraints; ■ = number of jobs; a = restructuring and philosophical change in the leisure department [January 1994]; b = implementing the use of champions/buddies [November 1994]; c = decentralization of the transportation department [April 1997].)

ber of jobs performed in this last phase reached a peak of 45. This change represents a 320% increase from baseline and a 160% increase from the previous phase. During the first months of this phase, a downward trend began in the percentage of people restrained, with subsequent rates of emergency physical restraints remaining relatively low but variable. The mean percentage of people who received an emergency physical restraint dropped from 17% during the "restructuring vocational services" phase to 10% (range 10%–16%) during the "restructuring vocational services and revising the motivation system" phase. This represents a 68% reduction from baseline and a 41% reduction from the previous phase.

Figure 4.1 indicates an inverse relationship between September 1991 and October 1994: As the number of jobs increased, the use of emergency physical restraints decreased. It is important to note that emergency physical restraints were not simply replaced by more restrictive behavior reduction procedures. Figure 4.2 shows that the percentage of individuals with planned restrictive behavior reduction procedures peaked at 22% in 1990, then decreased to a low of 10% in 1999. This indicates the decrease in emergency restraints was not due to an increase in the use of restrictive behavior reduction procedures.

Another factor that could have reduced the percentage of people receiving emergency physical restraints was the implementation of contingent restraint procedures. If a programmatic restraint procedure was implemented for an individual, then the restraint would not be measured as an emergency physical restraint. During the analysis period a mean of only 5% (range 3%–7%) of individuals received programmatic restraints, which cannot account for the decrease in emergency physical restraints.

Figure 4.3 compares the percentage of individuals on various types of restrictive behavior reduction procedures in December 1990 and in December 1999. The census in 1990 was 266 and in 1999 it was 185. This graph shows a distinct trend. In December 1990, nine types of restrictive behavior reduction procedures were implemented. These programs consisted of programmatic restraint, response–cost programs (this does not include the number of individuals on the Teaching Family Motivation Program, which also had a response–cost component), exclusionary time-out, nonexclusionary time-out, protective devices, visual screening (a mask over the eyes), compliance training, contingent oral stimulation (lemon juice squirted into the mouth), and contingent electric shock. By December 1999, four categories of restrictive behavior reduction procedures had been eliminated: visual screening, compliance training, oral stimulation, and contingent electric shock. Further examination of the programmatic restraint programs

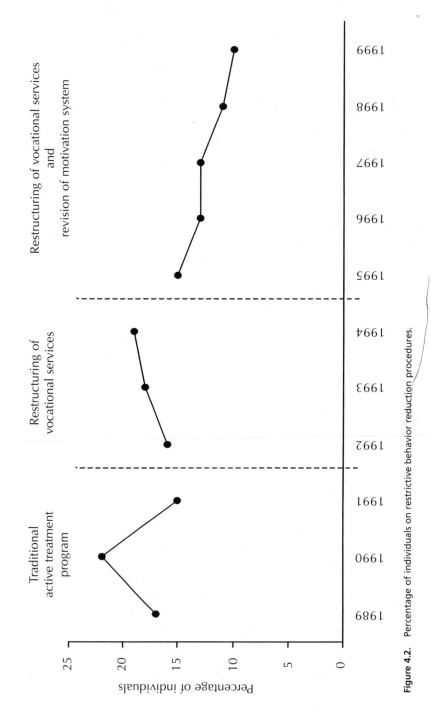

Figure 4.2. Percentage of individuals on restrictive behavior reduction procedures.

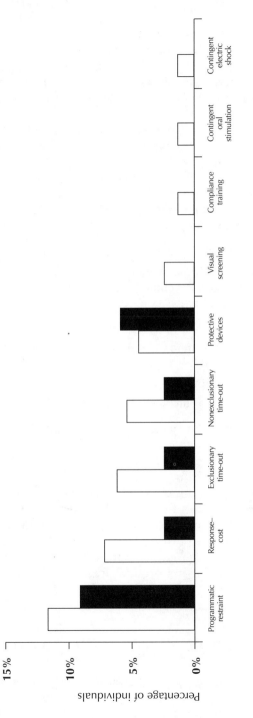

Figure 4.3. Percentage of individuals on various types of restrictive behavior reduction procedures. (*Key:* □ = December 1990; ■ = December 1999.)

implemented in 1999 showed that these type of restraints were not used as an immediate consequence for the targeted behavior but were used after other redirection strategies failed to stop a behavior that put people at risk. Together, Figures 4.2 and 4.3 show that the percentage of individuals on restrictive behavior reduction procedures dropped considerably during the 1990s.

Another possible explanation for the reduction in the use of emergency restraints and restrictive behavior reduction procedures is that the individuals admitted to the facility during the period in which data were collected may have had fewer challenging behaviors and required fewer restrictive procedures. To evaluate this alternative explanation, the files of all admitted individuals were examined for seven categories related to challenging behavior:

1. Exhibited physical aggression to others or to property
2. Was diagnosed with a psychiatric condition as defined by the DSM-IV (American Psychiatric Association, 1994)
3. Engaged in self-injurious behavior
4. Received a behavior modifying drug
5. Received poly pharmacy (receiving multiple behavior modifying drugs)
6. Committed a criminal act
7. Exhibited inappropriate sexual behavior

Table 4.1 shows the percentage of individuals admitted to the facility who exhibited evidence of challenging behaviors. These data indicate that the percentage of individuals in each category generally remained stable across time. In addition, during the 10-year analysis period, the percentage of individuals on behavior modification drugs remained between 26% and 33%, which suggests that the reduction in challenging behavior was not due to increased medication usage. Thus, the characteristics of the individuals admitted during the analysis phase did not change in an appreciable manner and would not account for the reduction in restraints or restrictive behavior reduction procedures.

CASE STUDY: PERSON-CENTERED PLANNING WITH SUSIE

Because person-centered planning builds on preferences specific to each individual, it seems appropriate to provide examples of changes that we observed after person-centered services were implemented for

Table 4.1. Percentage of people admitted to Parsons State Hospital and Training Center who exhibited challenging behaviors

	Percentage of individuals in each category related to challenging behavior						
Year	Exhibited physical aggression	Had a psychiatric diagnosis	Engaged in self-injurious behavior	Received a behavior modifying drug	Received poly pharmacy	Committed a criminal act	Exhibited inappropriate sexual behavior
1989	87	74	13	65	22	35	4
1990	80	60	30	30	0	20	20
1991	93	70	42	84	44	9	9
1992	33	67	0	50	50	33	33
1993	67	67	33	33	0	0	0
1994	75	50	75	25	0	0	25
1995	80	50	60	55	40	15	20
1996	93	93	60	93	80	20	20
1997	52	57	30	48	48	9	13
1998	94	76	53	100	65	35	35
1999	73	67	33	80	47	33	13
Overall percentages	75	66	39	60	36	29	17

a particular person. Due to severe aggression, Susie had lived in institutions since childhood. Once considered extremely dangerous, she
had severely injured others (e.g., concussions, broken bones) over the
years. Because of her aggression, she lived in isolation and spent a
majority of time in mechanical restraint (immobilizing her arms
through the use of a special jacket or tying all four limbs to a bed),
sometimes as long as 2 weeks at a time.

Numerous interventions based on functional assessments were
ineffective in reducing her aggression. Due to the ineffectiveness of less
restrictive procedures, the long periods of time that she spent in
restraints, and the severe harm that she caused others, a contingent
electric shock program was implemented in 1987. The program consisted of 1) brief, nontissue-damaging, electric shock applied when she
engaged in aggression, 2) positive and negative reinforcement of compliance with or resistance to staff demands and requests, and 3) functional communication training. The program was effective in reducing
aggression from a mean of nearly eight aggressions per hour (range
4–10) during baseline to a mean of 0.35 per hour (range 0–4). As a result
of reduced aggression, mechanical restraint was no longer used for
Susie. During the years in which the shock program was used, she was
also able to live with other people, attend school, ride in a car safely, go
shopping, and eat at restaurants.

Although substantial decreases in aggression occurred with the
use of contingent shock, Susie still engaged in periodic episodes of
intense aggression. As a safeguard in the program, a limit was set on
the number of contingent shocks that could be administered within a
specific period. When this number was reached, Susie was placed in
mechanical restraint. Susie also began requesting restraint through sign
language. She received the restraints on request. The contingent shock
was not used during this time, and her treatment team implemented
strategies to safely terminate the restraint.

Attempts at eliminating the shock program were unsuccessful.
When the shock program was stopped, the frequency and intensity of
aggression returned to the preshock baseline levels. An Essential
Lifestyle Plan was developed in an attempt to eliminate the contingent
electric shock program.

The focus of the plan was to learn what was important to Susie,
then help her attain her preferences in a safe manner. A primary issue
was whether we could stop administering contingent electric shock
and still keep others safe. We began the ELP process with Susie, shifting our focus from her bad reputation to her lifestyle preferences. As
Smull and Burke Harrison (1992) pointed out, "severe reputations"
occur when others try to fit people into available programs that do not

accommodate them. (Because it is beyond the scope of this chapter to describe the ELP process in detail, readers are referred to material by Smull & Burke Harrison, 1992.)

First, we had to understand what constituted quality of life improvement from Susie's perspective. For example, we learned how important closure was to Susie. It also became apparent that she created her own routines and decided when it was time to modify, change, or stop them (e.g., emptying all the food from serving dishes or emptying a trash can, even when it contained a single piece of paper). She would do whatever she could to maintain this control, including exhibiting aggression when others interfered with her routines (e.g., stopping her from finishing a routine, trying to change the way she did the routine).

Next, we reallocated our resources to better fit Susie's values. For example, both her love of food and her determination to finish anything she started (in this case, emptying the serving bowl) often resulted in Susie's attacking others at mealtime. When Susie served herself first, she tried to empty the serving bowl, leaving no food for others. When staff intervened, she became aggressive. This conflict became less problematic after the team recognized Susie's perspective and made slight modifications. Today, staff ask her whether she wants to dine alone or with others. When Susie chooses to dine with others, the serving bowls are passed around the table, and she serves herself last. In this way, Susie is free to take all of the food left in the bowl without others interfering or anyone going hungry. Some team members were concerned that respecting Susie's desire to eat this way might result in an unhealthy weight gain. However, monthly monitoring of her weight showed that excessive weight gain did not occur.

Aggression was often the only way that Susie could maintain control when others tried to interfere with her routines. We stopped trying to impose existing programs on Susie and focused on finding ways to accommodate what was important to her while still keeping others safe. Due to the numerous injuries Susie inflicted on others, her support team maintained the contingent shock program for a period of about 4 months after the Essential Lifestyle Plan was implemented. As the team identified other ways to help Susie obtain what was important to her, they gained confidence that the shock program could be discontinued without sacrificing the safety of other people.

From January 1997 to December 1997, while the contingent shock procedure was used, the number of minutes in mechanical restraints increased across time. The amount of time that Susie was in restraints peaked at nearly 23,000 minutes in September 1997, then stabilized at approximately 17,000 minutes for October through December 1997 (see

Figure 4.4). When ELP was implemented in conjunction with the shock procedure, the number of minutes of restraint began to rapidly decline and stabilized at approximately 4,000 minutes in April 1998. After termination of the shock procedure and continuation of the Essential Lifestyle Plan, mechanical restraint dropped to 0 and remained at that level for 15 months.

When we began the ELP process, our initial efforts focused on discontinuing shock and restraint while protecting Susie and others. Susie is a complex person, and she does things we still do not understand. The support team continues to struggle with these issues. Despite these ongoing challenges, there is little doubt that discontinuing the shock program and eliminating mechanical restraint, while keeping aggression low, has improved her quality of life. Other subtle, informal observations indicate that Susie's quality of life has improved since the Essential Lifestyle Plan began. For example, she seeks the company of others more often (e.g., sitting with others at mealtimes, handing out presents at Christmas) and has more privacy because it is no longer necessary to have staff in close proximity to monitor her. We are currently addressing numerous other aspects of Susie's life through ELP, such as family relationships, health, preferred staff, work, preferred learning style, likes and dislikes, and her dreams for the future.

CONCLUSION

At PSH&TC, moving from facility-based program services to person-centered services increased the number of job opportunities and was associated with a decrease in the use of restrictive behavioral procedures. Working at enjoyable jobs likely increased appropriate, prosocial behaviors and decreased both problematic behaviors and the need for restrictive procedures. Indeed, research has demonstrated that providing choices about work preferences increases on-task behavior (Parsons, Reid, Reynolds, & Bumgartner, 1990). In addition, providing choices about academic tasks to students with challenging behaviors increases academic behaviors while producing collateral decreases in problem behaviors (Dunlap et al., 1994; Dyer, Dunlap, & Winterling, 1990).

Individuals at PSH&TC have also made a number of other choices that affect them in both small and large ways (e.g., how their day is organized, what they learn, how staff are hired). By decentralizing and individualizing services, PSH&TC staff are able to provide supports that give each person more control over personal preferences. This reduces the need for challenging behavior, which some in the field describe as "counter control" (Halle, 1995).

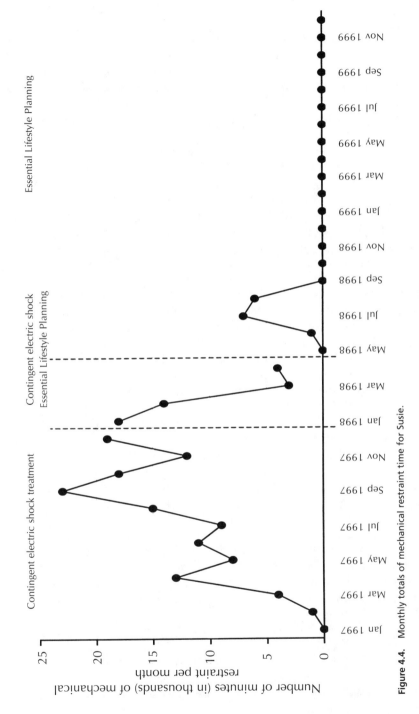

Figure 4.4. Monthly totals of mechanical restraint time for Susie.

According to Smull (1995), choice consists of three components: 1) preferences, 2) opportunities, and 3) control. *Preferences* are defined as what people want, including their dreams. *Opportunities* are an array of options about where, how, and with whom one will spend one's time. *Control* is the ability to act on an opportunity to satisfy a preference. Many instances of challenging behavior may result from individuals not having control over opportunities to fulfill preferences (Kearney, Durand, & Mindell, 1995; Mason, McGee, Farmer-Dougan, & Risley, 1989). There are legitimate concerns regarding control over decisions that may affect the individual's and others' health and safety. By addressing these concerns in a direct fashion with the individual and people who know and care about the person, however, choices are often available. These alternatives usually provide a reasonable degree of safeguards that are acceptable to the person but still address health and safety concerns (Wehmeyer, 1998). As the social services culture moves from a system-oriented, programmatic philosophy to a person-centered supports model that maximizes the individual's control, the responsibilities for staff shift from prescribing a daily schedule toward asking how they can honor choices in an alternative and safe way.

Cultural change is an ongoing process. If there is no support for person-centered services, they will fail. Not all staff members at PSH&TC have embraced person-centered approaches, nor do all staff actions reflect the cultural change. How to maintain cultural change in an organization remains a critical issue (Kotter, 1996). Without support from administration and direct-line supervisors, the cultural shift will not continue.

Administrative policies and decision making must be consistent with person-centered values. For instance, at one time, PSH&TC's hiring policies and practices for direct support and administrative positions (e.g., director of vocational services) did not include residents on the interview committee. Without their input, we were missing valuable perspectives regarding characteristics that are important for supporting these individuals. In September 1998, we began including residents on interview committees. Reports indicate that such resident input has 1) identified important applicant characteristics and 2) conveyed the message to applicants that the resident is the ultimate customer.

It is also important that day-to-day supervisors maintain a commitment to a person-centered service philosophy. It is necessary to continue training in person-centered services and administrative support that prompts and reinforces supervisors for making person-centered decisions. Without this training, supervisors will come under the control of system-oriented contingencies.

Person-centered approaches have been labeled as the latest *faux fixe* in the developmental disability field (Osborne, 1999). Osborne has labeled person-centered approaches as antiscientific and destructive in that they may replace proven behavior analytic methods of behavior change without empirical support. Any service delivery approach should conduct an evaluation to determine its effectiveness in improving quality of life and decreasing aberrant behavior. For person-centered planning to become a prevalent approach, future research is needed to examine the direct effects of this approach for individuals with and without challenging behavior. Multiple baseline and multiprobe designs would be ideal for such a controlled analysis. Unfortunately, until such analyses are conducted, many behavior analysts who work in programs that serve individuals with disabilities will not attempt to implement these strategies to improve individuals' lives.

Finally, we do not suggest that person-centered planning will completely eliminate the need to use traditional behavior analytic technologies. When large-scale system changes do not decrease or eliminate challenging behavior, we rely on behavior analytic technologies to address the behavior (Risley, 1996). Before behavioral technologies are applied, however, a critical question should be asked, "Am I trying to alter a behavior that is representative of the individual's value?"

REFERENCES

American Psychiatric Association. (1994). *Diagnostic and statistical manual of mental disorders* (4th ed.). Washington, DC: Author.

Axelrod, S., & Apsche, J. (1983). *The effects of punishment on human behavior.* San Diego: Academic Press.

Bair, H.V. (1958). Mental deficiency: A psychiatric problem. *Mental Hospital, 9,* 62–65.

Dunlap, G., de Perczel, M., Clarke, S., Wilson, D., Wright, S., White, R., & Gomez, A. (1994). Choice making to promote adaptive behavior for students with emotional and behavioral challenges. *Journal of Applied Behavior Analysis, 27,* 505–518.

Dyer, K., Dunlap, G., & Winterling, V. (1990). Effects of choice making on the serious problem behaviors of students with severe handicaps. *Journal of Applied Behavior Analysis, 23,* 515–524.

Girardeau, F.L., & Spradlin, J.E. (1964). Token rewards in a cottage program. *Mental Retardation, 2,* 345–352.

Halle, J.W. (1995). Innovations in choice-making research: An editorial introduction. *Journal of The Association for Persons with Severe Handicaps, 20,* 173–174.

Health Care Financing Administration. (1988, June 3). 42 CFR Parts 431, 435, 440, 442, and 483 Medicaid program: Conditions for intermediate care facilities for the mentally retarded: Final rule. *Federal Register, 53*(107), 20492–20505.

Kearney, C.A., Durand, V.M., & Mindell, J.A. (1995). It's not where but how you live: Choice and adaptive/maladaptive behavior in persons with severe handicaps. *Journal of Developmental and Physical Disabilities, 7,* 11–24.

Kotter, J.P. (1996). *Leading change.* Boston: Harvard Business School Press.

Lent, J.R., LeBlanc, J., & Spradlin, J.E. (1970). Designing a rehabilitative culture for moderately retarded adolescent girls. In R.E. Ulrich, T. Stachnik, & J. Mabry (Eds.), *The control of human behavior* (Vol. II, pp. 121–135). Glenview, IL: Scott Foresman.

Mason, S.A., McGee, G.G., Farmer-Dougan, V., & Risley, T.R. (1989). A practical strategy for ongoing reinforcer assessment. *Journal of Applied Behavior Analysis, 22,* 171–179.

Mayer, M.A. (1997). Introduction to dual diagnosis. In M.A. Mayer, A. Poindexter, & E. Gabriel (Eds.), *Multi-media self-instruction program series on mental and behavioral disorders in people who have mental retardation* (pp. 1–35). Durham, NC: TheraEd.

Mount, B. (1994). Benefits and limitations of personal futures planning. In V.J. Bradley, J.W. Ashbaugh, & B.C. Blaney (Eds.), *Creating individual supports for people with developmental disabilities: A mandate for change at many levels* (pp. 97–108). Baltimore: Paul H. Brookes Publishing Co.

Osborne, J.G. (1999). Renaissance or killer mutation? A response to Holburn. *The Behavior Analyst, 22,* 47–52.

Parsons, M.B., Reid, D.H., Reynolds, J., & Bumgartner, M. (1990). Effects of chosen versus assigned jobs on the work performance of persons with severe handicaps. *Journal of Applied Behavior Analysis, 23,* 253–258.

Phillips, E.L., Phillips, E.A., Fixsen, D.L., & Wolf, M.M. (1972). *The teaching-family handbook.* Lawrence: The University of Kansas, Bureau of Child Research.

Risley, T. (1996). Get a life! Positive behavioral intervention for challenging behavior through life arrangement and life coaching. In L.K. Koegel, R.L. Koegel, & G. Dunlap (Eds.), *Positive behavioral support: Including people with difficult behavior in the community* (pp. 425–437). Baltimore: Paul H. Brookes Publishing Co.

Smull, M.W. (1995). Revisiting choice–Part 1. *AAMR News and Notes, 8,* 2–3.

Smull, M.W., & Burke Harrison, S. (1992). *Supporting people with severe reputations in the community.* Alexandria, VA: National Association of State Directors of Developmental Disabilities Services.

Wehmeyer, M.L. (1998). Self-determination and individuals with significant disabilities: Examining meanings and misinterpretations. *Journal of The Association for Persons with Severe Handicaps, 23,* 17–26.

5

A Plan Is Not Enough

Exploring the Development of Person-Centered Teams

Helen Sanderson

This chapter identifies critical issues in a team's implementation of Essential Lifestyle Planning (Smull & Burke Harrison, 1992) for two people with profound and multiple cognitive disabilities. The action research[1] took place over the course of 2 years in a cognitive disability service, where I served as a development worker. The model of action research occurred in two phases of initial idea, reconnaissance (fact finding and analysis), planning, implementation, reconnaissance (evaluation), revision, amending the plan, implementation, and reconnaissance (evaluation) (Elliot, 1991).

There were many positive outcomes from developing the Essential Lifestyle Plans. After 4 months, however there was a lull in activities and monitoring. Effective implementation was limited, as the Essential Lifestyle Plans were not integrated within the team's culture and process. Job supervision, team meetings, and team days were redesigned to incorporate the Essential Lifestyle Plans. The research concluded that simply having a plan is not enough to ensure that people's lives continue to change. The plan needs to be viewed as part of the team's culture—"the way that we do things around here"—rather than seen as an extra piece of work. On the basis of this research and under the influence of the Team Performance Model (Drexler, Sibbet, & Forrester, 1994), the end of this chapter identifies six key questions for teams that want to develop a person-centered focus and to implement person-centered plans.

---

[1]For more details about the research, please refer to the following: Sanderson, H. (2000). *Critical issues in the implementation of Essential Lifestyle Planning within a complex organisation: An action research investigation within a learning disability service.* Unpublished doctoral dissertation, Manchester Metropolitan University, United Kingdom.

INITIAL IDEAS: PLANNING

A social service department and a Community National Health Service Trust provide a joint service to people with cognitive disabilities who live in a particular English city (Burton & Kellaway, 1998). This residential service (called "the service" throughout this chapter) supports people in group homes of two, three, or four people.

In the early 1990s, attempts were made to improve individualized planning in the city by revising paperwork and producing standards. However, these strategies did not produce lasting change. The Planning Action Group formed to improve individualized planning across the service. The group began by evaluating the content of goals set in individualized planning sessions. This evaluation revealed that 37% of the people who used the service did not have any form of plan or goal; 56% had three or four short-term goals but did not have any long-term goals. The highest number of goals were for improving health (21%) and skill building (16%). The lowest were related to relationships (2%) and work (1%). The goals-setting standard was very poor, with few goals having the characteristics recommended by Sigafoos, Kigner, Holt, Doss, and Mustonen (1991): specific, measurable, achievable, realistic, and timelined.

This analysis shows that staff were emphasizing the more traditional individual program planning (IPP) goals of improving skills and maintaining health, instead of the goals articulated by the service's mission statement of promoting communication, autonomy, relationships, and community integration. Recognizing this mismatch, the senior managers wanted to explore person-centered planning and emphasize increased community involvement and relationships (Hagner, Helm, & Butterworth, 1996; Malette et al., 1992; Mount, 1987). Again, the desire to improve planning and make it more person centered led to the senior managers' commissioning the Planning Action Group.

Various members of the Planning Action Group were trained in the following person-centered planning approaches to begin exploring how to introduce person-centered planning in the city:

- Essential Lifestyle Planning (ELP; Smull & Burke Harrison, 1992)

- MAPS (Making Action Plans, formerly known as the McGill Action Planning System; Pearpoint, Forest, & O'Brien, 1996)

- PATH (Planning Alternative Tomorrows with Hope; Pearpoint, O'Brien, & Forest, 1993)

- Personal Futures Planning (Mount, 1987)

The group members applied each planning process to their own lives to better understand the different styles and to select the appropriate one for the city. ELP was chosen for two reasons: 1) it provides detailed day-to-day information about what is important to the individual and 2) it specifies what support the individual needs. At that time, the service held mainly clinical information about people; although this information was useful for supporting people, it did not acknowledge what the service's users considered important in their lives. ELP was originally designed for use in residential services, unlike the other planning styles (Mount, 1990; O'Brien & Lovett, 1992; Lyle O'Brien, O'Brien, & Mount, 1997).

In the service, innovation was traditionally disseminated through an initial training course, followed by cascade training. In the case of IPP, however, new forms were given out. No training in goal planning was provided, although staff generally rate such training as a high priority (see Raynes & Sumpton, 1987; Sturmey, 1992). The service relied on the distribution of these 10 forms to complete. Complicated paperwork was a frequent staff criticism of the IPP process (de Kock, Saxby, Felce, Thomas, & Jenkins, 1988; Fleming, 1985, 1988; Humphreys & Blunden, 1987; Sutcliffe & Simons, 1993; Wright & Moffat, 1992). This issue and anecdotal comments from staff that were reported back to the Planning Action Group suggested difficulties with how information on IPP was disseminated.

THE AIM OF THE RESEARCH

Although I had been trained in ELP, members of the Planning Action Group were concerned that simply providing training and materials was insufficient due to the "uncharted" nature of implementing person-centered planning. Little was known about individual implementation (Marrone, Hoff, & Helm, 1997), and even less was known about organizational implementation. Even skilled facilitators faced difficulties and dilemmas in implementing planning. The group decided that further research was required before implementation could begin. Hagner and colleagues called for discovering "strategies for maintaining energy and commitment" before wider implementation could take place (1996, p. 170). This move suggested that learning about implementation from a small number of people might be helpful before the organization embarked on wider implementation.

The service has a history of making quick, poorly thought-out changes to practice and procedure. Thus, in-depth research and action was required to begin learning how to implement ELP. It was necessary to gather rich data that focused on a team and its complexity over time. This element also rendered the research "bottom up" in response to a "top-down" research brief and for greater participation to be introduced (Whyte, 1991). A longer, more detailed process of implementation was required. The research was therefore focused on an in-depth case study.

After a discussion, the Planning Action Group and senior managers agreed on a research aim: to explore critical aspects of implementing a style of person-centered planning (ELP) within a complex organizational context. As a result, a research methodology that focused on learning through action was required, and action research was selected—working with two people who have significant disabilities.

THE METHODOLOGY: ACTION RESEARCH

Argyris (1983), Hart and Bond (1995), Shani and Bushie (1987), and Susman and Evered (1978)—among others—provided detailed descriptions of the shared features of action research. Elliot described *action research* as "the study of a social situation with a view to improving the quality of action within it" (1991, p. 69). The group's research followed two cycles of Elliot's action research process, which consists of the following steps:

1. Initial idea
2. Reconnaissance (fact finding and analysis)
3. Planning
4. Implementation
5. Reconnaissance (evaluation)
6. Revision
7. Amending plan
8. Implementation
9. Reconnaissance (evaluation)

The Planning Action Group was concerned with the difficulties of planning with people who have profound and multiple cognitive disabilities and do not use language. Literature that specifically addresses the issues related to effectively involving people with profound and multiple cognitive disabilities in planning is scant (Sanderson, Kennedy, & Ritchie, 1997). This reflects the broader problem of how important issues in the lives of people with profound and multiple cognitive disabilities are "under-debated" and points to the "significant gap" between the knowledge provided by research and the reality of what services provide (Hogg, 1998). People with profound and multiple cognitive disabilities are also regularly excluded or left out until the last step in major service developments.

Based on this research, which matched their local issues, the Planning Action Group made a decision to positively focus on planning with people with significant disabilities. Therefore, the group's research aimed 1) to evaluate the process of implementing ELP within a team supporting two people with profound and multiple cognitive disabilities and, from this, 2) to identify the implications for implementation within a service context.

People Involved in the Research

The research focused on Kath and Derek, who lived together in a shared house as part of the residential service.

Kath   Kath was a single woman who was in her early thirties. She had a sister, an aunt, and a niece. Her parents lived approximately 30 miles from Kath's council house. She stopped living with her parents when she was 3 years old, as they "could not cope" with her disabilities. She then lived in a children's home. When she became an adult, Kath moved into the local social services hostel. The hostel was the subject of an investigation and subsequently closed amid a scandal of poor conditions and abuse. Five years later, the service workers selected Kath to live with Derek, and together they moved into the council house as tenants. Kath attended the "special needs" section of a local adult training center during the week. In addition to having profound cognitive disabilities, Kath had poor vision.

Derek   Derek was also single and in his early thirties. He had no contact with his parents. They had physically abused Derek, so he was removed from them by social workers when he was a baby. He had at least one brother, but there were no details of other relatives. He lived in children's homes before being moved to the hostel and then to the group home that he shared with Kath at the time of the study. Derek attended the "special needs" section of the same adult training center during the week. In addition to having profound cognitive disabilities, Derek exhibited challenging behavior.

The Team   Kath and Derek were supported by a team of six staff. An Assistant Network Manager (ANM) led the staff team. She was supervised by the Network Manager (NM). The team was comprised of six members—three females and three males.

As the task was to eventually implement ELP across the service, it was important to learn about the local critical issues that needed to be considered when planning a more extensive implementation. In accordance with this requirement, I planned to work alongside the ANM and the team as an active participant observer to facilitate the two Essential Lifestyle Plans. In this way, and in keeping with the principles of participatory (or collaborative) action research, the team, the manager, and I would learn together about how to implement planning.

FIRST PHASE OF THE RESEARCH: DEVELOPING AND IMPLEMENTING THE ESSENTIAL LIFESTYLE PLANS

The research began by spending time with Kath and Derek and their support team. Participant observation and semistructured interviews were used to learn about their lives. Table 5.1 is a summary of the aims, researcher's roles and methods, and outcomes of the first phase of research.

Developing the Plans

I began by spending time with Kath and Derek at their home and talking with each team member individually to create a picture of Kath's and Derek's lives. I found that Kath and Derek were viewed as and, thus, treated as a couple. Little was known about them as individuals, and they were perceived as having few interests. They spent much of their time watching TV when they were not at the adult training center. They received inconsistent support, and their team had low morale and poor communication.

I worked with the team to map out Kath's and Derek's relationships. I then spent time with each person on the relationship map to gather information for the plans (see Smull, Sanderson, & Allen, 2001, for a full description of this and other processes that are used in ELP). The ELP meetings were arranged once the plans had been drafted and checked.

The team members wanted to change the meetings to make them more accessible. They invited everyone on Kath's and Derek's relationship maps to the meetings. Invitations to Kath's meeting were sent on colored paper and written by a team member on Kath's behalf, and the recipient was instructed to reply to Kath. This was in stark contrast to previous planning meeting, for which typed letters were sent from the office with a tear-off slip to return to the NM. Kath's meeting took place during the evening at her church's hall. A buffet dinner was arranged to occur partway through the meeting. Kath's aunt talked about how included she felt.

Derek's meeting took place in his local pub's function room. The room had a door that led to the beer garden, where Derek could

Table 5.1. Summary of the first phase of research

Aim	Researcher's roles and methods	Outcomes
Meet Kath and Derek	Engaged in participant observation	Gathered information about Kath and Derek: • Both Kath and Derek communicated non-verbally. The team members did not agree on how Kath and Derek communicated. • Their living environment was well furnished and appropriate for their age, with photographs on the wall and other personal effects. • Kath and Derek watched TV during the researcher's visits, and there was little evidence (other than Kath's keyboard) of other activities. • The staff generally interacted with them in a warm and positive way.
Develop relationships with the team and an understanding of how the team functioned	Conducted semistructured interviews Engaged in participant observation during support team meetings Formulated a documentary analysis	Gathered information about the support team: • The team members viewed Kath and Derek as a couple; they knew little about Kath and Derek as individuals. • Kath and Derek were not involved in many community activities. (The team's explanation for this was the poor winter weather and a lack of drivers.) • Communication within the team was generally poor, and team meetings focused on administration. • There was little structure, organization, or clarity of team roles.

(continued)

Table 5.1. (continued)

Aim	Researcher's roles and methods	Outcomes
Develop separate Essential Lifestyle Plans for Kath and Derek	Developed relationship maps Talked with people who were identified on the relationships maps Drafted plans and shared them with the team	Kath and Derek had individual Essential Lifestyle Plans, which revealed what was important to them, their wide range of interests, and the support they required. The team now saw Kath and Derek as individuals with different interests.
Hold individual Essential Lifestyle Planning meetings for Kath and Derek	Planned the meetings with the team Facilitated the meetings	Kath's meeting: • Kath seemed to enjoy her meeting, as she sat with people who cared for her and ate from a buffet that included her favorite foods. • Actions were set at the meeting to ensure that Kath had what was on her plan. Derek's meeting: • Derek stayed for the whole meeting, wandering into the pub's beer garden during breaks, and he seemed to enjoy the meal afterward. • Actions were set at the meeting to ensure that Derek had what was on his plan.
Have an implementation meeting	Facilitated the meeting	An implementation plan was developed that described each staff member's role on a flexible, monthly basis. Each person agreed to check and sign off on an activity after it had been completed.

	The keyworkers agreed to provide a monthly summary that compared the Essential Lifestyle Plans with what actually happened during that month.
Evaluate the process and the outcomes	Conducted semistructured interviews
	Formulated a documentary analysis
	Engaged in participant observation
	The team members reported
	• An appreciation of the opportunity to stop and reflect
	• Improved structure to their work but with flexibility
	• An increase in morale and job satisfaction
	Kath and Derek experienced various individual outcomes.[a]

[a]See Table 5.2 for more details about Kath's and Derek's individual outcomes.

wander as he wished. It was held during the morning, and then everyone had lunch together in the pub. All who attended the meeting commented on how it differed in tone and content from Derek's IPP meetings. Several people said that they were surprised that Derek stayed at
the meeting and was apparently happy, as he always became restless
and distressed at previous meetings.

Implementing the Plans

The team held an implementation meeting 2 weeks after the ELP meetings. At this meeting, team members reviewed Derek's and Kath's
Essential Lifestyle Plans and determined whether each element needed
to happen on a daily, weekly, or monthly basis. Then, the team members and I discussed how much work-week structure we wanted to
achieve these goals. The team indicated a preference for a flexible
weekly structure. The team and I translated the daily, weekly, and
monthly information onto a monthly plan. Some activities, such as
Derek's swimming, had to be allocated to a day when Derek was not at
the adult training center. Other activities, such as Kath's foot spa and
foot massage, needed to take place twice per week but did not need to
happen on a particular day. Therefore, these activities were attributed
to sometime during the week and people were able to fit this in at their
discretion depending on what else was happening and their assessment of how Kath was feeling.

Once the implementation plans were completed, the team and I
discussed how to record and monitor each plan. People suggested that
monitoring the implementation plan would be a good role for the key-
worker, who could provide a monthly summary if people checked and
signed off on the activities that they had completed. The team could
then compare this checklist to what the team had set out to do, according to Kath's and Derek's Essential Lifestyle Plans.

Finally, the team members discussed whether they had learned
anything about each other through the team day that could influence
who supported Kath and Derek for particular activities. Several suggestions were made. For example, one team member was a keen gardener and agreed to support Derek in his gardening-related activities.
Another member was a Catholic and wanted to take the lead in supporting Kath's going to church. The team then discussed the logistical
steps to make these things happen. The plans were then put into action.

Outcomes

To evaluate the process and outcomes, I interviewed each team member and examined the documentation over this period. The evaluation

focused on outcomes for Kath and Derek, outcomes for the team, and difficulties in implementing the plans.

Outcomes for Kath and Derek Implementing the Essential Lifestyle Plans resulted in significant changes for Kath, Derek, and the team. The main changes for Kath and Derek were that they were seen as individuals with various individual interests who were given support to participate in a greater range of activities. They also received more consistent and individual support from the team in pursuing these activities. As one person noted,

> It has gone well: Kath and Derek are now being seen more individually and they are engaged in more activities than they were—different activities as well. Before, I'd say about this time last year, they were not doing anything at all really.

The activity charts that were completed following the ELP also indicated this change, which contrasted to the information that was gathered before the research began. Table 5.2 provides specific examples of these outcomes.

Handy (1981) stated that within various organizational settings, the most common impact of objective setting is that it raises standards. It could therefore be argued that any procedure that sets objectives could result in similar effects. If this was the case for Kath and Derek's team, then its previous IPP processes would have had similar outcomes; however, feedback from the team indicated that this did not occur. Kolb, Rubin, and McIntryre (1971) found that when business school students participated in selecting a goal rather than having it imposed on them, and when they also got more feedback from each other, the number of successful students rose from 5% to 61%. Thus, team member support of Kath's and Derek's goals may have contributed significantly to the team's improved working.

Another possible explanation is that the increase in activities resulted from my observation of the team and that positive change would happen regardless of any planned intervention (i.e., the "Hawthorne effect"). However, the activities that actually increased were those specified in Kath's and Derek's Essential Lifestyle Plans, not those in a range of unconnected activities. Equally different activities increased for Kath and for Derek, suggesting they were no longer seen as a couple but were now seen as individuals. Thus, it seems that generalized improvement occurred rather than an increase in activities because of external interest.

Outcomes for the Team The team said that ELP gave them the opportunity to stop and reflect on what they were doing rather than to continue with routines or the behavior of more established

Table 5.2. Kath's and Derek's experiences before and after Essential Lifestyle Planning

Before Essential Lifestyle Planning	After Essential Lifestyle Planning
Kath and Derek were viewed as a couple: • They were often supported in doing the same activities at the same time; even their dental checkups were booked together. • The priest from the local church had been invited to become both Kath's and Derek's advocate, even though Derek did not go to church. Little was known about them as individuals, and they were seen as having few interests: • Staff did not know who the people were in photographs on Kath's wall. • One staff member said, "Some staff come to me and say, 'What do you think about Kath doing this or Derek doing that?' and it is like they still do not properly know them—even though they have been working with them for a long time." Decisions were made based on what staff thought was good for Kath and Derek, the weather conditions, and staff preferences: • One staff member remarked about a co-worker, "She came in at 3 P.M., and I said to her, 'While you are catching up reading the books, I will bang a curry in and, as it is a lovely day, we can take Kath and Derek out for a couple of hours while it cooks. What would you like to do in the evening?'"	Kath and Derek were seen as individuals with a wide range of interests. After ELP was implemented, Kath • Was supported in seeing her aunt every 2 months • Went to concerts and clubs • Went to Mass regularly • Had her favorite "tipples" (i.e., drink) on a Friday • Had aromatherapy and massage every fortnight • Used a foot spa every week • Had facials and manicures every 2 weeks • Went to spa baths every month • Was involved in cooking and baking every week • Used her keyboard Although Kath loved loud music and bustling places, Derek preferred quieter activities such as • Going out in the car every day • Going swimming every week • Walking in the country, in wide open spaces • Eating out (preferably a curry dish) each week • Going to the local, quiet pub each week Decisions were made based on what staff knew was important to Kath and Derek, as recorded in their Essential Lifestyle Plans: • One staff member noted, "Kath and Derek are now seen as individuals. . . . Staff are seeing Kath and Derek as individuals rather than as a couple because they're talking about their individual interests rather than seeing them as a couple. It feels like staff know Kath

Kath and Derek were not involved in household or leisure activities:

• Staff collected Kath's benefits on her behalf.

• Derek was left with an agency staff member while another team member had the tire changed on Derek's and Kath's car. (Going out in the car was "most important" to Derek.)

• The house diary for a particular week did not list any activities for Kath and Derek other than their attending the adult training center. Also, the most frequently recorded item during the previous 6 months was, "Derek had a good bowel movement." The support team attributed this lack of various activities to poor weather and the fact that only two staff could drive.

• Kath and Derek spent a lot of time watching TV.

Kath and Derek received inconsistent support:

• One staff member put Kath on the treadmill to help Kath get more fit, but another staff member did not do so because she thought that Kath did not like the treadmill.

• The team supported Derek for three morning routines. Some days he would undress in the bathroom, some days in his bedroom—depending on the team member supporting him.

• Staff had different ideas about what and how Kath and Derek communicated.

and Derek much more—in their interests in what makes them happy, what makes them sad, etc.'"

Kath and Derek were more involved in household activities:

• They both collected their benefits themselves, on different days.

• They went shopping on different days.

• Kath was involved in baking and cooking.

Kath and Derek received more consistent and individual support:

• Both of their morning and evening routines were recorded and consistently followed.

• Both had communication sections, and staff used these to respond to their communications.

team members. Another benefit was the improved structuring of their work, in which important routines were clearly documented so that everyone could follow them in the same way. Nonetheless, the new structure also left room for flexibility and spontaneity within the parameters of the activities identified in the plans. Many team members attributed to ELP an improvement in morale and communication within the team and an increase in individual job satisfaction.

Barriers and Solutions

Implementing the Essential Lifestyle Plans was largely successful, yet there were still barriers. The amount of flexibility that could be created in a rota of six staff was a barrier. The evaluation also identified a lull in activity and monitoring, and some activities stopped happening as frequently as specified in the plans. This finding extended to the monitoring of activities, which happened on an ad hoc basis. The evaluation suggested that it was very positive to give the team a chance to stop and think about 1) Kath and Derek, 2) the team's role in their lives, and 3) the way that the team worked together. The evaluation also indicated that the team members were in danger of thinking that this learning and reflection was complete once ELP was finished.

It is clear that strategies were required to keep the plans alive. During ELP, the team reflected on what they were learning, and they problem-solved together. Later, however, the Essential Lifestyle Plans were not having any impact on job supervision or team meetings. Although implementing the plans resulted in the team's restructuring their time and decision making, this reorganization needed to be further embedded within the team culture. This would involve the Essential Lifestyle Plans' influencing the support and supervision that team members receive, thereby integrating the plans into team meetings to become part of "the way we do things around here." Therefore, a second phase of action research was required to embed the Essential Lifestyle Plans within the team's culture and process.

SECOND PHASE OF THE RESEARCH: EMBEDDING ESSENTIAL LIFESTYLE PLANNING INTO THE TEAM'S CULTURE

The team needed to agree on not only how plans would be implemented and monitored, but also how they could be "kept alive." If plans were not embedded into existing team processes, then they ran the risk of being seen as additional to, instead of central to, the team's work. Incorporating ELP into job supervision and team meetings meant that the plans could start becoming part of the team's work culture rather than being considered mere planning. Team days incorporated ELP in addition to six monthly reviews of the plans with all the people who participated in the original planning. Overall, this fostered a theme of continuous learning and review, a feature of the modern "learning organization" that "lies at the heart of individual growth and of corporate success" (Handy, 1994, p. 48). Figure 5.1 provides a graphic summary of the changes the team made, and Table 5.3 is a summary of the second phase of research.

Changing Team Meetings, Team Days, and Supervision

I suggested restructuring team meetings to provide opportunities for members to identify and celebrate what had worked in the plan implementation and to identify and rectify what had not worked so well. During meetings, team members considered whether they had learned anything new about Kath or Derek that would require amendments to

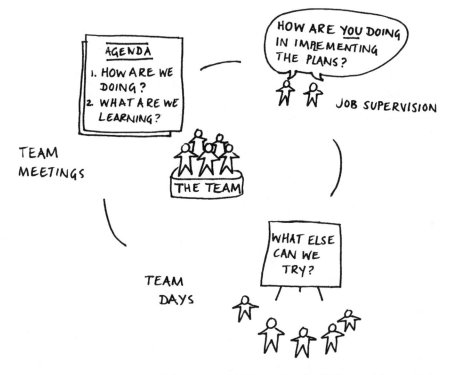

Figure 5.1. Graphic summary of making Essential Lifestyle Planning (ELP) part of the way that a team works.

Table 5.3. Summary of the second phase of research

Aim	Researcher's roles and methods	Outcomes
Change the team meetings to focus on Essential Lifestyle Plans	Facilitated the meetings Served as a mentor for the team leader Engaged in participant observation	Two team meetings were held each month: • The first meeting was shorter and focused on administration issues. • The second meeting focused on what worked and did not work during the previous month in relation to the implementation of the Essential Lifestyle Plans. It included celebrating successes, rectifying problems, and determining what had been learned about Kath and Derek. The plans were amended as necessary.
Develop team days to emphasize ongoing learning about Kath and Derek	Facilitated the meetings Served as a mentor for the team leader Engaged in participant observation	Three team days were held throughout the year: • Two days were spent learning about Kath and Derek in new ways (e.g., using maps from Personal Futures Planning, working on relationships). • One day was spent learning more about the way that the team worked together, developing and amending the Essential Team Plan, and developing a team mission statement. • Actions were set at each team day. These actions were reviewed during the monthly team meetings. The team put in place support for Kath and Derek to have new opportunities and to meet people more regularly.[a]

| Change job supervision to focus on Essential Lifestyle Plans | Served as a mentor for the team leader | Supervision focused on
 • Assessing how well team members implemented the plans
 • Problem-solving any difficulties
 • Identifying what support was required
 • Reviewing any issues arising from the Essential Team Plan
 • Addressing administration issues |
| Evaluate the process and outcomes | Conducted semistructured interviews
 Formulated a documentary analysis
 Engaged in participant observation | Kath and Derek experienced various individual outcomes.[a] |

[a]See Table 5.4 for more details about new opportunities for Kath and Derek.

their Essential Lifestyle Plans. ELP also became a strong focus of job supervision.

In addition to these changes, team meetings and team days provided opportunities to explore values issues and ways to increase the team's understanding of Kath and Derek, as well as to clarify and improve how members of the team work together. For example, the team developed an Essential Team Plan that was similar to an Essential Lifestyle Plan: It recorded what team members needed to do to support each other successfully, as well as their expectations about working together. The team also wrote a mission statement.

The team sought to learn more about Kath and Derek and their community, as well as to expand the opportunities available to them. For example, during a team day, members brainstormed with questions such as, "What might be typical and valued for a man or woman of Kath's or Derek's age who does not have a disability and lives in the same community?" The team set in place support for Kath and Derek to try some of these experiences or activities. During additional development days, team members used some of the maps from Personal Futures Planning to examine community mapping.

ADDITIONAL CHANGES FOR KATH, DEREK, AND THE TEAM

To evaluate the process and outcomes of this second phase of research, I interviewed each team member at the end of the team days. In addition, I interviewed each team member closer to the end of this stage. I also examined the documentation of this period.

The findings from this phase of the research suggested some positive changes in team involvement and in linking planning to activity through incorporating Essential Lifestyle Plans within job supervision, team meetings, and team days. The team evaluated and found beneficial strategies such as the Essential Team Plan and creating actions to increase opportunities for Kath and Derek. These outcomes led to other outcomes for Kath and Derek regarding increased support for relationships outside of the team and new activities. Team members reported that refocusing job supervision and team meetings on the Essential Lifestyle Plans helped them keep Kath and Derek at the center of their work rather than caused them to be "swamped in administration issues." (Table 5.4 provides a summary of the additional changes for Kath, Derek, and the team after this second phase of the research.)

Therefore, implementing ELP for Kath and Derek required the team to also develop an implementation plan that addressed how the plans would be put into practice, how they would be monitored, and

Table 5.4. Additional changes for Kath, Derek, and the team

Additional changes for Kath and Derek	Additional changes for the team
Seeing other people more regularly: One team day focused on how the team could support existing relationships and enable Kath and Derek to develop new relationships. As a result, the number of non-staff people whom Kath and Derek saw doubled.	Improving team meetings: • The team members found that restructuring their meetings generally made it easier to focus on the Essential Lifestyle Plans. • Team members commented that the meetings were more interesting now. They also appreciated the approach of continually trying new things, reflecting on what had been working, and having an opportunity to discuss issues.
Trying new activities in the community: Kath and Derek were given opportunities to try new activities.	Working together better with clearer responsibilities: • Responsibilities were now spread across the team and not left to keyworkers. One team member viewed this change as having a very positive effect: "The team works much better together—in the past, keyworkers got left to do everything—now it's the team working together."
In a month, Kath tried the following new activities: • Using a Jacuzzi • Using a sauna • Eating Thai food	• Setting goals clarified staff's responsibilities. A team member commented, "We tried out what worked and what did not. How else can you know what people may enjoy unless you try? . . . It's much more interesting now—you know what to do and make sure it happens."
In a month, Derek tried the following new activities: • Flying a kite • Using a computer	Improving supervision: • Job supervision focused on staff members' progress in supporting Kath and Derek and in implementing the plans, as well as what staff support (e.g., training) was required to do both more effectively. • Personal development and administration issues were important, but an attempt was made to reestablish these within the framework of how well staff were following the plan and working for Kath and Derek rather than in isolation.

(continued)

Table 5.4. (continued)

Additional changes for Kath and Derek	Additional changes for the team
	Establishing clearer expectations and more consistent teamwork:
	• The team viewed the Essential Team Plan as a useful tool for reviewing how team members worked together, fostering greater consistency, and enabling team members to speak up more easily about issues. A team member remarked, "The Essential Team Plan is definitely a living plan. . . . It's definitely ongoing for the people who were involved in it."
	• Some team members reported that the Essential Team Plan gave them more confidence to deal with staff issues. One staff member believed that she could tackle issues with a fellow team member because of the team plan, and the plan gave her more confidence at team meetings.

how the team would continue to learn and review its work. Implementing ELP in this way required embedding it within the existing team processes of job supervision and team meetings, as well as focusing team days on finding different ways to learn more about Kath and Derek and how the team worked together. One staff member summed up the impact that she thought the research had:

> When we first started, I thought it was crazy. I thought that Kath and Derek could not even communicate and it would have been better to have done it [the research)] with people less disabled. I thought "What more can they do?" I have been amazed at what more they could do. Now, it feels like they were just doing the bare necessities for existing. I was very wrong—they have so many interests and preferences. The sheer joy of trying things out and finding out that they enjoy it.

KEEPING PLANS ALIVE AND ENCOURAGING CONTINUOUS LEARNING

Through this research, Kath and Derek received more consistent support to obtain what was identified as being important to them, and they were given increased opportunities. The research process that was used to develop the team corresponds with some stages for team development in the Team Performance Model (Drexler et al., 1994). This chapter uses the term *person-centered team* for what the Team Performance Model calls a *semi-autonomous team*. A person-centered team sees its purpose as supporting people to achieve their desired lifestyle as part of their local community, and its members are characterized by their willingness to continually listen and learn and their high value on personal commitment and relationships with the people whom they support. Mount (1990) coined the term *person-centered team*, yet it still is not widely used, and no literature is available on how to develop and support a person-centered team. The assumption appears to be that if you have a person-centered plan, then it just needs to be implemented. However, the research presented in this chapter has demonstrated that this is not a simple equation. Work needs to be done with teams to support them to embed the plan within the team's culture and processes and to provide structured opportunities for reflection. The research discussed in this chapter, as well as the influence of the Team Performance Model, led me to identify six key questions that serve as a model for working as a person-centered team and implementing person-centered plans. I acknowledge that the model is a simplification of team development. Also, the questions are not in chronological order because each question may need to be revisited several times during a team's "life." For example, when team members leave and new people replace them, the first two questions will need to be revisited. Person-centered planning begins to be addressed in the model's third question. Figure 5.2 provides a graphic summary of the stages. The outer circle represents the first two questions, as the team needs to revisit them continually.

Question 1: "Why am I here?"

This question is about team membership and acceptance, and it begins to clarify team values and direction. O'Brien and Lyle O'Brien saw this as a key issue for effective organizations:

> The support worker has to be clear about the ways in which his or her personal preferences and values may differ from those of the person supported and keep re-creating ways to avoid imposing on that person without compromising his or her own integrity. (1994, p. 122)

As part of addressing individual values, each team member needs to consider why the team exists, whether he or she wants to be part of it, and whether he or she finds personal meaning in what the team is doing. This stage reflects the importance of a clear organizational mission statement and shared values (Emerson et al., 1993; Kotter, 1996; Peters & Waterman, 1982; Senge, 1990), so the team members do not simply ask this question about the team but also about the service.

This first question, like the questions that follow it, needs to be revisited continually. This action allows team members to add depth to their understanding of values and how this understanding affects their work. It is also one of the team leader's key roles. O'Brien and Lyle O'Brien stated that "An effective staff team leader collaborates with team members to develop, renew, and deepen commitment to the values and direction the . . . agency stands for" (1994, p. 123).

Question 2: "Who are you, and how can we work together?"

The second question focuses on building trust within the team because answering the question, "Who are you?" also means answering the hidden question, "What will you expect from me?" Without trust, the flow of information on the task and goals is threatened, and information may be withheld and distorted (O'Brien & Lyle O'Brien, 1994). The amount of trust will vary across members and over time.

Research on trust and familiarity between team members indicates that lower levels of familiarity were associated with lower levels of productivity (Watson, Kumar, & Michaelson, 1993). Handy stressed the

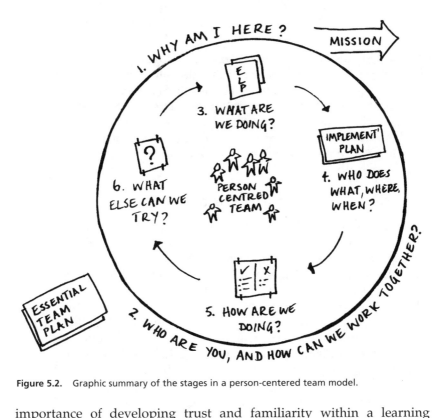

Figure 5.2. Graphic summary of the stages in a person-centered team model.

importance of developing trust and familiarity within a learning organization:

> Today we are seeing an increasing number of organizations made up of shifting 'clusters' of teams that share a common purpose. The need for togetherness, both to get things done and to encourage the kind of exploration that is essential to any growing organization, creates the conditions for trust. Trust, in turn, improves togetherness. (1994, p. 48)

However, some research indicates that for teams that have worked together for more than 3 years, familiarity may become detrimental to group performance (Katz, 1982). Developing trust and familiarity is important, but in the longer term, attention needs to be given to any possibly negative effects (e.g., complacency).

The initial analysis of Kath's and Derek's team showed some trust among certain team members. Yet, some people also distrusted a particular team member's motivation, suggesting that he withheld information and dominated decision-making processes. A significant part of building trust is being clear about people's support needs and how to meet them. Thus, by working with the team and directly addressing how the team members would support each other through the Essential Team Plan, some of these issues were addressed. Formal team as-sessment processes can be used in this stage to increase interpersonal understanding, such as Belbin's Team-Role Self-Perception Inventory (1981) or the Team Performance Inventory (Drexler et al., 1994).

Over time, this question can be revisited to add depth to team members' understanding of each other. Revisiting this question also helps team members discover who the other team members are and what support they need.

Question 3: "What are we doing?"

The task of Question 3 is to clarify as precisely as possible what the team must do and which roles the individual team members take to accomplish it. This task is informed by the answers to Question 1, "Why are we here?" At this point, Question 3 needs to be contextual-ized to the specific issues facing the people whom the team supports. A broad question in person-centered planning is, "Who are the people whom we are employed to support, what is important to them, what support do they want/need, and what is our role in providing this?" Person-centered planning, and in this case ELP, is the central mecha-nism for answering such questions. Research demonstrates that com-pared with the absence of group goals (or the presence of ill-defined ones), setting specific group goals raises group performance on dimen-sions that reflect the quality of the goals (Weldon & Weingart, 1993). Goals raise team member effort (Weldon, Jehn, & Pradhan, 1991) and stimulate cooperation and communication within teams (Locke & Latham, 1990). Drexler and colleagues stated that

> When a group can define its agenda clearly and achieve some consensus on it, and agree on the roles demanded by its goals, it has a common basis to guide the organization of its work. Its energies can thus be directed out-ward toward the task, setting the stage for both structure and creativity. (1994, p. 15)

Question 4: "Who does what, where, when?"

This question takes the person-centered plan and its goals and asks, "Who needs to do what, where, when?" to make the plan happen. It also returns to what was learned from Question 2 about team mem-bers, so the interests and talents of team members can be used to sup-port the individuals who receive services. Active Support (Jones et al., 1997) provides specific procedures for implementing plans and can be used to address Question 4.

The question also needs to address issues of the team's individual and collective power in making changes. Staff must be clear about what they can change and what they cannot change. The emphasis must be on giving power to the lowest level possible within the organization—the direct support staff—wherever possible. This is a key characteristic of a learning organization and is encapsulated in the word *subsidiarity*, meaning giving away power (Handy, 1994).

Giving away power or sharing power is managed by clearly defining job boundaries within the context of a person's plan. Handy (1994) stated that there are two boundaries. The "inner boundary" defines the essential core of the job. In the context of this chapter, the inner boundary means the issues that the Essential Lifestyle Plan classifies as Most Important, Second in Importance, and Third in Importance. This part of the job is clearly defined with specific roles and responsibilities, as identified by the Essential Lifestyle Plan and the implementation plan. If these jobs are not done, then the team has failed to implement the plan, and this failure must be addressed. Handy defines the "outer boundary" as "the limits of discretion." Therefore, this definition presents scope for initiative and personal responsibility.

As cited in Handy (1994), Gore made an eloquent distinction between the two boundaries. He suggested that there are experiments above the water line, which do little harm if they go wrong, and there are experiments below the water line, which might sink the ship. He suggests that "The former are encouraged; the latter are outlawed" (p. 50).

In many traditional organizations, there is limited space for initiative and control is tight. In a learning organization, the space between the two boundaries needs to be enlarged because not every aspect of a job can be prescribed in advance (Handy, 1994). This is the case in person-centered planning. This approach—specifying with team members at the time of plan implementation exactly how they can use their initiative and what is below the water line—would have been very useful for the team featured in this chapter. As the values were not sufficiently clarified and these boundaries were not discussed, the team members learned about the difference by default. One example occurred when a team member supported Kath to go for a walk on a Sunday morning instead of attending Mass. This team member was an atheist and did not personally value attending Mass. Mass was on Kath's "most important" list and, therefore, was below the water line. Although this was not below the water line for the organization in general, it was for Kath per her Essential Lifestyle Plan. The team members had not fully explored the ways in which their values might differ from those of the people whom they supported and the issue of when it was acceptable to use initiative and when it was not. Therefore, such mistakes occurred. If the stages of the person-centered team development model had been effectively implemented, then this incident could have been avoided.

Based on Handy's (1994) ideas, Smull devised the "donut exercise" in 1997 to help lifestyle planning teams examine these issues based on an Essential Lifestyle Plan. The exercise consists of three concentric circles. The first circle is identified as Core Responsibilities, the second as Requiring Creativity and Judgment, and the third as Not Our Paid Responsibility. He encouraged teams to consider how each item from an Essential Lifestyle Plan would be placed in the three circles. For example, team members would consider whether an item is part of their core responsibility (i.e., below the water line) or whether it is an area that requires creativity and judgment (i.e., above the water line). This exercise may be useful in completing this stage of team development.

Question 5: "How are we doing?"

This question involves evaluating how the plan is being implemented and how the team is working in general. This evaluation is conducted by considering what is working and what is not working, then celebrating or problem solving regarding these points. It also requires the team members to ask what else they are learning about the people whom they support and how the plan may need to be adapted to reflect that. This reflection needs to happen both on a daily basis by individual team members and in more formal and structured ways (e.g., individual supervision, team meetings, planning review meetings).

"How are we doing?" needs to be asked on a continual basis through a cycle of learning. This learning extends to the team leader's giving team members feedback about individual job performance. Evidence suggests that performance improves in relation to the quantity of feedback received: The absence of feedback is accompanied by high hostility and low confidence, whereas a high level of feedback, good or bad, fosters high confidence levels and friendly attitudes (Leavitt & Meuller, 1951). Setting goals, roles, and responsibilities and then forgetting about them only produces frustration and inefficiency (Handy, 1981). In addition, research has found that including some goals that specifically relate to self-improvement significantly improves the number of overall goals achieved (Kay, French, & Myer, as cited in Handy, 1981).

Question 6: "What else can we try?"

In addition to reviewing existing goals and processes, the team must use other methods to discover more about the person whom they support, specifically by using different ways of thinking about the person's life. For example, the team in this chapter used and based actions on maps from Personal Futures Planning. By building this step into a stage of team development, ELP can extend opportunities rather than only support existing ones. As Smull and Danehey suggested,

> Person centered planning efforts simply provide a structured process by which this understanding can be achieved. However, doing a good person centered plan once is essential but insufficient. Continuous active treatment should be replaced with continuous active listening. Facilitating changes in whom the individual lives with, what the individual does during the day, or daily routines, and so forth should be seen as the norm rather than the exception. (1994, p. 67)

Team competence is important, but team members also must be curious to keep learning and then offer forgiveness if something goes wrong or celebration if it works (Handy, 1994). Handy identified a "learning wheel" as a way of doing this:

> The wheel has four quadrants that, ideally, rotate in sequence as the wheel moves. The first quadrant consists of questions, which may be triggered by problems or needs that require solutions. The questions prompt a search for possible answers or ideas, which must pass rigorous tests to see if they work. The results are then subjected to reflections, until we are certain we have identified the best solution. Only when the entire process is complete can we truly say that we have learned something. There are no short cuts. (1994, p. 48)

For the team presented in this chapter, team meetings changed from focusing on administrative issues to focusing on what Handy termed *incidental learning*. Team days also changed from emphasizing administrative issues to team building (i.e., building trust and togetherness per Question 2); conducting critical incident analysis (Question 6); and going through the learning circle, then focusing on one particular question (Question 6). Incidental learning incorporates many elements of action research; therefore, it was a familiar process for the team.

Incidental learning is vital when dealing with divergent problems that, unlike convergent problems, do not have "right" answers. Rather, they require the application of principles to a particular situation at a particular time.

Mount (1987) and O'Brien and Lovett (1992) indicated that problems in implementing person-centered planning tend to be divergent; therefore, explicit values need to guide problem solving. This factor emphasizes the importance of making values and issues clear in Question 1. In practice, the team needs to consider what it has learned about the service user after each session of incidental learning. Consequently, the team must decide whether anything needs to be added to or taken away from the person's Essential Lifestyle Plan.

CONCLUSION

The research presented in this chapter aimed to evaluate the process of implementing Essential Lifestyle Plans within a team that supported two people with profound and multiple cognitive disabilities. From this evaluation, the research aimed to identify the implications for implementation within a service context. The outcomes for Kath and Derek and the team were positive; however, difficulties were initially experienced in maintaining and monitoring the activities and support identified in the plans. A further phase of action research focused on embedding the Essential Lifestyle Plans within existing team processes (job supervision and team meetings) and team days. I found that the Essential Lifestyle Plans provided direction for the team and clarified expectations for team members. Through this research and under the influence of the Team Performance Model, six key questions were identified for teams that want to implement person-centered plans and to develop as a person-centered team. These questions acknowledge a trilogy of learning that is required to support people in obtaining desired lifestyles. The continual learning took three directions: 1) what the team members were learning about Kath and Derek and their community; 2) the way that they were implementing the plans; and 3) how they worked together as a team.

As Smull stated, the plan is not the outcome. Indeed, the plan is not the outcome, nor is it enough. The plan is a vehicle for recording our learning and acting on it. The challenge for teams is to identify how this learning can be kept alive and meaningful, and the six questions identified in this chapter provide a framework for addressing this issue.

REFERENCES

Argyris, C. (1983). Action science and intervention. *Journal of Applied Behavioral Science, 19,* 115–140.

Belbin, R.M. (1981). *Management teams.* London: Heinemann.

Benne, K.D., & Sheats, P. (1948). Functional group members. *Journal of Social Issues, 4,* 41–49.

Burton, M., & Kellaway, M. (1998). *Developing and managing quality services for people with learning disabilities.* Aldershot, United Kingdom: Ashgate.

de Kock, U., Saxby, H., Felce, D., Thomas, M., & Jenkins, J. (1988). Individual planning for adults with severe or profound mental handicaps in a community based service. *Mental Handicap, 16,* 152–154.

Drexler, A., Sibbet, D., & Forrester, R. (1994). *The team performance model.* San Francisco: The Grove Consultants International.

Elliot, J. (1991). *Action research for educational change.* Buckingham, United Kingdom: Open University Press.

Emerson, E., McGill, P., & Mansell, J. (1993). *Severe learning disabilities and challenging behaviours: Designing high quality services.* London: Chapman & Hall.

Fleming, I. (1985). Individual programme planning. *Senior Nurse, 3,* 20–21.

Fleming, I. (1988). Making individual plans for change. *Mental Handicap, 16,* 77–79.

Hagner, D., Helm, D.T., & Butterworth, J. (1996). This is your meeting: A qualitative study of PCP. *Mental Retardation, 34,* 151–171.

Handy, C. (1981). *Understanding organisations.* London: Penguin.

Handy, C. (1994). *Managing the dream.* London: Hutchinson.

Hart, E., & Bond, M. (1995). *Action research for health and social care.* Buckingham, United Kingdom: Open University Press.

Hogg, J. (1998). Competence and quality in the lives of people with profound and multiple learning disabilities: Some recent research. *Tizard Learning Disability Review, 3,* 6–14.

Humphreys, S., & Blunden, R. (1987). A collaborative evaluation of an individual plan system. *The British Journal of Mental Subnormality, 33,* 19–30.

Jones, E., Perry, J., Lowe, K., Felce, D., Toogood, S., Dunstan, F., Allen, D., & Pagler, J. (1997). *Opportunity and the promotion of activity among adults with severe learning disabilities living in community housing: The impact of training staff in Active Support.* Cardiff, United Kingdom: Welsh Centre for Learning Disabilities, University of Wales College of Medicine.

Katz, R.L. (1982). The effects of group longevity on project communication and performance. *Administrative Science Quarterly, 27,* 81–104.

Kolb, D.A., Rubin, I.M., & McIntyre, J.M. (1971). *Organizational psychology.* Upper Saddle River, NJ: Prentice Hall.

Kotter, J.P. (1996). *Leading change.* Boston: Harvard Business School Press.

Leavitt, H.J., & Meuller, R.A.H. (1951). Some effects of feedback on communication. *Human Relations.*

Locke, E.A., & Latham, G.P. (1990). *A theory of goal-setting and task performance.* Upper Saddle River, NJ: Prentice Hall.

Lyle O'Brien, C., O'Brien, J., & Mount, B. (1997). Person-centered planning has arrived . . . or has it? *Mental Retardation, 35,* 480–483.

Malette, P., Mirenda, P., Kandborg, T., Jones, P., Bunz, T., & Rogow, S. (1992). Application of a lifestyle development process for persons with severe intellectual disabilities: A case study report. *Journal of The Association for Persons with Severe Handicaps, 17,* 179–191.

Marrone, J., Hoff, D., & Helm, D.T. (1997). Person-centered planning for the millennium: We're old enough to remember when PCP was just a drug. *Journal of Vocational Rehabilitation, 8,* 285–297.

Mount, B. (1987). *Personal futures planning: Finding directions for change* (Doctoral dissertation, University of Georgia). Ann Arbor: University of Michigan Dissertation Information Service.

Mount, B. (1990). *Imperfect change: Embracing the tensions of person-centered work.* Manchester, CT: Communitas Communications.

O'Brien, J., & Lovett, H. (1992). *Finding a way toward everyday lives: The contribution of person centered planning.* Harrisburg: Pennsylvania Office of Mental Retardation.

O'Brien, J., & Lyle O'Brien, C. (1994). More than just a new address: Images of organization for supported living agencies. In V.J. Bradley, J.W. Ashbaugh, & B.C. Blaney (Eds.), *Creating individual supports for people with developmental disabilities: A mandate for change at many levels* (pp. 109–140). Baltimore: Paul H. Brookes Publishing Co.

Pearpoint, J., Forest, M., & O'Brien, J. (1996). MAPS, Circles of Friends, and PATH: Powerful tools to help build caring communities. In S. Stainback & W. Stainback (Eds.), *Inclusion: A guide for educators* (pp. 67–86). Baltimore: Paul H. Brookes Publishing Co.

Pearpoint, J., O'Brien, J., & Forest, M. (1993). *PATH (Planning Alternative Tomorrows with Hope): A workbook for planning positive futures.* Toronto: Inclusion Press.

Peters, T., & Waterman, R.H. (1982). *In search of excellence: Lessons from America's best-run companies.* New York: Harper & Row.

Raynes, N.V., & Sumpton, R.C. (1987). Training needs of community staff: What do they want? *Mental Handicap, 15,* 95–96.

Sanderson, H., Kennedy, J., & Ritchie, P. (1997). *People, plans and possibilities: Exploring person centred planning.* Edinburgh, United Kingdom: SHS Ltd.

Schwartz, P. (1991). *The art of the long view.* New York: Currency Doubleday.

Senge, P.M. (1990). *The fifth discipline: The art and practice of the learning organization.* New York: Doubleday.

Shani, A.B., & Bushie, G. (1987). Visionary action research. A consultation process perspective. *Consultation, 6,* 3–19.

Sigafoos, J., Kigner, J., Holt, K., Doss, S., & Mustonen, T. (1991). Improving the quality of written developmental policies for adults with intellectual disabilities. *British Journal of Mental Subnormality, 37*(Part 1, No. 72), 35–46.

Smull, M.W., & Burke Harrison, S. (1992). *Supporting people with severe reputations in the community.* Alexandria, VA: National Association of State Directors of Developmental Disabilities Services.

Smull, M.W., & Danehey, A.J. (1994). Increasing quality while reducing costs: The challenge of the 1990s. In V.J. Bradley, J.W. Ashbaugh, & B.C. Blaney (Eds.), *Creating individual supports for people with developmental disabilities: A mandate for change at many levels* (pp. 59–78). Baltimore: Paul H. Brookes Publishing Co.

Smull, M.W., Sanderson, H., & Allen, B. (2001). *Essential lifestyle planning: A handbook for facilitators.* Whalley, United Kingdom: North West Training and Development Team.

Sturmey, P. (1992). Goal planning for adults with a mental handicap: Outcome research, staff training and management. *Mental Handicap Research, 5,* 92–107.

Susman, G., & Evered, R. (1978). An assessment of the scientific merit of action research. *Administrative Science Quarterly, 23,* 582–603.

Sutcliffe, J., & Simons, K. (1993). *Self-advocacy and adults with learning difficulties: Contexts and debates.* Leicester, United Kingdom: National Institute of Adult Continuing Education.

Watson, W.E., Kumar, K., & Michaelson, L.K. (1993). Cultural diversity's impact on interaction process and performance: Comparing homogeneous and diverse task groups. *Academic Management Journal, 36,* 590–602.

Weldon, E., Jehn, K.M., & Pradhan, P. (1991). Processes that mediate the relationship between a group goal and improved group performance. *Journal of Personal Sociology and Psychology, 61,* 555–569.

Weldon, E., & Weingart, L.R. (1993). Group goals and group performance. *British Journal of Sociology and Psychology, 32,* 307–334.

Whyte, W.F. (1991). *Participatory action research.* Thousand Oaks, CA: Sage Publications.

Wright, L., & Moffat, N. (1992). An evaluation of an individual programme planning system. *British Journal of Mental Subnormality, 18*(2), 87–93.

6

Overcoming the Barriers

Moving Toward a Service Model that
Is Conducive to Person-Centered Planning

Darlene Magito-McLaughlin,
Thomas R. Spinosa, and Michael D. Marsalis

Quality of life represents an important goal for service providers in the field of developmental disabilities (Schalock, Keith, Hoffman, & Karan, 1989). As of 2002, a variety of person-centered approaches have been developed not only to describe the lifestyle desired by a person, but also to describe the supports that are required to assist a person in achieving a quality lifestyle. Personal Futures Planning (Mount, 1994), Life Quilters (Kincaid, 1996), Essential Lifestyle Planning (Smull, 1999), and Group Action Planning (Turnbull & Turnbull, 1994) are examples of person-centered approaches. Out of these efforts, many service providers have developed a new vision for service delivery, designed to promote "essential" lifestyle outcomes (Kincaid, 1996; OBrien, 1987). These outcomes have been described in the literature as guiding principles of person-centered planning. They include increased community access and inclusion, relationship development, increased opportunities for choice, valued and respected roles, and enhanced personal competencies.

In the research literature, a growing interest in quality of life enhancement has been accompanied by a focus on conceptualizing, defining, and measuring these essential outcomes. For example, researchers have measured 1) physical inclusion, the number of activities experienced in the community; 2) social inclusion, the number of activities experienced with people other than program staff and participants; 3) independence, progress on instructional objectives from the individualized support plan; 4) variety, the number of different activities experienced; and 5) preference, the number of valued or preferred activities experienced. In addition, there has been an increased focus on improving service delivery systems to assist people in achieving these outcomes (Newton, Ard, Horner, & Toews, 1996).

BARRIERS TO PERSON-CENTERED PLANNING IN LARGE, TRADITIONAL SERVICE MODELS

Despite the previously described advances, there is widespread recognition among service providers of the continued presence of barriers to person-centered planning in typical service delivery models. These barriers, which can ultimately compromise the attainment of valued outcomes, are described in detail next.

Managing Conflicting Priorities

Person-centered planning creates opportunities for flexible supports and stable funding so that needed and desired services can be rendered safely, reliably, and flexibly in home and community environments (Allen & O'Dell, 1997). Typically, person-centered plans are developed collaboratively by the person and his or her circle of support, including friends, neighbors, paid staff, and co-workers. Directions are built around a person's areas of strength and interest rather than around his or her areas of weakness. In the person-centered planning approach, priorities include tailoring supports to individual needs, desires, and preferences and fostering choice, empowerment, and inclusion.

In large, traditional service models, service delivery systems such as intermediate care facilities and day treatment programs are often built around regulatory compliance issues and the establishment of broad, systemic treatments that impose rigorous standards of care to meet licensure requirements. Comprehensive rehabilitation "packages" are developed by teams of agency clinicians and administrators and then applied to individuals based on their assessed needs and type of disability. Because the stability of funding is based largely on the agency's consistent service provision, top priorities often concern compliance with regulatory standards rather than attainment of individually desired outcomes or inclusion (Magito-McLaughlin & Spinosa, in press).

Individualizing Plans While Serving Large Numbers of People

Person-centered planning creates opportunities for supports and services to be individually tailored to meet each person's lifestyle preferences and needs. Critical to the design of these supports is attention to each person's

1. History and experiences
2. Health and well-being
3. Important relationships and social contacts
4. Community life
5. Preferences
6. Rituals and routines
7. Communication strategies
8. Aspirations and fears
9. Reputation
10. Level of self-determination

In large, traditional service delivery systems, the number of people served (often up to several hundred in well-established agencies) can be a barrier to planning and providing individualized supports. For many of the larger providers, serving hundreds of people simultaneously results in overcrowding in living environments (where 10 or more people typically live together) and in day program environments (where 15 or more people typically attend class together). Overcrowding can result in frequent exposure to nonpreferred people, standardized activities, and inattention to the important details of a person's life plan. These factors have the potential to compromise the integrity of the individualized supports and services that a person with disabilities receives.

Providing Adequate Staffing

Person-centered planning creates opportunities for a person's circle of support to be highly active and responsive to the elements of an individualized plan. For many people with disabilities, direct care staff are important members of the person's circle of support, and they are often relied on for successful implementation of the person-centered plan.

In large, traditional service delivery systems, limitations in staffing resources can be a barrier to person-centered planning. Typically, direct care staff are given different assignments, based on the overall number of people served and on the availability of enough staff to provide coverage across program sites. Often, staff are assigned to groups of people or programs (e.g., group homes, buildings, regions, units, classrooms) rather than to individuals. As delegates of an agency, staff can be called on to provide coverage in different parts of the agency, to support a greater number of people on any given day, or to support people other than those with whom they are typically assigned to work. As a result, many people who receive services fail to receive the level of

intensive staffing and instructional support that they need to participate fully in the general community. Direct support staff, who may
become frustrated with their inability to effect change, often respond
by moving on and changing jobs. This creates an instability in the work
force that can ultimately compromise the successful implementation of
even the best person-centered plans.

Ensuring Adequate Transportation

Person-centered planning creates opportunities for each person to gain
access to public or private transportation that allows him or her to plan
an individualized day. Adequate transportation gives the individual
the flexibility needed to gain access to a wide array of inclusion opportunities, such as paid jobs, volunteer work, and preferred leisure and
recreational events.

In large, traditional service delivery systems, transportation
resources typically consist of large agency vehicles designed to transport groups of people to and from central locations, such as group
homes or day treatment centers. Vehicles are often dispatched with
prearranged drivers, at prearranged times, and to and from prearranged destinations. The high demand for vehicles often results in
their overuse. Thus, vehicle breakdowns, scheduled servicing, and
needed repairs lead to further vehicle shortages. Many times, the varied needs and preferences of those receiving services cannot be accommodated because either too few vehicles are available or too many limitations are placed on vehicle usage. In addition, the fear of liability and
high agency insurance premiums often limit the number of available
drivers and prohibit staff members from using their own private vehicles to support community inclusion. Although public transportation
may be an option in some communities, many people with disabilities
require total support when traveling on buses, on trains, or in taxicabs.
As noted previously, staffing ratios often do not support this intense
level of intervention. Furthermore, public transportation can impose
limitations on flexibility and can limit the overall number of transition
opportunities in the day. These factors have the potential to compromise the integrity of a person-centered plan, particularly when movement to multiple locations or different activities is an integral part of
someone's day.

Coordinating Services
Across Teams and Environments

Person-centered planning creates opportunities for supports that are
global and comprehensive. Supports are effectively and harmoniously

implemented by several people, across home, work, and community environments, 24 hours per day, 7 days per week. This approach requires synchrony and coordination: Directions and supports that are required for each person hinge on successful integration of lifestyle elements across environments, social circles, and daily rhythms.

In large, traditional service delivery systems, ineffective service coordination can be a barrier to person-centered planning. Typically, people with disabilities are provided separate supports by separate providers in distinctly different physical and social environments. Support staff in day treatment programs, day habilitation programs, or supported work programs typically are not those who assist in the evening or on weekends in a group home or family home. Furthermore, services may be provided by two or more agencies and by two or more teams of clinical, administrative, and direct support staff—each of which receive different training, supervision, and oversight. Such arrangements necessitate that teams spend a great deal of time meeting to coordinate plans so that services can be duplicated across multiple environments. If team members are unavailable to meet on a consistent basis, then treatment fidelity can be lost in the process and valuable resources can be wasted on rescheduling. These factors have the potential to limit not only the integrity of the person-centered planning process, but its outcomes as well.

A SERVICE MODEL THAT IS CONDUCIVE TO PERSON-CENTERED PLANNING

Recognizing the challenges that are inherent in the larger, more traditional program models, we set out to create an alternative model of support in the agency that would be more conducive to person-centered planning. We developed a small pilot program, designed to minimize the barriers described, with the hope of enhancing the attainment of valued outcomes for the participants. We then conducted a program evaluation study to compare important quality of life indicators in the two models of service delivery.

Creating a Model of Service Based on Essential Outcomes

In the alternative model, individuals were provided with opportunities for flexible supports and stable funding through New York state's Medicaid waiver program. Thus, staff were able to prioritize individualization (instead of standardization) in the planning process. In place of a traditional needs assessment, the alternative model established person-centered planning as the starting point for each person's individualized support plan. Staff were trained to observe and interact with the people they supported to gain ongoing feedback regarding the activities that each person enjoyed. Data were routinely collected on a simple, five-point Likert-type rating scale. These data then served as the basis for uncovering new interests and identifying future programming directions. Each person's residential and day supports were developed with the goal of achieving five essential outcomes (community inclusion, relationships, choice, respected roles, and personal competencies). The following subsections describe changes that the alternative model made to foster these essential outcomes. (See Magito-McLaughlin & Spinosa, in press, for a more detailed account of the curriculum used in the alternative model program.)

Providing a Smaller Residential Environment and Community-Based Day Supports   The alternative model gave four people access to a new living opportunity at a small four-bedroom home, termed an *individualized residential alternative (IRA)*. In the new home, each person had his or her own bedroom and shared a bathroom with one other housemate. These living arrangements markedly reduced the overcrowding that was typical in larger living environments. Furthermore, adequate personal space in bedrooms and bathrooms ensured each persons privacy and selfhood. As part of the waiver option, day treatment "slots" were converted to individualized, community-based day supports, wherein each person's activities were individually developed and planned around his or her interests. We felt that when the group size was limited to four people, standardized activities would be less likely to occur. The creation of smaller, individualized living and work opportunities gave providers the opportunity to attend to the important details of each person's life and his or her life plan. Thus, each person's supports and services could be individually tailored according to the person's individual lifestyle preferences and needs.

Offering One-to-One Support During "Peak" Periods of the Day   Each person was afforded the opportunity to receive 6 hours minimum of one-to-one instructional support from a staff member who was assigned as that person's primary staff. Because staff worked directly with each person in the community, they were rarely pulled away to provide coverage at other program sites. This arrangement afforded staff members the opportunity to provide intensive, flexible, individualized supports that enabled each person to participate more fully in the community.

Providing Individualized Transportation   Each person had access to his or her own vehicle—a small, leased car. These compact cars were more fuel efficient and cost effective than larger vans, and they allowed each person to travel in a more typical manner—with one other person. Vehicles were driven by primary staff members and were available at all hours of the day and night. Because vehicles were assigned to a single person, breakdowns rarely occurred, and there were generally few limitations on vehicle usage. These individualized transportation arrangements were designed to readily accommodate the varied needs and preferences of the four people living in the IRA. They provided increased flexibility so that someone could make an immediate departure if an urgent or even a capricious need arose. Furthermore, they facilitated opportunities to gain access to multiple community locations, leisure activities, and work activities in a single day. This was seen as a critical component of successful inclusion.

Using a Single Team of Clinical, Administrative, and Support Staff A single team of clinical, administrative, and direct care staff was employed in the day and in the evening, across all environments (i.e., home, work, and community). The net cost savings for not having to duplicate teams allowed each team member to carry a smaller caseload; thus, clinical and administrative staff had the opportunity to provide more in-depth, comprehensive supports. To facilitate consistency and treatment fidelity across environments, team members all received identical training, supervision, and oversight.

Conducting the Program Evaluation Study

Eight people with developmental disabilities and their support staff participated in a program evaluation study aimed at evaluating the methods and outcomes of two different program models in the agency where the study was conducted. Four of the eight participants experienced traditional residential and day treatment program supports. They lived in either an intermediate care facility for people with mental retardation (ICF/MR) or in an IRA that adhered to the ICF/MR service model. Participants in this traditional model typically lived in larger group homes and attended a traditional day treatment program, where their services were based on identified needs and type of disability. Participants in this model experienced varied staffing ratios, shared vehicles, and two separate teams of administrative and clinical supports. The remaining four participants were those who experienced the previously described alternative service model. They lived in the small four-person IRA where community-based day supports were offered as part of their continuous service plan. All goals and activities were coordinated throughout the day and evening and were designed to achieve the five essential outcomes of person-centered planning. Participants in the alternative model group participated in person-centered planning meetings and received individualized staffing and transportation, which were coordinated by a single team of administrative, clinical, and support staff.

Selecting and Matching Participants   The participants were three women and five men between the ages of 37 and 41 years. Each participant had mental retardation in addition to autism and/or a secondary psychiatric diagnosis, including schizophrenia, anxiety disorder, and mood disorder. Four of the participants (Carl, Molly, Ed, and Sam) previously lived in an institution and demonstrated profound deficits in daily living skills, communication, and socialization. The remaining four participants (Mark, Jen, Jake, and Bonnie) previously lived at home with their families and demonstrated severe to moderate deficits in adaptive skills areas. All participants demonstrated severe challenging behavior, including aggression, self-injury, and property destruction. One participant displayed pica, and three participants frequently eloped. Table 6.1 summarizes participant characteristics and identifies in which of the two service models the participants were involved.

Participants in the alternative model group had previously been on the agency's waiting list and were identified to move into the new IRA program. Two of the participants had lived in institutional settings previously and this was their first opportunity as adults to live in a community environment. The other two participants lived at home and attended a traditional day treatment program prior to moving into the new IRA program. Participants in the traditional model group were

Table 6.1.   Participant characteristics and service models

Participant	Age	Background	Disabilities	Service model
Molly	40	Institution	Autism, profound mental retardation, schizophrenia	Alternative
Sam	38	Institution	Autism, profound mental retardation	Alternative
Jen	40	Community	Autism, severe mental retardation	Alternative
Bonnie	37	Community	Autism, moderate mental retardation, anxiety disorder	Alternative
Ed	37	Institution	Autism, profound mental retardation	Traditional
Carl	41	Institution	Autism, profound mental retardation	Traditional
Jake	37	Community	Autism, moderate mental retardation, schizophrenia	Traditional
Mark	39	Community	Autism, moderate mental retardation, mood disorder	Traditional

randomly selected from existing agency programs, and they were matched to the alternative model participants on the basis of age (within 2 years) and similar residential history (i.e., previous institutional versus community living arrangement).

Data Collection   We created a data collection system in which direct care staff recorded continuous data on the activities underway during all waking hours (7 A.M.–10 P.M.). Figure 6.1 shows the daily activity data sheet that was used for data collection. For each activity initiated, staff recorded the following:

- Type of activity initiated
- Purpose or objective of the activity (e.g., community participation/inclusion, relationships, choice, respected roles, skills/competencies)
- Whether the activity involved informal or formal instruction
- Time of day
- Total number of minutes spent on the activity
- Location of the activity (e.g., home, inclusive environment, segregated setting, travel)
- Person's preference for the activity (based on a five-point rating scale in which staff judged the person's apparent enjoyment of the activity)
- Whether the activity involved paid staff or unpaid, natural supports (e.g., friends, neighbors)
- Whether challenging behavior occurred during the activity (e.g., aggression, property destruction, self-injury, elopement, pica)
- Comments, if clarifying information was necessary

Research Design and Data Analysis   A matched group comparison design was employed in the study. Direct care staff who were naïve to the study served as primary observers and collected continuous direct observation data as part of their usual work responsibilities. Data were collected for a period of 5 weeks in all relevant environments (i.e., home, work, community). Because each day represented 900 minutes of coded direct observation data for each participant, on any given day, 7,200 minutes of data were available for the eight participants. This resulted in nearly 252,000 minutes of activity data in a 5-week period (35 days of data collection). To make this rather large data set meaningful, a single week-long period was randomly assigned to each pairing for analysis (i.e., Carl and Molly [Week 3], Ed and Sam [Week 1], Mark and Jen [Week 4], Jake and Bonnie [Week 5]). This allowed us to use a typical week as a meaningful unit of analysis when comparing the two program models.

Person: _____   Home: _____   Day/Date: _____

Activity	Activity catalog — Domain (1-4)	Activity catalog — Area (1-26)	Activity catalog — Type	5 essential areas (A, B, C, D, E)	Activity type (P/I)	Start time	End time	Total minutes	Location of activity	Location of activity (H, CI, CS, T)	Preference (1-5)	Paid staff/other (P, U)	Problem behavior (A, PD, SI, E, P)	Comments
Shift totals: Page ___ of ___	Domain: 1 = 2 = 3 = 4 =			Freq. A = B = C = D = E =	P = I =			Min.		Min. H = CI = CS = T = Total =	Freq. 1 = 2 = 3 = 4 = 5 =	P = U =	# Intvls. PB	

Figure 6.1. Sample daily activity data sheet. (Key: **5 Essential areas:** A=community participation/inclusion, B=relationships, C=choice, D=respected roles, E=skills/competencies. **Activity type:** P=participation, I=instruction. **Location of activity:** H=home, CI=community integrated, CS=community segregated, T=travel. **Preference:** 1=loved, 2=enjoyed, 3=neutral, 4=disliked, 5=hated. **Paid staff/other:** P=paid staff, U=unpaid person. **Problem behavior:** A=aggression, PD=property destruction, SI=self-injury, E=elopement, P=pica.)

136

For two of the four matched pairs (Ed and Sam, Jake and Bonnie), a typical week consisted of a sequential, 7-day period, from Saturday through Friday. For the remaining two matched pairs, typical weeks were shortened to 5 or 6 days, because portions of the data set had missing or incomplete information. For Carl and Molly, the typical week was Sunday through Friday, because data were missing for Carl on Saturday. For Mark and Jen, the typical week was Monday through Friday, because weekend data were not consistently recorded at Mark's house.

    Reliability   Given the extensive time periods involved in data collection, it was not feasible to collect reliability data at the time data were recorded by staff. Because it was not possible to achieve reliability sampling of observational data, reliability measures were collected on permanent product data that were available. For the purpose of analysis, activity data were coded, using the coding categories available in *The Activities Catalog* (Wilcox & Bellamy, 1987). Two raters independently reviewed the data sheets and examined recorded data in three areas: type of activity, duration, and location. Agreement was defined as 1) perfect agreement between both raters on activity code (i.e., domain, area, and type of activity); 2) agreement on the amount of time spent on the activity within 1 minute, based on recorded start and end times; and 3) perfect agreement on location code (i.e., home, community integrated, community segregated, or travel, based on actual location data reported). Interrater reliability was calculated by dividing the number of agreements by the number of agreements plus disagreements and then multiplying this figure by 100%. Using this formula, interrater reliability was 84%.

Evaluating Essential Outcomes in the Two Service Models

Table 6.2 presents a summary of essential outcomes across participants in each grouping during a typical week. The following subsections detail the findings for each outcome.

    Community Participation/Inclusion   With the right type and amount of supports, person-centered planning assumes that all people, regardless of the nature or severity of their disabilities, can lead normalized lives in the general community (Carr et al., 1999). To measure community presence across the two different models of service delivery, we calculated the number of places visited (e.g., shopping mall, movie theater, house of worship) by participants in each model, as well as the total variety of activities performed during the course of a typical week. In addition, using the location code (Figure 6.1), we determined the amount of time that each person spent in community inclu-

Table 6.2. Summary of essential outcomes across participants in a typical week

Essential outcome	Measure	Traditional model		Alternative model	
		Across participants	Mean (range)	Across participants	Mean (range)
Community participation/ inclusion	Number of places visited	20	5 (4–6)	86	22 (17–26)
	Number of different activities	80	20 (15–28)	121	30 (19–43)
	Time spent in inclusive settings	47 hours	12 hours (5–20 hours)	158 hours	40 hours (26–48 hours)
	Time spent in segregated settings	101 hours	25 hours (14–32 hours)	25 hours	6 hours (4–8 hours)
Choice	Percentage of preferred activities	42%	(28%–58%)	67%	(46%–75%)
Relationships	Number of participants with unpaid contacts	1	—	3	—
	Number of unpaid contacts	11	3 (0–11)	14	4 (0–7)
	Duration of unpaid contacts	9 hours	2 hours (0–9 hours)	9 hours	2 hours (0–4 hours)
Respected roles	Number of activities associated with problem behavior	34	9 (0–33)	5	1 (0–3)
	Number of participants involved in jobs/community service activities	3	—	4	—
	Number of job/ community service activities	19	5 (0–9)	25	6 (1–11)
	Time spent in jobs/ community service activities	22 hours	6 hours (0–13 hours)	9 hours	2 hours (1–5 hours)
Personal skills/competencies	Percentage of activities involving formal instruction	17%	(5%–61%)	2%	(0%–2%)

Note: All values have been rounded to the nearest whole number.

sive environments (i.e., where the majority of the people in the setting did not have a disability) and in community segregated environments (i.e., where the majority of the people in the setting had a disability).

The results showed that in the traditional model, across the four participants, a total of 20 places were visited in the sample week-long period. This represents a mean of 5 places per participant over the course of a typical week (range 4–6). In the alternative model, participants visited a total of 86 places in the community, representing a mean of 22 places per participant over the course of a typical week (range 17–26).

Individual program data showed that participants, who were matched for age and residential background, had substantially different inclusion experiences, depending on the program model in which they were enrolled. For example, Carl, a 41-year-old man with a long history of institutionalization, lived in a traditional group home and attended a traditional day treatment program. During his typical week, Carl had a total of four community experiences: he spent time in his day treatment unit, went on a van ride to see circus animals (although he did not exit the vehicle), practiced street crossing, and had his picture taken at a department sore. His matched partner, Molly, a 40-year-old woman who had moved out of the institution less than 1 year prior to the study, experienced a total of 21 community experiences in the alternative model. During the same week, she visited several friends' homes, went to several parks, worked in a greenhouse, went to convenience stores, went food shopping, ate out at an ice cream parlor, walked along the waterfront, went to a movie, watched a softball game, and spent time at the beach. For the matched pairs with a community background, a similar pattern occurred. For example, Jake, a 37-year-old man who lived with his family prior to moving to a traditional group home nearly 5 years prior to the study, attended day treatment program on a full-time basis. During his typical week, Jake had a total of five community experiences: he spent time at day treatment, walked on the grounds of the day treatment center, went to two parks, and visited the waterfront. Jake's matched partner, Bonnie, a 37-year-old woman who also lived at home prior to her move to the alternative program, had a total of 26 community experiences in the alternative model. During the same week, Bonnie visited several friends' homes, went to convenience stores, did her own banking, visited her family's home, walked on a track at two local colleges, went out for coffee, shopped at a clothing store, went on a picnic, had ice cream at an ice cream parlor, ate out at several fast-food restaurants, saw a movie, and did gardening.

Data on variety of activities indicated that across the four participants in the traditional model, a total of 80 different activities took place over the course of the week, representing a mean of 20 different activities per participant (range 15–28). In the alternative model, 121 different activities were recorded, representing a mean of 30 different activities for each participant over the course of a typical week (range 19–43).

Figure 6.2 presents data on the average number of hours participants spent on various activities over the course of a typical week in the different program models. Individual program data showed that in the traditional model, participants were more likely to participate in games, craft activities, and hobbies (e.g., puzzles, bowling), as well as in work activities involving distribution jobs (e.g., counting, sorting, grouping, straightening) and domestic and building services (e.g., trash removal, maintenance). "Down time" activities, such as relaxing, people-watching, and hanging out, were salient features in the traditional model. On average, participants spent more than 25 hours per week engaging in these activities.

In the alternative model, participants often attended special events (e.g., sporting events, movies, nature parks) and engaged in personal management activities (e.g., self-care, personal business, management of space and belongings). Their most common work activities involved agriculture and natural resource activities (e.g., groundskeeping, animal care) and office and business services (e.g., copying, recycling). Active recreational activities, such as playing sports and attending scheduled events in the community, were salient features in the alternative model. On average, participants spent nearly 15 hours per week engaging in these active recreational activities, nearly double that of the traditional group. The two models were similar in their focus on food-related activities (e.g., meal preparation, eating), fitness activities, and socialization (e.g., visiting others).

Participants in the traditional model spent a total of 47.3 hours (32%) in inclusive environments and 100.5 hours (68%) in segregated environments, such as all-purpose rooms and segregated workshops, gymnasiums, and classrooms. Thus, the people served in traditional programs spent about two-thirds of their time in segregated environments. Individual program data suggested that in many cases, the people in traditional programs frequently went on van rides to "practice" prerequisite community skills (e.g., buckling seatbelt, sitting quietly, following directions) without ever actually reaching a community destination. Participants in the alternative model spent a total of 158.2 hours (86%) in inclusive environments and 24.8 hours (14%) in segregated environments. Individual program data showed that the rela-

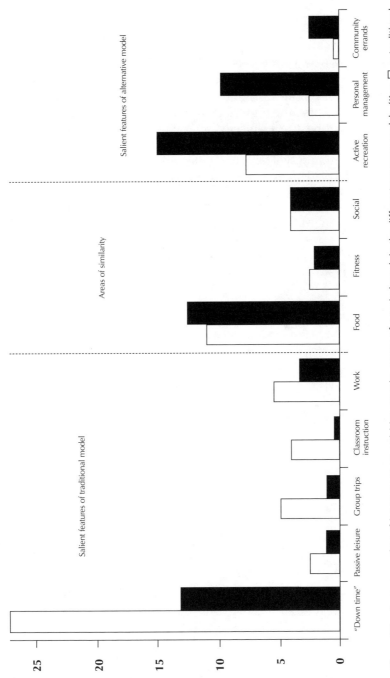

Figure 6.2. Average number of hours spent on activities over the course of a typical week in the different program models. (*Key:* □ = traditional model; ■ = alternative model.)

tively few segregated activities usually occurred during scheduled medical appointments in the agency's clinics or in building-based cafeterias and in vending areas during lunchtime.

Figures 6.3 and 6.4 represent community inclusion data for the matched pairs. The data in Figure 6.3 show that for participants who previously lived in an institution (i.e., those who demonstrated profound skill deficits), the traditional model offered fewer opportunities to become involved in inclusive environments. The circles show that participants in the traditional model consistently spent 0–2 hours per day in the community. The squares show that participants in the alternative model had more access to inclusive environments, spending 4–10 hours per day in such environments. Similar but less pronounced differences were observed in matched pairs who previously lived in community environments (i.e., those who demonstrated severe to

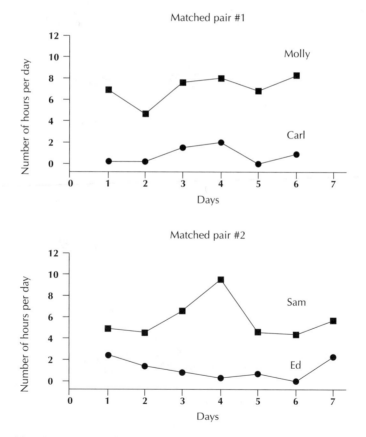

Figure 6.3. Time spent in inclusive environments for individuals with an institutional background. (*Key:* ● = traditional model; ■ = alternative model.)

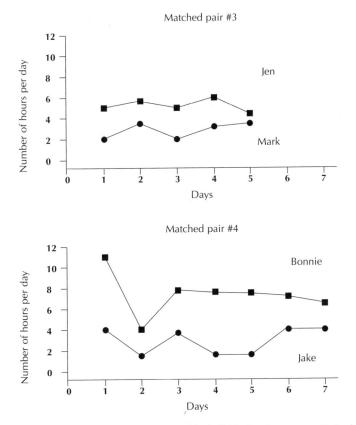

Figure 6.4. Time spent in inclusive environments for individuals with a community background. (*Key:* ● = traditional model; ■ = alternative model.)

moderate skill deficits), as shown in Figure 6.4. Again, the circles show that traditional model participants consistently spent 2–4 hours per day in inclusive environments. The squares show that alternative model participants spent 5–8 or more hours per day in inclusive environments. These findings were particularly robust in that differences in inclusion opportunities were found across all four matched pairs and on all days of the week in which data were examined.

Choice Choice is a second essential outcome in person-centered planning (Dyer, Dunlap, & Winterling, 1990). One of the goals of person-centered planning is to diligently and respectfully work with a person and his or her family to fully understand and provide whatever personalized supports are desired and needed, as well as to maximize the person's level of enjoyment and involvement in decision making. To quantify choice in the study, each activity received a preference rating based on a five-point Likert-type scale, ranging from highly preferred

(1 = "loved") to highly nonpreferred (5 = "hated") (see Figure 6.1). Ratings were based on staff's judgment of the person's affect and involvement in the activity underway. An activity was considered preferred if it was rated 1 or 2 on the Likert scale, it was considered neutral if it was rated 3, and it was considered nonpreferred if it was rated 4 or 5. Frequencies of assigned ratings were converted to percentages to determine the relative proportion of activities occurring in each category.

The results showed that across the four participants in the traditional model, 198 of 476 activities (42%) recorded during the week were rated as preferred or highly preferred. Of the remaining 278 activities, 245 (51%) were rated as neutral, and 33 (7%) were rated as nonpreferred or highly nonpreferred. Thus, more than half of the activities of the four participants receiving traditional services were rated as neutral or nonpreferred. In the alternative model, across the four participants, 453 of 680 activities (67%) recorded during the week were rated as preferred or highly preferred, whereas 211 (31%) were rated as neutral, and 16 (2%) were rated as nonpreferred or highly nonpreferred. Thus, the majority of the activities experienced in this group were activities that the participants enjoyed.

Individual program data revealed an important finding. In the traditional model, only one of the four participants, Carl, engaged in activities at home that were rated as being "highly preferred." The remaining three, all of whom lived in larger group homes, had *no* recorded instances of highly preferred activities in the home over the course of a typical week. In contrast, in the alternative model, three of the four participants engaged in activities at home that were rated as being "highly preferred." Highly preferred activities in the home included relaxing, dining, watching television, helping with chores, showering, and taking a bath. This finding suggests that in traditional program models, people with disabilities may have difficulties finding enjoyment in their typical routines. Although activities such as dining, relaxing, or bathing represent important quality of life elements (Smull, 1999), staff consistently reported that traditional model participants did not show a preference for these activities.

Relationships   Relationships represent a third essential outcome of person-centered planning (Amado, Conklin, & Wells, 1989). Recognizing that the overall number and quality of relationships influence a person's health, happiness, and quality of life, an important goal of person-centered planning is to support each person in establishing and maintaining a network of social supports. To measure relationships, we counted the number of participants who engaged in social contacts with people who were not being paid to provide support over the course of a typical week. We also measured the number of social contacts that occurred and the total duration of these contacts.

The results showed that in the traditional model, across all four participants, there were 11 social contacts with two people who were not being paid to provide support. Only one of the four participants had unpaid social contacts, and the total duration of these contacts was 9.1 hours during the week. Ten of the eleven contacts involved a peer with disabilities in the person's classroom unit at day program. The remaining contact involved a housemate in the person's group home. In the alternative model, there were 14 social contacts with five people who were not being paid to provide support. Three of four participants were involved in these unpaid contacts. Although the total duration of these contacts was similar to that in the traditional model group (9.2 hours), the nature of the contacts differed in several ways. In the alternative model, 10 of the 14 contacts were with family members of support staff, three contacts were with peers who did not have disabilities (i.e., friends of support staff), and the remaining contact was with a peer with disabilities from a different group home.

Individual program data showed that in the traditional model, social contacts with unpaid others typically revolved around "down time" activities, such as choosing reinforcers at bonus time, eating lunch, going on a van ride, or taking a break. In the alternative model, however, unpaid social contacts typically revolved around planned social activities such as exercising, playing cards, having dinner, and going to the movies.

Respected Roles   Respected roles represents a fourth essential outcome of person-centered planning (Smith, Belcher, & Juhrs, 1995). The ability to establish a positive reputation in one's community is widely recognized as a critical component of successful inclusion for people with developmental disabilities. Because poor reputations can result from socially unacceptable behavior, one measure of respected roles involved examining the number of activities that were associated with the occurrence of challenging behavior. The results showed that in the traditional model, across the four participants, a total of 34 activities were associated with severe challenging behavior. Challenging behavior involved three of the four participants and occurred in nine different contexts: food preparation and eating, bathing and washing, dressing, transportation, TV viewing, medication time, community trips, prevocational work, and arrival at a day program. In the alternative model, across the four participants, only five activities were associated with challenging behavior. These activities with challenging behavior occurred in three different contexts (food preparation and eating, using the bathroom, and transportation) and involved two of the four participants. Thus, although all eight participants in the study had a history of severe challenging behavior, participants in the alternative model demonstrated fewer incidences of socially unacceptable behavior, which also occurred in fewer contexts.

Person-centered planning also strives to assist people in developing positive reputations through meaningful, respected roles, such as volunteer work, paid work, neighborhood watch programs, beautification projects, and so forth. Thus, a second measure of respected roles involved determining the number of participants who engaged in activities that were focused on such activities—specifically job development, volunteer work, or community service. We also measured the number of respected roles activities that occurred and the total duration of these activities.

In the traditional model, a total of 19 activities involved job development or community service, an average of 4.8 activities per participant during the week. Respected roles activities occurred on 12 of 25 days (48%), by three of four participants, for a total of 21.9 hours (range 0–13.3 hours per participant). In the alternative model, 25 of the recorded activities involved job development or community service, an average of 6.3 activities per participant during the week. Respected roles activities occurred on 11 of 25 days (44%), by all four participants, for a total of 9.4 hours (range 1–5.2 hours per participant).

Individual program data showed that in the traditional model, participants tended to participate in distribution and domestic jobs (e.g., packaging, custodial work), whereas in the alternative model, work activities varied (e.g., horticulture, office services). In addition, in the traditional model, participants engaged in work-related activities for sustained periods of time, whereas in the alternative model, participants had a tendency to "job sample." They engaged in several different job activities for short periods of time, in an apparent effort to identify work preferences.

Personal Skills/Competencies   Personal competencies represents the fifth essential outcome of person-centered planning (Evans & Scotti, 1989). In a person-centered approach, each person is afforded an opportunity to learn and grow and to acquire new skills that are not based exclusively on need, but on personal interest as well. To measure personal competencies, we calculated the number of activities that included a formal instructional component, relative to the number of activities in which the individuals participated. Although individual task analysis data were collected as a measure of skill acquisition in both environments, these data were not considered in the comparison due to the brief 5-week period of the study.

The results showed that in the traditional model, 81 of 482 activities (17%) recorded during the week involved formal, goal-based instruction. More than 80% of the recorded teaching trials were conducted with the two participants who lived in ICFs/MR, where regulations specifically focus on the attainment of rehabilitation objectives. In the alternative model, 708 activities were recorded; however, only 11 (2%) were reported as being goal based. An analysis of the types of skills that were taught indicates that in the traditional model, goal activities appeared to be systems driven (e.g., showering, toothbrushing, fire safety, prevocational task training). They were carried out during multiple trials in the day, and the same goals were implemented nearly every day. In the alternative model, goal activities were often based on self-determination activities (e.g., self-administration of medication, communication, banking and money management). Goals were carried out on an intermittent and varied basis, as needs arose (e.g., taking an analgesic when in pain, cashing a paycheck on payday). Hence, in the alternative model, participants experienced more activities but fewer teaching trials overall.

CONCLUSION: PUTTING IT ALL TOGETHER

Service providers widely recognize the presence of barriers to person-centered planning, particularly in large, traditional service models. These barriers include managing conflicting person-centered and system-centered priorities, individualizing plans while serving large numbers of people, providing adequate staffing and transportation supports, and coordinating services across teams and environments. In an effort to overcome these barriers, we created an alternative model of service delivery that was designed to be more conducive to person-centered values, methods, and outcomes. Program evaluation data suggested that participants achieved a variety of valued outcomes if they experienced 1) a smaller residential environment with community-based day supports; 2) a single team of clinical, administrative, and direct support staff; and 3) enhanced transportation and staffing supports. Participants who received traditional supports and services achieved traditional outcomes.

In the area of community participation, data on physical inclusion showed that participants in the alternative model visited many places in the community, experienced a wide array of activities, and consistently spent a greater proportion of their time in inclusive (versus segregated) environments. It is important to note that people with severe needs who had previously lived in institutional settings achieved consistent access to the community, even though they were at the greatest disadvantage for inclusion. In the area of choice, preference data indicated that alternative model participants engaged in many activities that were judged to be preferred, both at home and in the community. These data suggest that essential lifestyle elements were in place across environments. In the area of relationships, alternative model participants experienced planned, organized social contacts outside of their immediate peer group (i.e., with peers who did not have disabilities), although the overall number of unpaid contacts was limited. Further research in this area is needed to address this challenge. In the area of respected roles, alternative model participants demonstrated few challenging behaviors overall, suggesting that they responded well to the individualized supports that were available. Furthermore, all four participants in the alternative model were afforded diverse opportunities for job development and community service activities. Finally, in the area of personal competencies, teaching occurred in typical environments and at natural times in the alternative model. The participants had frequent access to experiential learning and incidental teaching opportunities (i.e., they participated in nearly 50% more activities overall than participants in the traditional model); however, given the low number of formal instructional activities recorded, it remains unclear whether staff routinely attended to these opportunities by offering instruction. Further research is needed in this area to ensure that staff who are working in inclusive environments are promoting skills that ultimately teach each person to participate fully in improving his or her quality of life.

The program evaluation study presented in this chapter has several limitations. First, the investigation was conducted in a naturalistic environment, and it was designed to capture "typical" activities in service delivery locations. Paid staff members served as primary observers and collected direct observation data as part of their usual work responsibilities. This resulted in two important confounds: 1) missing data, which prevented us from looking at a full, 7-day week for two of the four matched pairs, and 2) the absence of observational reliability, which prevented us from making convincing statements about the findings. A second limitation is that as a quasi-experimental design, the study lacks the rigor and control of a true experiment that are necessary to make causal statements about the results. In the absence of a more rigorous test, it is possible that some of the outcomes observed are attributable to factors other than those that were formally considered. Although participants in the two program models were matched for age and residential background, they were not directly matched for other factors, such as skill level and challenging behavior, that indeed could have affected the outcomes. A third limitation of the study is that the results reflect a brief, 1-week time period that may not necessarily be representative of long-term gains. Because individual person-centered plans were not specifically examined in the study, it remains unclear to what extent individually valued outcomes were actually achieved for each participant. Finally, because the study includes a multicomponent intervention (i.e., different curriculum, program size, staffing pattern, transportation arrangements, administrative oversight), further research is needed to determine whether a single component or some unique combination of components might have achieved similar results.

Despite the study's shortcomings, the investigation represents an important attempt to merge science with the policy and practice of person-centered planning. The study suggests practical and feasible strategies for measuring broad, systemic variables and for altering valued outcomes at a molar level. Most important, the study identifies ways of evaluating and improving service delivery models to further enhance the attainment of valued outcomes.

REFERENCES

Allen, D.R., & O'Dell, K.E. (1997). *The key to individualized services in the home and community based waiver: A provider guide.* Albany, NY: Office of Mental Retardation and Developmental Disabilities.

Amado, A.N., Conklin, F., & Wells, J. (1989). *Friends: A manual for connecting people with disabilities and community members.* St. Paul, MN: Governor's Planning Council on Developmental Disabilities.

Carr, E.G., Levin, L., McConnachie, G., Carlson, J.I., Kemp, D.C., Smith, C.E., & Magito-McLaughlin, D. (1999). Comprehensive multisituational intervention for problem behavior in the community: Long-term maintenance and social validation. *Journal of Positive Behavior Interventions, 1*(1), 5–25.

Dyer, K., Dunlap, G., & Winterling, V. (1990). Effects of choice-making on the serious problem behaviors of students with severe handicaps. *Journal of Applied Behavior Analysis, 23,* 515–524.

Evans, I.M., & Scotti, J.R. (1989). Defining meaningful outcomes for persons with profound disabilities. In F. Brown & D.H. Lehr (Eds.), *Persons with profound disabilities: Issues and practices* (pp. 83–107). Baltimore: Paul H. Brookes Publishing Co.

Kincaid, D. (1996). Person-centered planning. In L.K. Koegel, R.L. Koegel, & G. Dunlap (Eds.), *Positive behavioral support: Including people with difficult behavior in the community* (pp. 439–465). Baltimore: Paul H. Brookes Publishing Co.

Magito-McLaughlin, D., & Spinosa, T.R. (in press). Individualized waiver services: Working methods. In J. Jacobsen, J. Mulick, & S. Holburn (Eds.), *Dual diagnosis service models.* New York: The National Association for the Dually Diagnosed.

Mount, B. (1994). Benefits and limitations of personal futures planning. In V.J. Bradley, J.W. Ashbaugh, & B.C. Blaney (Eds.), *Creating individual supports for people with developmental disabilities: A mandate for change at many levels* (pp. 97–108). Baltimore: Paul H. Brookes Publishing Co.

Newton, J.S., Ard, W.R., Horner, R.H., & Toews, J.D. (1996). Focusing on values and lifestyle outcomes in an effort to improve the quality of residential services in Oregon. *Mental Retardation, 34,* 1–12.

O'Brien, J. (1987). A guide to life-style planning: Using The Activities Catalog to integrate services and natural support systems. In B. Wilcox & G.T. Bellamy (Eds.), *The Activities Catalog: An alternative curriculum for youth and adults with severe disabilities* (pp. 175–189). Baltimore: Paul H. Brookes Publishing Co.

Schalock, R.L., Keith, K.D., Hoffman, K., & Karan, O.C. (1989). Quality of life: Its measurement and use. *Mental Retardation, 27,* 25–31.

Smith, M.D., Belcher, R.G., & Juhrs, P.D. (1995). *A guide to successful employment for individuals with autism.* Baltimore: Paul H. Brookes Publishing Co.

Smull, M. (1999, March). *Essential lifestyle planning.* Seminar presented by the New York State Association for Community and Residential Agencies, New York City.

Turnbull, A.P., & Turnbull, H.R. (1994). *Group action planning as a strategy for getting a life.* Lawrence: The University of Kansas, Beach Center on Disability.

Wilcox, B. & Bellamy, G.T. (1987). *A comprehensive guide to The Activities Catalog: An alternative curriculum for youth and adults with severe disabilities.* Baltimore: Paul H. Brookes Publishing Co.

7

Lifestyle Quality and Person-Centered Support

Jeff, Janet, Stephanie, and the Microboard Project

Paul H. Malette

In existence since the early 1970s, a continuum of residential and vocational services provided in the least restrictive environment (LRE) remains the predominant support structure in aging, mental health, and disability support. The LRE concept was created in response to public opposition to the dehumanizing conditions of large state-run institutions. It consists of an array of services such as long-term care facilities, group homes, day activity centers, sheltered workshops, and supported employment. Although it was a forward-looking concept for its time, the disability field is moving away from the LRE (Racino & Taylor, 1993). Characterized by conceptual and programmatic flaws, the concept of LRE sanctions infringements on people's rights, supports the primacy of professional decision making, and directs attention to physical settings rather than to the services and supports that people need to be included in their communities (Taylor, 1988). As of the late 1980s, the disability field has been exploring more flexible and individualized approaches under the rubric of person-centered planning and support (Malette, 1996; Mount, 1987; Mount & Zwernik, 1988; O'Brien, 1987; Racino & Taylor; 1993).

Person-centered planning is based on the assumption that people with disabilities have the right to direct their own lives. Coordinated efforts among formal and informal supports are necessary components of successful planning, as well as the achievement of a quality life in

I am grateful to Janet, Jeff, and Stephanie for welcoming me into their lives. I also thank members of the microboards, Vela Microboard Association, and Services for Community Living Branch for opening up their files and hearts to me.

the community for the focus person. Planning identifies the strengths and capacities of the individual to build a desirable future. However, planning alone is not sufficient to enable people with disabilities to direct their own lives. Person-centered support structures are also needed, and they include three defining characteristics. First, housing and support services are separated, enabling people to obtain necessary supports wherever they live. People with disabilities are not viewed as having different housing needs than people without disabilities. Person-centered support allows people with disabilities to lease, rent, and personally or cooperatively own homes. Second, support strategies vary for each individual and reflect a unique combination of services; adaptations; and assistance from friends, family, paid staff, and neighbors to enable people to live in homes of their choosing. Finally, person-centered support advocates choice in all aspects of a person's life (Racino & Taylor, 1993).

Although the disability field is beginning to examine creative housing and support options for people with disabilities, there has been little research on these emerging practices. Both in research and practice, the disability field is just beginning to examine these new strategies to see how or if they have a positive impact on the lives of people with disabilities (Racino & Taylor, 1993). The shift to more inclusive supports for people with disabilities requires research methodologies that attempt to understand life in the community from the perspective of people with disabilities and to capture their impressions of lifestyle quality. In this context, ethnographic research strategies such as interviews and participant observation techniques are useful (Bogdan & Biklen, 1982; Nisbet, Clark, & Covert, 1991).

The study detailed in this chapter is a qualitative investigation of a person-centered approach known as microboards. A *microboard* is a small group of committed family and friends who join together with a person to create a small nonprofit society to address the person's support needs in an empowering and customized fashion. The broad purposes of the study are to provide a comprehensive description of the lives of three people with complex needs who are living in homes of their own and to examine how these lives came to be. Following a description of research methods, this chapter introduces an overview of the role and function of microboards and two organizations responsible for introducing the microboard concept to the study participants. Personal histories and perspectives on quality of life for each study participant are then explored. The chapter concludes with a discussion of the major themes that emerged in the study, which are framed within the emerging paradigm of person-centered planning and support.

METHOD

Participants and Setting

The study was conducted in 1996 in the city of Vancouver and the nearby city of Richmond, both growing urban centers on the west coast of British Columbia, Canada. The study participants were Jeff, Janet, and Stephanie. They formed a diverse group of young adults who lived in subsidized and cooperative housing projects in Vancouver and Richmond. Their housing and paid supports were facilitated by their microboards. Prior to the microboard project, Janet and Jeff were living in group homes and Stephanie was living in her mother's home. Janet, Jeff, and Stephanie had cerebral palsy and required 12- to 24-hour support daily. Given the need for individual perspectives of quality of life in person-centered approaches (Nisbet et al., 1991; Walker, 1999), the study in this chapter used a "purposeful sampling technique" (Taylor & Bogdan, 1984). The study participants were specifically chosen because they believed that they had achieved quality lives in the community through the microboard project.

Jeff   Jeff was 27 years old. He was a bright young man with many interests, including hockey, soccer, wheelchair bocci ball, and parasailing. He primarily used speech to communicate, and his written communications were facilitated with the use of a computer and a head stick. Jeff received 12 hours of daily support—including assistance with bathing, eating, and dressing—and had a team of five support providers, each of whom he interviewed and hired. Jeff joined the microboard pilot project in 1991, and his microboard consisted of his brother, his sister-in-law, his aunt, and two friends.

Janet   Janet was 26 years old. She was a social woman who enjoyed wheelchair soccer, crafts, eating at a favorite restaurant, listening to Michael Jackson's and Madonna's music, visiting with friends, and shopping. Her dream was to be reunited with her birth mother, whom she located during the study. Janet used an electric wheelchair with a joystick. She communicated primarily by pointing to the letters of the alphabet, which were pasted to a lap tray attached to her wheelchair. Janet had a voice output communication device, but she did not routinely use it. Janet required 24-hour care for assistance with eating, bathing, cooking, cleaning, shopping, and so forth. Her in-home support network comprised five people. For her daytime supports, she contracted with an agency. Janet's microboard was composed of her foster mother and four friends.

Stephanie   Stephanie was 25 years old. She was a gentle, patient woman who loved life. She was part of a close and caring family, whom she saw often during the study. Stephanie enjoyed fashionable clothes, and she was a fan of basketball, baseball, football, and hockey. Stephanie was nonverbal and responded to questions with a head nod. She used vocalizations and body gestures to communicate discomfort, anxiety, and pleasure and used photographs for scheduling and making choices. Her paid supports comprised a network of six people. This network, which provided 24-four hour care, was hired by Stephanie and her microboard. Stephanie's microboard comprised her mother, her brother, her sister-in-law, her sister, and two friends.

Setting   A micro-macro technique similar to that of Mehan, Hertweck, and Meihls (1986) was employed in the study. The micro research strategy was to develop a detailed understanding of the lives of the study participants and their perceptions of lifestyle quality. To understand the roles and organizational characteristics of key formal support agencies, two agencies central to the microboard project were also a target of study: 1) Vela Microboard Association and 2) Services for Community Living Branch. Vela Microboard Association and Services for Community Living Branch initiated the microboard pilot project in British Columbia and introduced person-centered planning and support to the study participants. The methodology and data collection procedures of the study were both structured and open ended, following a reflexive approach (Hammersley & Atkinson, 1983; Taylor, Bogdan, & Racino, 1991). Four themes, or foreshadowed problems, comprised the structured component of inquiry: 1) the values and philosophy of organizational support, 2) the structure and nature of organizations, 3) the nature of relationships between formal and informal supports, and 4) a focus on the individual's quality of life (Racino & Taylor, 1993; Taylor et al., 1991).

Participant Observation

I functioned as a participant observer. Guiding principles for my observations were O'Brien's (1987) five essential lifestyle accomplishments: 1) community presence, 2) choice, 3) competence, 4) respect, and 5) community participation. A rotating schedule of observations across contexts was employed to record and describe important aspects of the participants' daily lives and interactions with the community and formal and informal support systems (Salisbury, Palombaro, & Hollowood, 1993). I spent 50–100 hours in each participant's home, as well as in a variety of community settings, such as microboard meetings, parties, family events, college classes, wheelchair bocci ball, wheelchair soccer, swimming, eating at restaurants, and visiting the local pub. Over time, I was increasingly included in day-to-day interactions and functions with Janet, Jeff, and Stephanie; I eventually joined Stephanie's microboard as a full participating member during the course of the study.

Interviews

Semistructured and unstructured interviews occurred throughout the 18-month research period. The participants were interviewed, as were their support staff, microboard members, friends, family members, neighbors, members of Vela Microboard Association, and members of Services for Community Living Branch. Interviews ranged from 1 to 4 hours, as determined by participants. Semistructured interviews were audiotaped, transcribed verbatim, and incorporated into a chronological database. The goals of the interviews with Janet, Stephanie, and Jeff were 1) to develop a framework of personal background, including biological, educational, medical, and residential history; and 2) to explore their perceptions of quality of life in the microboard project. The interview goals with members of the three microboards, Vela Microboard Association, and Services for Community Living Branch were to develop an understanding of the underlying values, purpose, history, and structure of these organizations.

Permanent Products

Written materials from individual microboards, as well as materials from Services for Community Living Branch and Vela Microboard Association, were collected over the course of the study. These materials included philosophy statements, monitoring tools, and newsletters. The information was dated, its source and context were identified, and it was entered into the chronology for that week and month. These written materials provided a framework to evaluate and link each organization's mission with each participant's lifestyle outcomes.

Data Analysis and Validity

The main purposes of the data analysis were to identify themes that emerged from the data concerning the quality of life of the study participants and to frame these themes within the emerging paradigm of person-centered planning and support. Rotating schedules of observation, coupled with ongoing interview schedules, provided the opportunity to discuss trends, affirm perceptions, and evaluate the data (Taylor & Bogdan, 1984). All field notes, permanent products, and interviews were sorted and transcribed in chronological order. Final data analyses involved the identification, coding, and categorizing of primary patterns in the data. These patterns were then cross-referenced with relevant literature regarding the emerging characteristics of a person-centered approach. Finally, meetings were held with the participants, microboard members, and members of Vela Microboard Association and Services for Community Living Branch to share the emergent themes of the research and supporting evidence.

Triangulation was used to validate the data and process of analysis (Borg & Gall, 1989). First, triangulation of data sources was employed. I reviewed each microboard's written philosophy statements and principles and functions. I then interviewed individual microboard members about their perceptions of roles and procedures; observed how these procedures actually occurred in Jeff's, Janet's, and Stephanie's lives; and solicited the three participants' perceptions. Second, analytic triangulation was employed. Data were sorted into categories and themes. These themes were then reviewed by those being studied (i.e., the three participants, their microboard members, and members of Vela Microboard Association and Services for Community Living Branch) and were affirmed, revised, and finally validated by these members. This "member check" (Salisbury et al., 1993, p. 78) served to reduce the potential bias that might arise from my perspective as a full participant in Stephanie's microboard, and it served to further ensure that the findings reflected the perceptions and experiences of the study participants. Third, as patterns emerged from the interviews and observations, these themes were considered in the context of traditional models of disability support and person-centered approaches to community living. This process of triangulation identified consistency and congruency in practice and procedure. Finally, the period of observation and my participation in Stephanie's microboard contributed to greater assurance that in-depth collection of evidence would be possible and that data were accurately interpreted.

ROLES AND FUNCTION OF MICROBOARDS, VELA MICROBOARD SOCIETY, AND SERVICES FOR COMMUNITY LIVING BRANCH

In broad terms, a microboard is a nonprofit society comprised of the focus person and a small group of committed individuals. Typically, family and friends make up a microboard. Microboards are formed to direct funding and decision making about housing and support to people with disabilities and their valued relationships. Microboard members are not paid for their services. Specific functions of microboard members include the following:

- Assist with lifestyle planning
- Identify and prepare requests for housing and support funds

- Identify and negotiate services with service providers
- Monitor services
- Honor the legal requirements of the provincially legislated Societies Act, which governs nonprofit support associations in British Columbia (a microboard is considered a nonprofit society)

A microboard needs at least five members to meet the requirements of the Societies Act (Vela Microboard Association, 1995). Depending on the individual needs of the focus person, microboards may meet as frequently as once per month or as infrequently as four times per year. Specific principles guide microboards:

- All people are assumed to have the capacity for self-determination.
- Services must be based on need rather than on available services.
- Housing and support must be separate.

These principles, which are not legislated, are the defining feature of microboards (Vela Microboard Association, 1995; Women's Research Centre, 1994).

At the time of the study, 35 microboards were operating in British Columbia. Following the innovative work of David and Faye Wetherow, Vela Microboard Association introduced microboards to British Columbia and study participants. Vela Microboard Association was partially funded by the British Columbia Ministry of Health. Its primary role was to support the growth and development of individual microboards so that they were ready to enter into a contract with a governmental funding agency. Vela Microboard Association was qualified for this support role because of its expertise and experience with person-centered planning, the legal requirements of the Societies Act, and the funding and fiscal responsibilities required by the provincial government. Vela Microboard Association did not provide funding to microboards; rather, it prepared microboards for a funding agreement with the provincial government's funding agency, Services for Community Living Branch. Vela Microboard Association offered specific support services: 1) disseminating information, easing anxiety, and fostering relationships with individual microboards; 2) assisting individuals and their microboards to build a vision of a quality life in the community; 3) assisting in the logistics of developing a microboard, including budgeting, hiring staff, and setting up a payroll; and 4) public education, training of government personnel, and advocacy with government on behalf of microboards (Women's Research Centre, 1994). At the time of the study, Vela Microboard Association had seven board members and four paid support staff. Vela Microboard Association did not negotiate with the government on behalf of microboards.

Its goal was to assist microboards in becoming autonomous in their negotiations and functioning. Procedurally, this was highly individualized and reflective of the needs of the three participants and their emerging microboards. The study participants and their microboards relied on Vela Microboard Association to provide extensive support to enter into a contract with Services for Community Living Branch.

Services for Community Living Branch served people with complex physical and health care needs throughout the province. They provided funding for housing and support. Two senior members guided the work of 13 service coordinators, who assisted human service agencies and microboards to plan, coordinate, and monitor quality supports for people with disabilities. Services for Community Living Branch had three primary roles in the microboard project: 1) partially fund Vela Microboard Association to support the development of microboards, 2) fund individual microboards and develop contracts for support, and 3) monitor supports and quality of life via a service coordinator. Figure 7.1 illustrates the funding and support relationships of each partici-

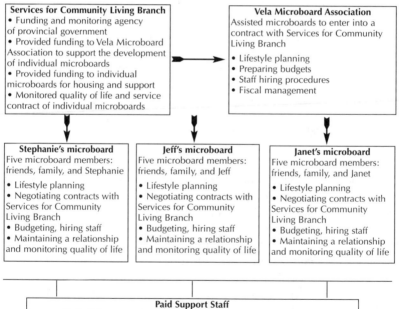

Figure 7.1. Organizational relationships of Services for Community Living Branch, Vela Microboard Association, and individual microboards.

pant's microboard, Vela Microboard Association, and Services for Community Living Branch.

WELL-BEING: JEFF'S STORY

The youngest of five children, Jeff was born in Halifax, Nova Scotia, on April 20, 1968. The notion of family elicits strong positive images for Jeff. Photographs of Jeff as a young child showed him smiling and involved in family functions. Yet, not all members of his extended family shared the inclusive attitudes of his immediate family. Jeff's brother explained,

> When Jeff was born we had relatives that said forget about him . . . put him in an institution; it's the best thing that you can do. . . . I was 7 years old. I will never forget that, and I have never forgiven those relatives.

In 1972, Jeff and his family moved to Edmonton, Alberta, where he first experienced segregation. Jeff described his school experience in a hospital setting of 200 people:

> I felt it wasn't fair. . . . It was really sterile. It was by a mall. We hung out at the mall a lot. One part of the school was like a jail for juvenile delinquents. One of the teachers at my brother and sisters' school wanted me to go to a regular elementary school. It was two blocks away, but the government said no.

In 1985, Jeff and his mother moved and found an apartment in Central Vancouver. He was enrolled in a disability program at a secondary school. Jeff enjoyed life in Vancouver and met his future bride, Janet, while attending high school. Jeff's most influential contacts with the disability culture and the continuum model of residential support occurred in 1987, when he turned 19 and his mother and personal care attendants were no longer able to meet his support needs. Jeff and his mother were confronted with limited options; they could either choose a group home or a hospital. Jeff discussed his reaction to these restrictive options, "I did not want to leave my mom's house. It's like they were telling me where to live. I had to choose between the lesser of two evils." When Jeff turned 19, he moved into a group home with five other people with disabilities whom he did not know. Jeff's impressions of life in the group home were explicit:

> I moved in on my 19th birthday at noon. I will never forget that birthday. I cried, I didn't want to leave my mom's house. . . . Get up, watch TV, eat, watch TV—that's what we did. . . . I couldn't do what I wanted . . . so I lost

interest. In a word, living in a group home was hell. I know all about abuse. There was a person that tried to sexually assault me in the shower . . . I experienced everything. . . . I was punched in the stomach. . . . One guy took money from me. There were 64 people in 4 years that took care of me.

Involvement in the Microboard Pilot Project

While living in the group home, Jeff became reacquainted with Janet, who was living in another group home. Janet and Jeff's relationship grew and they became engaged. Janet initiated the microboard concept with Services for Community Living Branch. Janet and Jeff's joint microboard was formed in 1992. The couple married and moved into a home of their own in August of that year. Their microboard, Vela Microboard Association, and Services for Community Living Branch facilitated the transition from living in a group home to living in a home of their own. After living together, Jeff and Janet found they were not as well suited to one another as they had thought. In March 1995, they separated and Janet moved to Richmond. For the first several months, Jeff and Janet shared the same microboard, which was comprised of members of Jeff's family, Janet's family, and mutual friends. Eventually, Jeff and Janet developed separate microboards consisting of their respective family members and personal friends. Jeff lived in a subsidized housing cooperative in the south section of Vancouver. He chose the apartment and was simply another member of the cooperative. All people in Jeff's building were renters; however, they were an autonomous group and shared in running the cooperative. Initially, Jeff was on the board of directors but opted out. Jeff had a three-bedroom apartment that was modified for a person in a wheelchair. Jeff's support network consisted of an array of formal and informal supports. These included his microboard, his personal friendship circle, five direct support staff, and his community-based physical and medical support staff.

Jeff's closest ties were with his brother, Joe. According to Jeff, "I don't know what I would do without him; he has been there since day one." Jeff's brother was similarly emotive, "Jeff has always added more to any environment than he has ever taken from it. No one has ever bought that 'put him away, he will be such a burden bullsh__.' " At the time of the study Jeff and his brother had regular telephone contact and got together for dinner or a beer approximately once per week. Jeff maintained regular telephone contact with other members of his family who lived outside of Vancouver. Jeff's microboard met approximately three times per year and assisted him with lifestyle planning, hiring staff, and negotiating with Services for Community Living Branch.

An innovative feature of Jeff's formal support network was that he hired all of his own staff. Jeff received 12 hours of support per day. He hired the people whom he felt were best suited for the job. His daily agenda was therefore set by him rather than by an agency. Other innovative features of his support network included supports and services that were community based rather than facility based. These services included Jeff's wheelchair mechanic, his physiotherapist, and his occupational therapist.

Jeff's schedule, lifestyle, and home were highly personalized. Jeff usually rose between 9:30 A.M. and 10:30 A.M. A support person arrived at 10:00 A.M. and waited until Jeff called for assistance. Jeff chose his own menu. After breakfast, Jeff and his support person decided what to do until late afternoon. A board mounted on a wall of his living room listed the days of the week and selected activities. Important appointments were placed on the board, but Jeff did not always use it: "I usually keep my schedule in my head." Jeff was not rigid about his day and stated, "I like it loose; I hate formal." During the study, Jeff enrolled in two courses at a local college and worked with a governmental steering committee on disability issues. Jeff's support network was an intricate balance of family, friends, and paid supports. The roles and relationships within Jeff's support network evolved naturally and were not constrained by a rigid, prescribed support model. Jeff did not have a job description for his paid supports. It was negotiated. According to Jeff, "I don't like it formal; if somebody prefers doing laundry, then they do laundry." A common theme throughout Jeff's support structure was a desire to honor and support him in his quest for a quality life in the community. The blurring of lines between support and friendship were openly discussed and related back to Jeff's desires and wishes about the types of relationships that he valued and wanted.

Quality of Life

According to Jeff,

> Respect is most important to me. . . . [With the microboard,] I am respected. I have more say with the government. I don't think that I got asked in the group home. . . . I'm getting respect in restaurants, at the bar at the local video place.

The second most important dimension of a quality life for Jeff was choice and independence. Jeff was able to choose 1) where he wanted to live, 2) with whom he wanted to live, 3) the content of his apartment, 4) the members of his microboard, and 5) the structure and people that composed his paid support network. Jeff and his support staff reported that he was taking much greater control over personal decisions in his life. There was also the realization that Jeff required support to become more assertive in this regard. Jeff noted,

> The most important choices to me are where I want to go, what I want to do, what I want to eat, what time I go to bed, and what time I get up. I have these choices now [in the microboard].

Jeff was well connected in his community and had a balance of paid supports, family, and friends. For example, he was present at microboard workshops, government forums, wheelchair bocci ball, and his local coffee shops and pub. Although Jeff had few positive experiences in the group home, he did make some personal connections with other people with disabilities who lived there. Jeff commented on meeting people and making personal connections:

> I look for people that have a sense of humor, that are intelligent, and interesting. Some friends I have met through my brother, others I have met at school, or in the group home, others I have met through the microboard. It just happens. You make connections.

Jeff's desire to be a participating member of the general culture drove him to assume risk and search for equal status and a quality life in the community. His strength, humor, and flexibility helped him to attract and maintain a group of supporters that shared his interests, appreciated his individuality, and viewed him as their friend. Jeff's close family ties were critical in helping him with the transition from the disability culture to the general community. Finally, the enabling and empowering structure of the people and policies at Vela Microboard Association and Services for Community Living Branch reduced many of the systemic barriers to a quality life in the community. In his words, "I'm feeling stronger about what I want. I'm still searching, but I'm getting there."

CHANGE: JANET'S STORY

Janet was born in West Vancouver, British Columbia, on March 15, 1969. Janet was adopted shortly after birth, as her biological mother was very young and was unable to care for her. At 7 months of age, with the onset of cerebral palsy, Janet's adoptive parents placed her in the care of the Ministry of Social Services. Janet lived in a hospital until 1972, when she moved in with her foster parents. Janet lived with her foster parents until she was 13. Janet spoke highly of Irene, her foster mother. Irene described her first meeting with Janet and her philosophy of support: "I went to see Janet and fell in love with her right away. We tried to normalize her life as much as possible, to keep her doing as many sports activities as she desired."

Janet initially received her schooling at a rehabilitation center. According to Janet, "I don't remember much. We did some reading and writing." Janet lamented the fact that literacy skills were not emphasized more during her childhood and adolescence. When Janet turned 16, she attended a general high school that included two classes for students with disabilities. Irene reported a lack of the necessary community-based supports for Janet to live at home, so in 1983, Janet moved into an adolescent group home with four other people with disabilities. Janet stated that she enjoyed the social aspects of living with peers her own age and the relationships that she had with some staff. Her negative recollections involved certain staff who she described as being mean. At the age of 19, Janet moved into an adult group home for people with disabilities. At this point, she was reacquainted with Jeff, whom she had met in high school. Her positive recollections involved the relationships that she developed with certain staff and the friends with disabilities whom she met. Her negative perceptions were once again related to "mean staff":

> I was upset. [*Sticks tongue out.*] [That group home] was bad. Bad staff. "C" was mean, "Z" was mean—made us go to bed at 8:00. [There were] two good staff. Helped. Helped to go out. Patty and Shelly [Janet's roommates] became my friends. I [began] dating Jeff.

Inspired by one of her roommates at the group home who was setting up a microboard, Janet contacted Services for Community Living Branch, and Janet and Jeff were put in touch with Linda Perry, a staff member at Vela Microboard Association. Janet and Jeff's microboard was formed in 1992, and they moved out of their respective group homes into a home of their own. In March of 1995, Jeff and Janet separated.

Life on Her Own with a Microboard

After the separation, Janet moved into a bright, new, two-bedroom apartment on the third floor of a housing cooperative in Richmond, British Columbia. Services for Community Living Branch provided the funding for housing and furnishings, and Janet chose the location and the content of her apartment. Janet's support network consisted of an eclectic mix of formal and informal supports. These included her microboard, a friend in her apartment building with whom she grew up, her wheelchair soccer team, friends from her previous adult group home, and her direct support staff. Janet's microboard played an active role in supporting her to develop a life on her own. Janet reflected on her support network and commented, "[My support situation] is good; it is better now. They help me." Janet relied heavily on the support of her foster mother, Irene, who was the chair of her microboard. Irene explained her role and the role of the microboard:

> I want Janet to be as autonomous and independent as possible and I want Janet's life to be as exciting and momentous as possible. I see the board's role as similar. I think that everyone on the microboard loves Janet and that love is reciprocated.

Although Irene supported the autonomy afforded to Janet in the microboard project, she found the intense level of support that Janet required to be stressful and compromising at times. Particular duties that she found difficult were coordinating the volunteers on Janet's microboard, arranging meetings, and ensuring that the fiscal responsibilities were met. It took Janet 18 months to recruit and hire home care staff with whom she felt comfortable. Janet was particular about the appearance of her apartment and required staff who were patient, who respected her needs, and who had a good work ethic. With the help of her microboard, she hired and fired her own home care support. Janet described her home support situation:

> It's great now. I have nice staff. They help me. [I want] people to look me in the eyes. [I need people] to respect me. [I had to] fire "D": She was doing her homework and not helping. "C" is strong; that's good.

Janet contracted with a community support agency, Daily Endeavors, for her daytime supports. Daily Endeavors provided an alternative to center-based day programs. The goal of Daily Endeavors was community inclusion and supporting individuals to be actively involved in their communities through one-to-one support. Janet did not hire her daily support staff, but she was consulted regarding this matter. Her daytime supports consisted of four people who provided a rotating schedule of one-to-one support. Janet commented, "I like them, they're good, if I need help, I go to Irene and DE [Daily Endeavors]." Janet formed strong relationships with members of DE during the course of the study. A DE support person described her personal philosophy of support and how she came to be involved with Daily Endeavors:

> I think most of us chose Daily Endeavors so that we can provide one-to-one support. You can build a strong relationship and really be there for the person. "What do you want to do with your life; how can I help you?" I

> believe that everyone has a strong life inside of them, and if you are prop-
> erly supported, all sorts of magical things can happen. For anyone, I mean
> anyone. Those beliefs came from being a misunderstood, whacked-around
> child. There is magic in every person, and so many people don't see it.

Janet enjoyed an active schedule, which included a mix of recreational activities, house maintenance, a college literacy course, and
social engagements. Although she was free to choose her daily schedule, Janet stated, "I need help planning my days." Janet typically rose
at approximately 9:00 A.M. Her overnight staff left at 9:30 A.M., when
her daytime support person from Daily Endeavors arrived. Janet preferred and requested a relaxing morning, as she did not like to be
rushed. She was most active between the hours of 11:00 A.M. and 5:00
P.M. One of her support staff described Janet's daily rhythm: "Janet's
attitude is, 'Let's get out in the sunshine; let's do something.'. . . Janet
wants to live." After a full day, Janet typically spent her evenings at
home watching television or a movie. A friend from her building came
over for dinner several times per month.

Quality of Life

During observations and structured and unstructured interviews, Janet
identified several of O'Brien's (1987) lifestyle accomplishments as
being most important to her quality of life: respect, choice and control,
community presence, community participation, and developing a relationship with her birth mother. Respect was paramount: "I want people to look me in the eyes." Janet described her apartment as "her
home," and she was the "boss." Janet's support structure encouraged
and respected her need for choice and control in both daily living matters and life-defining matters (i.e., with whom to live, where to live,
daily routines, and relationships). During the course of the study, Janet
expressed a desire to move from Richmond to Burnaby, an adjacent
suburb, to be closer to her friends. In the final months of the study,
Services for Community Living Branch provided her with the funds to
purchase a one-bedroom apartment in a new accessible complex in
Burnaby. In Janet's words, "Wow."

Janet's monthly activity schedule was reflective of her personal
preferences and desires. She enjoyed being in the community, and on a
daily basis, she shopped, visited parks, ate at restaurants, visited
friends, or paid her bills in person. She pursued a volunteer job with
Big Sisters, but her volunteer work had not yet started by the time the
study ended. An important goal for Janet was improving her literacy
skills. She enrolled in a literacy course at a local college for adults with
physical disabilities and was supported by her microboard and support staff to make the 4-hour return bus trip. By the end of the study,

Janet had located her birth mother and was fostering this relationship. With the help of her microboard, Janet was able to develop a group of paid supports that was best suited to her personality and station in life. Janet's strongest and most powerful relationship throughout the course of the study was with her foster mother. Irene reflected on Janet's quality of life in the microboard project:

> Janet should have as much peace of mind as possible . . . to be an autonomous adult who can live and love and go on with her life. I find in many ways the microboard can do that for her. I think her life is on a positive path at the moment.

IT'S ABOUT RELATIONSHIPS: STEPHANIE'S STORY

Stephanie was born in Lethbridge, Alberta, on June 14, 1970. She had microcephaly from brain damage that occurred at birth. At 12 months of age, Stephanie could sit up, had started to talk, and was breaking toys. She experienced her first seizure at age 2½ and was taken to the hospital. Her brother Ed recalled, "It was major, it happened in the middle of the night. I remember the sound of the ambulance. She was just a different person when she got out." Stephanie's mother, Jean, recalled with anger how Stephanie was viewed and treated in the hospital: "I was totally distraught. The doctor asked if he should do everything for her if something went wrong. Fortunately her father told the doctor, 'Do everything for her as you would any other child.' " Despite professional suggestions that Stephanie should be institutionalized, Stephanie's family resisted. They unanimously proclaimed that Stephanie enriched their home life.

Jean was committed to keeping Stephanie at home and sought various therapies and volunteers. At 4 years of age, Stephanie and her family moved to a suburb of Vancouver, British Columbia. Stephanie attended school in a treatment center with other children with severe disabilities until she was 7, when the treatment center deemed that she was "too handicapped" to benefit from schooling, and that "she was taking up room for someone who could make progress." For 2 years, Stephanie remained at home with no formal schooling. Once again, Jean was encouraged to institutionalize Stephanie. She recalled, "I did not institutionalize her at this time. The pressures were strong, Stephanie has given so much, a lot of joy." At 9 years of age, Stephanie was enrolled in a segregated day school comprised of students with severe cognitive and physical disabilities. There was little academic emphasis, but Jean noted that the teachers were committed and worked on communication. Stephanie began to respond favorably.

When Stephanie turned 11, the only respite service available to the family was at a hospital. While in respite care at the hospital, Stephanie broke her leg and it was 2 days before anyone noticed. Stephanie returned home with a cast, and her mother and siblings had to carry Stephanie up and down several flights of stairs. Jean recalled, "It was the second time I felt I was going to die. I had so much pressure. I felt like I was suffocating. I started looking into getting Stephanie into a permanent hospital residence." Later that year, Stephanie left her family home and moved into the hospital on a full-time basis, where she lived for 2 years. Jean discussed the factors influencing her decision, her relationship with staff at the hospital, and Stephanie's quality of life:

> It was horrible; it was the worst time in our lives. Stephanie fell out of bed, she cut her lip, and one of her ears was torn and bleeding. She also had a bad bruise on her neck. It was a big mystery; no one knew what happened. They can't love Stephanie like I do, but they can give better care than that. Over time Stephanie began coming home on weekends, and finally I said, "She is staying home."

When Stephanie turned 13, she and her mother moved to a new, subsidized housing complex in South Vancouver. Jean advocated strongly for home care and community support and developed a workable solution. Stephanie's sister, Alida, had moved out of the family home but was hired to provide home care. Alida explained,

> It was hard working for your mom and step dad [laughed]. I enjoyed being with Stephanie. I got a lot of peace and fulfillment working with her. But it was a lot of physical work, and it opened my eyes a bit more.

Stephanie continued her schooling in the hospital where she previously resided. She underwent successful hip surgery when she was 13, and at age 16, she had surgery on her back to treat scoliosis. During Stephanie's late teenage years, life had stabilized for Stephanie and her mother.

Good Fortune and the Microboard Pilot Project

In 1989, when Stephanie turned 19, her care was transferred to an adult service system. Stephanie and her mother could choose a group home or a hospital. Jean resisted and began exploring options and attended an adult support conference sponsored by The Association for Persons with Severe Handicaps. Jean described this fortuitous event:

> It was pretty emotional. They [some adult service providers] were talking about beds. One person got up and said that she never wanted to hear that

a place for her son to live was called a bed. I was inspired. I got up and spoke. I asked, "Why does Stephanie need to leave her home just because she turned 19?" I mean, Prince Charles lived at home until he was 35. I met Sally [Regional Coordinator of Services for Community Living Branch] there, and she was very supportive and connected me with Linda Perry of Vela [Microboard Association].

Linda facilitated Stephanie's microboard, which was named "The Stephanie Anne Friends Society," and planning began in September of 1990. In March 1991, The Stephanie Anne Friends Society received funding from Services for Community Living Branch and was officially recognized as a fully functioning microboard. Jean described her feelings when Stephanie's microboard was formed: "There was a big burden lifted off of my shoulders. . . . Now young people who cared about Stephanie were in her life. I felt a physical lifting; it wasn't just me."

Stephanie's support network consisted of both formal and informal supports. Her informal supports included her microboard, her neighbor, and Sonny and the "guys" who resided in a group home that Stephanie visited on weekends. Stephanie's formal support network consisted of five support staff whom she hired with the assistance of her microboard and her community-based communication, medical, and literacy supports.

Of her paid supports, her closest ties were with her direct support staff, on which she depended for all aspects of her daily living. Stephanie's home and community support workers were from the Philippines. Her sister, Alida, and friend, Angela (pseudonym; also a microboard member), assisted in the hiring and training of staff. Criteria for hiring included patience, kindness, respect, inclusive values, and community connections. The relationship that evolved with Stephanie and her support network was described as "family." A member of Stephanie's support staff explained,

> Part of our culture is close family ties. If there is a family affair, Stephanie is usually invited. Sally [pseudonym] used to work with Stephanie; if Sally has a party, she usually invites Stephanie. For Stephanie, I think she wants her workers to respect her: "Respect me, understand me, care for me, and work with me as a family."

Stephanie typically rose between 7:30 A.M. and 8:00 A.M. Her roommate supported her between the hours of 7:30 A.M. and 10:30 A.M. Stephanie's morning routine consisted of 1) stretching exercises in her bed, 2) being lifted and transferred to her couch in the living room, 3) general hygiene activities, 4) eating, and 5) dressing. Stephanie's day support staff (Maria) arrived at 10:30 A.M. and coordinated much of Stephanie's daily schedule. Stephanie's activity preferences were identified through lifestyle planning exercises by using the McGill Action Planning System (MAPS; Vandercook, York, & Forest, 1989) as well as discussions with Stephanie's microboard. Maria worked with Angela to develop activity preferences and choices for Stephanie. Typically, Stephanie had a choice of three or four activities per day, which were represented by photographs. She made choices by looking at the photographs and nodding her head for "yes" and shaking her head side to side for "no." Stephanie was very expressive, and she smiled, curled her tongue, and widened her eyes when she was happy and excited. She made a guttural sound when she was in discomfort or unhappy.

Stephanie was not employed, but her schedule was varied and reflective of her preferences. There was an effort to include a mix of daily living activities (e.g., shopping, going to the hairdresser, banking) and leisure-oriented activities in her monthly schedule (e.g., going to the park, going to a play or concert, swimming). Stephanie spent the majority of time in the community between 10:00 A.M. and 4 P.M. Stephanie's roommate supported her at home between 4 P.M. and 8 P.M. Stephanie typically relaxed during these hours while her roommate prepared Stephanie's meal and fed her. Stephanie's overnight support person worked from 7:30 P.M. to 7:30 A.M. A typical evening for Stephanie involved listening to the stereo, watching sporting events, or making crafts.

Quality of Life

Rigorous efforts were made to include Stephanie in all decisions related to her lifestyle; however, her limited expressive communication necessitated close monitoring and decision making with the support of her microboard and support staff. Stephanie's support network did not view Stephanie's lifestyle issues as being substantively different from their own. Her brother viewed intimate relationships as central to his quality of life and Stephanie's quality of life:

> The relationship is really kind of the key thing in terms of quality of life. And that's what's different about this [the microboard]. It's our life, it's our family relationships . . . which you can't put in a box. . . . There's love, there's commitment, and it's informal by nature.

Angela was interested in expanding Stephanie's community presence and worked closely with staff to ensure that Stephanie was included in all aspects of her daily living. Stephanie participated in daily living activities such as banking, shopping, and purchasing furnishings for her apartment. Stephanie had her own van for transportation and had access to a range of leisure activities that reflected her strengths and preferences. Respectful and caring relationships were observed throughout the study. The microboard ensured that Stephanie's support staff offered her choices and supported Stephanie to partially participate in all aspects of her daily life. Stephanie's staff was considerate of her need for patience and dignity regarding feeding, dressing, and bathing. Support people were also responsive to Stephanie's nonverbal communication and patiently waited for Stephanie to express herself.

Stephanie's microboard was directive when training support staff. The assumption of competence enabled Stephanie to participate in a range of meaningful activities. If documents needed to be signed, then Stephanie signed them with a stamp or was assisted with direct physical prompts. Stephanie's closest relationships were with her family, her direct support staff, and her friends. She developed a cordial relationship with a neighbor in her housing complex. A circle of support was created around Stephanie, and she was included in the social circle of her support staff. Her sister-in-law, Kim, commented, "She's been included in their [the support staff's] families, and it's a cultural thing, too. Stephanie is always included in christenings and weddings and stuff."

Stephanie was given the opportunity to make choices in all aspects of her daily living, including where to live, with whom to live, who to hire, what to wear, and where and with whom to spend time in the community. In April 1996, Stephanie was given the opportunity to move closer to her mother, who had moved from Vancouver and was living in Grand Forks, British Columbia. With the support of Services for Community Living Branch, Vela Microboard Association, and her microboard, she now owns her own condominium beside her mother in Grand Forks, British Columbia.

Jean initiated Stephanie's involvement in the microboard project, and throughout Stephanie's life, Jean challenged traditional support structures and believed in the principles of person-centered support. She enlisted the support of Stephanie's siblings and friends to form a microboard, and the relationships were voluntary; mutual; and rooted in love, reciprocity, and respect. Jean summarized Stephanie's life and her life in the microboard project: "[The microboard project] has been great for us. Not every family could do it, but my suggestion is not to be afraid. It has been wonderful for Stephanie."

DISCUSSION

Qualitative methods provide a portrait of the lives of the study participants. An analysis of the data reveals important personal characteristics of the participants and their microboards that contributed to a quality life in the community. These data also show that the enabling characteristics of Vela Microboard Association and Services for Community Living Branch played an important role in changing the lives of Jeff, Janet, and Stephanie. This section examines these themes and frames them within the emerging paradigm of person-centered support.

During the data analysis, three pivotal aspects of person-centered support were highlighted: 1) planning, 2) housing and support structures, and 3) formal organizations responsive to person-centered principles and practice. The emerging paradigm of person-centered support advocates a shift in thinking and planning from an emphasis on the degree and nature of disability to a focus on the personal preferences, strengths, hopes, and dreams of the individual (Kennedy, 1993; Moore, 1993; Mount & Zwernik, 1988; O'Brien, 1987).

A person-centered approach separates housing and support, enabling people with disabilities to obtain necessary supports wherever they live. Historically, housing and support for people with disabilities have been packaged together and have been owned and operated by disability support agencies. A person-centered approach assumes that people with disabilities have the same needs as all community members regarding safe, affordable housing. A person-centered approach extends the roles and rights of people with disabilities to those of tenants, homeowners, and cooperative members (Racino & Taylor, 1993). Traditional support structures for people with disabilities have focused on the amelioration of deficits and have been dominated by professional decision making (Mount, 1987). In contrast, support in a person-centered approach is focused on the hopes and dreams of the individual, and the goal of support is a quality life in the community. Choice in all lifestyle decisions is central to person-centered support. Support strategies vary for each individual and reflect a unique combination of services; adaptations; goods; and assistance from paid staff, neighbors, families, and friends (Racino & Taylor, 1993).

The unique combination of formal and informal support structures in person-centered support implies a change in the way that disability support organizations respond to the individual needs of people. Taylor and colleagues (1991) studied characteristics of responsive organizations in a person-centered approach. They found several attributes that define responsive organizations. First, responsive organizations are characterized by a belief system or values base that guides all elements of the staff's work as well as the organization as a whole. This philosophy statement is grounded in respect and the recognition that all people have unique traits and contributions. Second, responsive organizations do not rigidly adhere to specific models, programs, or approaches but adapt what they can learn from others to fit their own situations. Third, these organizations involve people with disabilities, their families, and their staff in decision making, and they tend to be either decentralized or small, with administrators who are deeply involved in the spirit of the organization. Finally, responsive organizations tend not to define themselves in terms of narrow service categories. Instead, they play more of an advocacy role that brings them into the broader community domain, addressing general community issues such as housing and poverty.

The next section illustrates how the person-centered concepts of planning, housing and support, and responsive organizations were evident in the lives of the study participants and the microboard project.

Personal Profiles of Study Participants

Interviews and observations with the participants revealed three people with a desire to express their individuality and to be recognized for their personal strengths rather than their perceived disabilities. They viewed disability not so much as a personal characteristic but as a set of attitudinal and opportunity barriers present in the disability system and society in general. Their interests reflected the culture of people without disabilities, and they described their self-concepts in terms of their strengths, preferences, and abilities. These positive self-images were evident throughout the study and were fostered and supported by their inclusive, respectful, and reciprocal family lives. These strong familial relationships were identified as a key factor that enabled participants to break free of traditional models of support and to develop microboards. These findings support the notion that people with disabilities and their families are no different than people without disabilities concerning a need for a safe, personalized home and supportive relationships (Kennedy, 1993; Moore, 1993; Mount & Zwernik, 1988; O'Brien, 1987).

Life in the Least Restrictive Environment

Again, a central tenet of a person-centered approach is that housing and support should be separate so that people can receive the support that they need wherever they live (Racino & Taylor, 1993). All three participants experienced life in conditions under the LRE concept prior to the microboard project, as they were unable to receive the services and supports that they needed within their family homes. They lived in hospitals and group homes and attended segregated schools. Despite their inclusive family lives and their positive self-images, all three participants felt that they had lost some of their personal ambition, assertiveness, and connection to their hopes and dreams while living in the LRE. Furthermore, Jeff and Stephanie reported incidents of abuse and neglect while residing in the LRE. Interviews and observations revealed that all three participants relied on their microboards and support staff to help them make choices in major and minor life decisions and to assert and "rekindle" their hopes and dreams. This finding is consistent with other self-reports from people with disabilities who have moved from institutional settings to the community and homes of their own (Goffman, 1961; Kennedy, 1993), and it confirms the need to separate housing from support so that people can attain the assistance that they need in homes of their choosing.

Quality of Life in the Microboard Project

During observations and interviews, it became evident that O'Brien's (1987) five essential lifestyle accomplishments of choice, competence, respect, community presence, and community participation were represented in the lives of the study participants. During observations and interviews, I observed and recorded how the principles and functions of microboards translated into choice and empowerment for the participants. A central enabling theme identified by participants and their microboards was that funding flowed directly to each microboard. With this direct funding, participants and their microboards were free to develop personalized living arrangements, support structures, and daily activity schedules. These choices in major life decisions were viewed as essential to lifestyle quality and as a defining feature of the microboard project. This finding is consistent with the emerging theory of person-centered support, in which choice is encouraged and honored in all aspects of a person's life (Racino & Taylor, 1993).

Direct Support Staff

Interviews and observations revealed that the ability to hire and define direct support structures was an enabling feature of the microboard project. These support structures reflected the participants' profiles and desires. Jeff's support network was loosely defined and he considered its members to be his friends. Janet's support network was more formal—a respectful employer–employee relationship in which Janet was the boss. Stephanie's support network was defined as familial and rooted in respect. These findings support the assertion that a person-centered approach implies a change in how people with disabilities are viewed, as well as a change in the relationships between people with disabilities and those supporting them. Prescriptive notions of support are giving way to individualized, reciprocal relationships that are dynamic and driven by the person receiving support (Racino & Taylor, 1993).

Role of the Microboards

Interviews, observations, and immersion into Jeff's, Janet's, and Stephanie's lives revealed that their microboards performed two distinct functions. The first was pragmatic, involving budgeting, record keeping, and contract obligations with Services for Community Living Branch. This function was closely aligned to the Societies Act, and the participants' microboards were required to meet the same standards of accountability as any other community support agency.

The second function involved support in hiring, lifestyle planning, and daily life. Each microboard in the study shared the same goals of autonomy, safety, respect, and opportunity for the focus person. There was considerable variability among the participants and their support needs. Each participant and his or her microboard defined the degree to which the microboard was involved in day-to-day affairs. Stephanie had the most intensive support needs and therefore received the most intensive support from her microboard, including help in hiring staff, training staff, developing activity schedules, budgeting, and so forth. Conversely, Jeff had the least extensive support needs, so his microboard met approximately three times per year and helped with lifestyle planning, budgeting, and contracting. They also performed informal monitoring, such as dropping by to watch a hockey game with Jeff or going out with Jeff for a beer or dinner. The study participants and their microboards viewed lifestyle planning procedures (Mount & Zwernik, 1988; O'Brien; 1987; Vandercook et al., 1989) as important tools to guide the quest for empowerment and quality of life.

Another important theme that emerged regarding relationships and quality of life was that the microboard project was not just enriching for the focus participants. A majority of microboard members expressed that their lives and worldview were enhanced by their roles as microboard members. The microboard project allowed participants, their families, and their friends to reconnect and rebuild their relationships. As Melzer noted, these findings contribute to a conceptualization of person-centered support that allows for variability in nonrestrictive intervention even when needs are complex and self-determination is low (Hasazi, 1991). These findings also confirm that mutually enriching relationships can emerge when the power and tools to define these relationships are placed in the hands of people with disabilities and their families (Racino & Taylor, 1993).

Enabling Characteristics of Vela Microboard Association and Services for Community Living Branch

Interviews, observations, and a review of documents from each organization revealed that the staff and organizational characteristics of Vela Microboard Association and Services for Community Living Branch substantially influenced the positive lives of Janet, Jeff, and Stephanie. Two central features of Vela Microboard Association and Services for Community Living Branch were congruent with a person-centered approach and responsive organizations: 1) the willingness to change and 2) the inclusion of people with disabilities and their families in the organization's philosophy statement and the day-to-day operations (Racino & Taylor, 1993; Taylor et al., 1991).

Prior to the microboard project, Vela Microboard Association was part of a traditional support agency that provided a continuum of residential and vocational services (e.g., group homes, semi-independent living, sheltered workshops). Board members at Vela Microboard Association recognized that a continuum model of segregated service was not empowering people to direct their own lives. A board member described this juncture: "We began to realize more and more clearly that what we were really interested in was not more physical structures but what we could do to support people to have maximum control over their lives."

Services for Community Living Branch was described as "grassroots developed." People with disabilities and their advocates were involved in the creation and philosophy of support at the Branch. Members were hired based on their inclusive values. Senior members of the Branch looked at their mission and purpose and recognized that four-bed group homes were not leading to quality lives for many people requiring support.

Through these reflections, Vela Microboard Association and Services for Community Living Branch began the microboard pilot project. Vela Microboard Association and Services for Community Living Branch were small, flexible, and creative formal support structures. Both organizations created philosophy and mission statements that explicitly stated the goals of person-centered support: choice; control; and empowerment regarding where to live, with whom, and with what nature of support. Both organizations committed themselves to support structures based on personal need rather than on organizational policy and procedures. All people, regardless of degree of disability, were seen as having the right and ability to direct their own lives. Another responsive organizational characteristic of Vela

Microboard Association and Services for Community Living Branch was the implementation of collaborative, nonhierarchical planning and implementation strategies. Both organizations maintained close ties with the people whom they served, and they valued and encouraged the input of families and people with disabilities to guide their practice. Success was measured by the degree of positive influence on the lives of people served.

LIMITATIONS

The results of this study must be interpreted in light of several factors. Participants were selected because of the positive nature of their support networks and lifestyle. This purposeful sampling was conducted to illuminate the factors that contributed to the positive lifestyles of the study participants. There are few such studies in the literature, so the study findings cannot be interpreted as representative of all microboard situations or outcomes.

Although the study illustrated exemplars of system and family support, the lives of the participants and the pragmatic demands of running a microboard were not without problems. The participants did not have full-time paid employment. Jeff was enrolled in some college courses and was thinking of a career as a disability consultant or a model. Janet was looking for volunteer work with Big Sisters, and Stephanie was not pursuing work at the time of the study. Factors involved in this lack of employment included personal choice and motivation, opportunity, community attitudes, and level of physical and cognitive disability.

During the course of the study, the participants were able to develop staffing and support structures that suited their personal preferences and needs and were reasonably stable. However, this does not mean that microboards are immune to staff turnover, staff abuses of power, and lack of respect for the individual's needs. For instance, Jeff and Janet had to fire several staff and roommates who did not listen to them and who were imposing their values and lifestyle standards. As previously mentioned, Jeff's support structure was the most loosely defined and he preferred it that way. Yet, this arrangement was not problem free. Some support staff felt that sometimes Jeff relied too much on his group of friends and did not take control. Initially, Jeff found it difficult to let his staff know when chores needed to be done and organization around the house was lacking.

During interviews with parents and members of Vela Microboard Association and Services for Community Living Branch, I explored some of the shortcomings of microboards. From the perspective of managers at Services for Community Living Branch, the microboards' fiscal and contractual obligations were not always in place. One person stated,

> If there has been a struggle, it hasn't been so much with the good intentions of the microboards regarding the service they want to provide, but we've certainly been concerned about their lack of understanding around the contract; we need to be more helpful here.

A member of Services for Community Living Branch also commented that in a few isolated cases, the focus person's self-determination was undermined by the values and lifestyle vision of his or her family.

To gain perspectives of successful and unsuccessful microboard situations, I interviewed Linda Perry of Vela Microboard Association, a key informant who was instrumental in facilitating the microboard pilot project and the microboards of the study participants. Specifically, I asked Linda which factors contributed to an unsuccessful microboard. She replied,

> There is only one board that has fallen apart, and time was not spent on developing relationships and taking responsibility. People need to take responsibility and take risks. If people want to play it safe, then microboards aren't the place to do it.

CONCLUSION

This study has contributed to a compelling body of research and perspectives that suggest restructuring disability support on person-centered rather than system-centered principles (Bellamy, Rhodes, Bourbeau, & Mank, 1982; Biklen, 1988; Hasazi, 1991; McKnight, 1977; Mount, 1987; Nisbet et al., 1991; Racino & Taylor, 1993; Taylor, 1988; Taylor et al., 1991). A central message of these studies and perspectives is that people with disabilities are no different than people without disabilities regarding the desire for safe, quality housing; inclusive valued relationships; and freedom and access to their communities. Person-centered planning and support are promising practices in this regard. The study in this chapter examined microboards, one option within the person-centered support paradigm. Microboards are suitable for any person who needs some type of support structure to achieve a quality life in the community. Essential characteristics for successful microboards are circles of support that are willing to be accountable, assume risk, and make a commitment to a person's life.

This study illustrated that a focus on individual need and capacity, a separation of housing and support, choice in all aspects of major and minor life decisions, direct access to funding, and responsive support organizations that embody these principles in their mission and functioning can contribute to quality lives in the community for people with complex support needs. Since the 1970s, disability support has been the era of the LRE. The time has come for the era of person-centered planning and support. Jeff, Janet, Stephanie, and the thousands of people who share their story are ready, willing, and able.

REFERENCES

Bellamy, T., Rhodes, L., Bourbeau, P., & Mank, D. (1982). *Mental retardation services in sheltered workshops and day activity programs: Consumer outcomes and policy alternatives.* Paper presented at the National Working Conference on Vocational Services and Employment Opportunities, Madison, WI.

Biklen, D. (1988). The myth of clinical judgment. *Journal of Social Issues, 44(1),* 127–140.

Bogdan, R., & Biklen, S. (1982). *Qualitative research methods for education: An introduction to theory and methods.* Needham Heights, MA: Allyn & Bacon.

Borg, W.R., & Gall, M.D. (1989). *Educational research. An introduction* (5th ed.). New York: Longman Publishing.

Goffman, E. (1961). On the characteristics of total institutions. *Asylums.* Chicago: Aldine.

Hammersley, M., & Atkinson, P. (1983). *Ethnography: Principles in practice.* London: Routledge.

Hasazi, S.B. (1991). An exchange on personal futures and community participation: An interview with John McKnight and Ronald Melzer. In L.H. Meyer, C.A. Peck, & L. Brown (Eds.), *Critical issues in the lives of people with severe disabilities* (pp. 537–541). Baltimore: Paul H. Brookes Publishing Co.

Kennedy, M.J. (1993). Turning the pages of life. In S.J. Taylor, J.A. Racino, & B. Shoultz (Series Eds.) & J.A. Racino, P. Walker, S. O'Connor, & S.J. Taylor (Vol. Eds.), *The community participation series: Vol. 2. Housing, support, and community: Choices and strategies for adults with disabilities.* (pp. 205–216). Baltimore: Paul H. Brookes Publishing Co.

Malette, P. (1996). *Lifestyle perspectives of persons with disabilities in a person-centered support paradigm.* Unpublished doctoral dissertation. University of British Columbia.

McKnight, J. (1977). The professional service business. *Social Policy, 8(6),* 110–116.

Mehan, H., Hertweck, A., & Meihls, J.L. (1986). *Handicapping the handicapped: Decision making in students' educational careers.* Stanford, CA: Stanford University Press.

Moore, C. (1993). Letting go, moving on: A parent's thoughts. In S.J. Taylor, J.A. Racino, & B. Shoultz (Series Eds.) & J.A. Racino, P. Walker, S. O'Connor, & S.J. Taylor (Vol. Eds.), *The community participation series: Vol. 2. Housing, support, and community: Choices and strategies for adults with disabilities* (pp. 189–204). Baltimore: Paul H. Brookes Publishing Co.

Mount, B. (1987). *Personal futures planning: Finding directions for change* (Doctoral dissertation, University of Georgia). Ann Arbor: University of Michigan Dissertation Information Service.

Mount, B., & Zwernik, K. (1988). *It's never too early, it's never too late: A booklet about personal futures planning* (Publication No. 421-88-109). St. Paul, MN: Metropolitan Council.

Nisbet, J., Clark, M., & Covert, S. (1991). Living it up! An analysis of research on community living. In L.H. Meyer, C.A. Peck, & L. Brown (Eds.), *Critical issues in the lives of people with severe disabilities* (pp. 115–144). Baltimore: Paul H. Brookes Publishing Co.

O'Brien, J. (1987). A guide to life-style planning: Using The Activities Catalog to integrate services and natural support systems. In B. Wilcox & G.T. Bellamy, *A comprehensive guide to The Activities Catalog: An alternative curriculum for youth and adults with severe disabilities* (pp. 175–189). Baltimore: Paul H. Brookes Publishing Co.

Racino, J.A., & Taylor, S.J. (1993). "People first": Approaches to housing and support. In S.J. Taylor, J.A. Racino, & B. Shoultz (Series Eds.) & J.A. Racino, P. Walker, S. O'Connor, & S.J. Taylor (Vol. Eds.), *The community participation series: Vol. 2. Housing, support, and community: Choices and strategies for adults with disabilities* (pp. 33–56). Baltimore: Paul H. Brookes Publishing Co.

Salisbury, C.L., Palombaro, M.M., & Hollowood, T.M. (1993). On the nature and change of an inclusive elementary school. *The Journal of The Association for Persons with Severe Handicaps, 18*(2), 75–84.

Taylor, S.J. (1988). Caught in the continuum: A critical analysis of the principle of the least restrictive environment. *The Journal of The Association for Persons with Severe Handicaps, 13*(1), 41–53.

Taylor, S.J., & Bogdan, R. (1984). *Introduction to qualitative research methods.* New York: John Wiley & Sons.

Taylor, S.J., Bogdan, R., & Racino, J.A. (Vol. Eds.). (1991). *The community participation series: Vol. 1. Life in the community: Case studies of organizations supporting people with disabilities.* Baltimore: Paul H. Brookes Publishing Co.

Vandercook, T., York, J., & Forest, M. (1989). The McGill Action Planning System (MAPS): A strategy for building the vision. *Journal of The Association for Persons with Severe Handicaps, 14,* 202–215.

Vela Microboard Association. (1995). *Vela Housing Society: Guiding principles and functions.* Vancouver, British Columbia, Canada: Author.

Walker, P. (1999). From community presence to sense of place: Community experiences of adults with developmental disabilities. *The Journal of The Association for Persons with Severe Handicaps, 24*(1), 23–32.

Women's Research Centre. (1994). *A report to Vela Housing Society by The Women's Research Centre.* Vancouver, British Columbia, Canada: Vela Microboard Association.

III

Preference Assessment and Program Evaluation

8

Person-Centered Planning with People Who Have Severe Multiple Disabilities

Validated Practices and Misapplications

Dennis H. Reid and Carolyn W. Green

Person-centered planning is becoming an increasingly popular means of designing and providing supports for people with developmental disabilities. As well illustrated in other chapters in this book, successful applications of person-centered planning have been reported in a wide variety of environments in which people with disabilities live, work, and play. The widespread interest in person-centered planning is a direct result of numerous reports on how person-centered values and tools can improve the quality of life of people with disabilities and their families (Browder, Bambara, & Belfiore, 1997; Holburn, 1997; Mount, 1994).

Although the reported benefits of person-centered planning have been many and varied, the benefits have not been realized proportionally across all people who have developmental disabilities. For the most part, applications of person-centered planning have involved individuals with mild and moderate disabilities. Much less attention has been directed to people who have more severe disabilities. There has been a particular lack of attention directed to person-centered planning with individuals who have severe multiple disabilities.

Providing supports to ensure that people with severe multiple disabilities experience a desirable lifestyle has consistently presented difficulties for service providers and family members. People with severe multiple disabilities have severe or profound mental retardation as well as highly significant physical challenges that seriously hinder or prevent ambulation. The cognitive and physical disabilities interfere with communication and other areas of adaptive functioning to the point that these individuals are very dependent on support from others for meeting basic needs (Reid, Phillips, & Green, 1991).

The severity of challenges that people with severe multiple disabilities face has hindered their social inclusion relative to the advances that other people with disabilities have made in attaining inclusive lifestyles. To illustrate, when compared with people who have less severe disabilities, people with severe multiple disabilities have not experienced nearly the degree of opportunity to live in typical community environments instead of institutional or other segregated, congregate settings (Lakin, Anderson, Prouty, & Polister, 1999). These individuals also have been generally excluded from opportunities for community-based, supported work relative to people with mild or moderate disabilities (Wehman, 1996).

The relative exclusion of people with severe multiple disabilities from the person-centered movement appears to be due in part to a lack of emphasis within the person-centered literature on people with the most significant disabilities. As a result, there is insufficient information about how person-centered approaches can be adequately adapted for these individuals. Furthermore, person-centered planning with people who have severe multiple disabilities frequently has not resulted in the expected benefits of person-centered approaches (Everson & Reid, 1999).

The purpose of this chapter is to discuss person-centered planning specifically for people who have severe multiple disabilities. A related purpose is to describe how person-centered planning tends to be misapplied with these individuals, with the ultimate intent of preventing future misapplications. Much of the chapter content stems from results of applied research aimed at validating various person-centered practices. However, because there has been relatively little research with person-centered planning in general (Hagner, Helm, & Butterworth, 1996; Whitney-Thomas, Shaw, Honey, & Butterworth, 1998) and even less with people who have the most significant disabilities (Reid, Everson, & Green, 1999), the content is also based on the authors' experience with person-centered planning. A final purpose is to call attention to areas of research that might enhance the degree to which people with severe multiple disabilities lead person-centered lifestyles.

The core values and tools that form the basis of person-centered approaches are well described in other chapters in this text (e.g., Chapter 2). In-depth descriptions of person-centered planning are likewise presented elsewhere (Everson & Reid, 1999; Kincaid, 1996; Whitney-Thomas et al., 1998). Consequently, an overview of person-centered planning is not provided here. Rather, discussion focuses on issues that are most relevant to the successful application of person-centered planning with people who have severe multiple disabilities. These issues relate to values that form the philosophical core of person-centered approaches and to the most common tools used to design and implement person-centered supports and services. Specific issues to address include 1) ensuring accurate identification of preferences as part of the person-centered process, 2) implementing person-centered planning in typical environments where people with severe multiple disabilities spend their time, and 3) ensuring adequate staff performance during the implementation of person-centered plans to effectively support people with severe multiple disabilities in attaining their desired outcomes.

ENSURING ACCURATE IDENTIFICATION OF PREFERENCES

In large part, the essence of person-centered approaches is determining the desires of an individual with a disability (i.e., the focus person) and then supporting that person in actually realizing those desires. Hence, a key foundation upon which person-centered planning is based is the initial, accurate identification of a focus person's desires, as well as what the person does not like. A number of person-centered tools are available to help an individual express important likes and dislikes (Everson & Reid, 1999), such as a variety of mapping procedures (Everson, 1996; Mount, 1997). As of 2002, however, descriptions of mapping and related procedures for identifying a person's desires have centered on people with disabilities who can express their likes and dislikes in relatively conventional ways. These individuals can, with varying degrees of support, express what they want and do not want in ways that are readily understood by other members of person-centered support teams.

When determining preferences—or likes and dislikes—of people who have severe multiple disabilities as part of the person-centered process, it becomes clear that alterations in the usual mapping and related procedures are necessary. Pronounced cognitive and physical disabilities often prevent expression of important preferences by these individuals. According to the person-centered literature, when a person cannot express important desires, the opinions of support team members who are most familiar with the person should be relied on for identifying the focus person's preferences (Kincaid, 1996; O'Brien, 1987).

Relying on the opinions of support team members who best know the person is a logical extension of person-centered procedures used with people who have less severe disabilities. However, reliance on support personnel for these purposes contradicts results of empirical research in this area. Investigations have repeatedly shown that caregivers of people with highly significant disabilities typically have opinions that are not accurate representations of the true preferences of these individuals (Favell & Cannon, 1976; Green et al., 1988; Windsor, Piché, & Locke, 1994).

During the same general time period that person-centered approaches were being developed and popularized (i.e., the 1990s), a behavioral technology was being developed for identifying the preferences of people with severe disabilities. The initial impetus for behavioral research on preference assessment was to identify items and activities that could be used as reinforcing stimuli to help teach adaptive skills to learners with severe disabilities (Green et al., 1988; Pace, Ivancic, Edwards, Iwata, & Page, 1985). Subsequently, research on methods for identifying preferences has expanded by demonstrating ways to enhance work performance (Parsons, Reid, Reynolds, & Bumgarner, 1990), reduce challenging behavior (Ringdahl, Vollmer, Marcus, & Roane, 1997), and improve overall life quality and enjoyment (Brown, Gothelf, Guess, & Lehr, 1998). The technology resulting from such research involves determining what an individual prefers by systematically presenting the individual with various items or situations and carefully recording how the individual responds. Depending on an individual's cognitive, communicative, and physical skills, observed responses may involve making a choice among items or activities when presented repeatedly with two or more options (Parsons et al., 1990), approaching or avoiding systematically presented items and activities (Pace et al., 1985), and indicating happiness or unhappiness (Green & Reid, 1996).

Due to the problems in relying on opinions of support team members to identify preferences among people with severe multiple disabilities and to the success of behavioral assessments for identifying preferences, a seemingly logical step is to supplement person-centered planning with systematic preference assessments. We have conducted two investigations with our colleagues that provide some support for the utility of supplementing person-centered planning with systematic preference assessments (Green, Middleton, & Reid, 2000; Reid et al., 1999). Within each investigation, person-centered plans were developed for a respective focus person by using mapping procedures. Subsequently, systematic preference assessments were conducted involving observations of participant approach and avoidance responses when the individuals were actually presented with items or activities that the person-centered plans reported as being preferred.

Combined results of the two investigations are presented in Figure 8.1. Figure 8.1 shows the percentage of preferences reported in person-centered plans for seven individuals with severe multiple disabilities that were subsequently identified through systematic behavioral assessments as being highly preferred, moderately preferred, and non-preferred. In accordance with standard procedure in preference assessment research (Fisher et al., 1992), criteria for the three types of preferences were that the items or activities were deemed highly preferred if they were approached on at least 80% of the presentations, moderately preferred if approached between 50% and 80%, and nonpreferred if approached less than 50%. For the four individuals who participated in the initial Reid and colleagues (1999) investigation, most preferences reported in the person-centered plans were highly or moderately preferred based on the systematic preference assessments (see data on the left side of Figure 8.1). However, for two of the individuals (Lance and

Type of preference based on systematic preference assessment

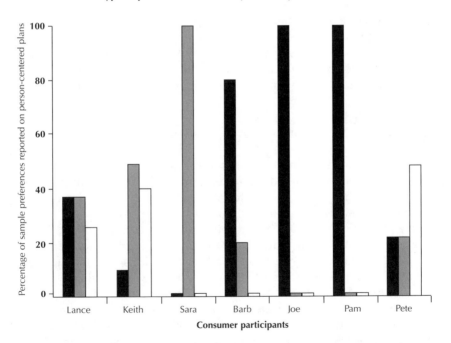

Figure 8.1. Percentage of sampled preferences reported on person-centered plans that were highly preferred, moderately preferred, and nonpreferred based on systematic preference assessments for seven individuals with severe multiple disabilities. Results for the first four people on the left side of the figure are drawn from Reid and colleagues (1999) and results for the last three people on the right side are drawn from Green and colleagues (2000). (*Key:* ■ = highly preferred; ▨ = moderately preferred; □ = nonpreferred.)

Keith), 25% and 40% of reported preferences, respectively, were non-preferred based on the systematic assessments. For the latter items or activities, the individuals did not approach the items or activities often when given the opportunity and sometimes avoided them. Similar results occurred in the subsequent Green and colleagues (2000) investigation in that 1) most preferences identified on person-centered plans were highly or moderately preferred during the systematic assessments (see data on the right side of Figure 8.1), but 2) for one of the three participants (Pete), 50% of the reported preferences in the plan were found to be nonpreferred when systematically assessed.

The primary conclusion from this research is that although person-centered planning resulted in a number of reported preferences that subsequently were empirically confirmed to be valid, person-centered planning also identified nonpreferred items and activities as preferences. Such a conclusion supports the previously noted research on staff opinion of consumer preferences, and it suggests that relying on staff opinion within the person-centered planning process is not likely to identify accurate preferences consistently. A second outcome of the research was the recommendation that person-centered planning tools be supplemented with systematic preference assessments when considering the preferences of individuals with severe multiple disabilities. The behaviorally based preference assessment procedures could help ensure the accuracy of preferences identified in the plans.

Special Considerations
for Research and Application

It should be noted that research that uses systematic preference assessments with person-centered planning is still in its initial stages. Additional investigations are needed to more definitively determine how to accurately identify the most important preferences of people with severe multiple disabilities as part of person-centered planning. When proceeding with research in this area, as well as in person-centered planning in general, several additional considerations warrant attention if person-centered planning is to truly enhance the lives of these people.

Careful Specification of What "Preference" Means   One problem that occurred repeatedly in our research was that a reported preference was not always well specified. What an individual was perceived to like by support team members frequently was not specified to a degree that could be validated by using preference assessments. For example, some plans reported that individuals liked anything social. What was meant by *social*—in terms of how to actually support a person—was not clear. Lack of specification led to different interpretations across support team members regarding what should occur when implementing person-centered plans; social activities meant different things to different team members.

At this point, it is not clear why some preferences identified in various person-centered plans lack sufficient specification to allow careful validation or implementation. Potential reasons for problems with specification include varying skills among support team leaders in facilitating person-centered planning meetings, differences in the efficacy of the various planning procedures used to identify preferences, and variations in skills and commitment among support team members within the planning process. The degree of severity and complexity of disabilities across focus individuals may also be a factor. Nevertheless, the primary point is that an important step in ensuring that truly valid preferences are identified, as well as appropriately attended to by support personnel while implementing person-centered plans, is to carefully articulate an individual's preference. It would be useful for investigations to demonstrate specific procedures within the person-centered planning process that result in clearly identified preferences of individuals with severe multiple disabilities.

Emphasis on a Focus Person's Most Important Preferences When considering the precise identification of preferences in person-centered planning as just summarized, a caution warrants mention. By requiring careful specification of preferences to allow validation through systematic preference assessments, a risk exists that person-centered plans will begin to focus on preferences that readily lend themselves to specification. Correspondingly, there may be a de-emphasis on what is most important for overall quality of life for the individual. In this regard, behavioral research that developed the assessment technology has been characterized as focusing on preferences that affect relatively small aspects of life for individuals with severe disabilities (cf. Newton, Ard, & Horner, 1993). Such research has tended to emphasize preferences for specific leisure items (e.g., Roane, Vollmer, Ringdahl, & Marcus, 1998; Zhou, Goff, & Iwata, 2000) or individual snack and food items (Roane et al., 1998; Roscoe, Iwata, & Kahng, 1999). Although these items are important, other areas can have a broader or perhaps more powerful impact on overall life quality, such as one's preference for where and with whom to live and how to spend one's day. The latter preferences are often reflected in person-centered plans of individuals with mild or moderate disabilities. Yet, plans for people with severe multiple disabilities sometimes lack these types of preferences or include them with questionable accuracy.

There are several reasons why the behavioral literature has not focused on assessing more life-encompassing preferences, relative to the typical focus on leisure and food items, among people with severe multiple disabilities. For one, the original intent of developing preference assessment procedures was to identify reinforcing items to use in programs to teach adaptive skills. In this area, the behavioral preference assessment research has been quite successful. Discrete items or snacks that are identified as preferred frequently have been used successfully as reinforcing agents in teaching and related programs (Green, Reid, Canipe, & Gardner, 1991; Green et al., 1988; Pace et al., 1985; Ringdahl et al., 1997). Another reason why the behavioral assessment literature has not targeted more life-encompassing preferences is that a technology for assessing and validating these types of preferences among people with severe multiple disabilities has not been developed. The latter preferences, ranging from with whom to live to where to obtain supported employment, do not readily lend themselves to the systematic, repeated presentation trials that are common in the behavioral research on preference assessment.

Using situational preferences as an alternative means of assessing and validating preferences may lend itself to more global preferences. Situational assessments involve arranging for people to experience different situations, such as going to various restaurants, and closely observing how they respond to each situation or asking them which situations they liked the most (Everson & Reid, 1997). As of 2002, most reported situational assessments have not involved people with severe multiple disabilities. As indicated next, however, initial research does suggest that situational assessments may also be used to verify global preferences identified in person-centered plans by focusing on indices of happiness and unhappiness.

Several investigators have evaluated preferences across different situations among people who have severe multiple disabilities by systematically observing indices of happiness (Favell, Realon, & Sutton, 1996; Ivancic, Barrett, Simonow, & Kimberly, 1997). To obtain information about which situations individuals enjoy, indices of happiness— which generally involve responses such as smiling or laughing—are behaviorally defined and systematically observed as the individuals participate in different situations. Happiness indices have been shown to occur more frequently with activities that have been validated as preferred through systematic preference assessments relative to activities that have been systematically assessed as being nonpreferred (Green, Gardner, & Reid, 1997). In addition, support personnel who are familiar with an individual tend to report that the person likes activities if the individual shows the specified happiness indices during the activities (Green & Reid, 1996). Nevertheless, using happiness indices for situational preference assessments has been investigated infrequently, particularly for helping to ensure the validity of global preferences identified in person-centered plans.

Considerable research is needed on how to accurately identify preferences that affect comprehensive aspects of the lives of individuals with severe multiple disabilities. Given the existing state of preference assessment technologies, cautious reliance on the consensus of support team members currently appears to be the best available approach for determining life-encompassing preferences within person-centered planning. In some ways, the behavioral preference research supports such a conclusion. Although investigations have repeatedly shown that the opinions of support personnel are not very accurate for identifying various preferences, the research has shown that opinions of support personnel are rather accurate for identifying the *strongest* preferences of a respective individual (Green et al., 1991; Parsons & Reid, 1990). That is, when faced with numerous items and activities, support personnel experience difficulty in accurately ranking the items and activities but they are usually accurate in identifying items and activities that are the *most* liked. Consequently, with respect to preference validity, an important part of person-centered planning for people with severe multiple disabilities is forming a consensus among support team members regarding an individual's *strongest* preferences.

Procedural Practicality   As recommended previously in this chapter, person-centered planning with people who have severe multiple disabilities should be supplemented with systematic preference assessments to ensure the validity of reported preferences, at least for those preferences that lend themselves to such assessments. A potential problem with this recommendation is that by adding systematic preference assessments to person-centered planning, the process requires more effort and time. Increasing the effort and time necessary to develop and implement person-centered plans can reduce the likelihood that the process will be conducted adequately by support team members. It is well established that the more effortful or time consuming a work responsibility becomes (e.g., implementing components of person-centered plans), the less likely it is that the work responsibility will be fulfilled adequately (Everson & Reid, 1999; Reid, Parsons, & Green, 1989). Hence, consideration should be given to the practicality of including preference assessments as part of the person-centered process.

Directing attention to the practicality of fulfilling work expectations of human service staff can be somewhat controversial when considering responsibilities associated with person-centered planning. Support teams involved in person-centered planning should be comprised of people who have a close relationship with the focus person

and a sincere interest in supporting the individual in fulfilling important dreams and desires (Lyle O'Brien, O'Brien, & Mount, 1997). It is
assumed that the relationships with and interest of support team members provide motivation to develop and implement a plan to make the
focus person's dreams and desires a reality (cf. Everson & Reid, 1999).
In some ways, relying on the special relationship between support
team members and a focus person to motivate successful development
and implementation of a plan represents the purest form of a person-
centered approach. In actual application, however, person-centered
planning is not conducted in its purest form in many human service
agencies.

As discussed in the next section, the environments in which people with severe multiple disabilities frequently live, work, and play
tend to mitigate against providing person-centered supports and services. In those environments, special care must be taken to ensure that
person-centered planning occurs in the intended manner. Paramount
to the approach's successful application is a work environment that
maximizes the probability that support team members adequately fulfill their duties associated with implementing person-centered plans.
As noted previously, the more complex or cumbersome staff responsibilities become in conducting person-centered planning—such as by
adding systematic preference assessments to the planning process—
the less likely it is that the responsibilities will be fulfilled and the
process will occur as intended. Hence, concern is warranted regarding
how efficiently preference assessments can be conducted.

Although some attention has been directed to conducting preference assessments in a time-efficient manner (e.g., Roane et al., 1998;
Windsor et al., 1994), the process typically requires support personnel to
give relatively significant time and effort. The amount of time involved
in conducting preference assessments can be a particular issue when
considering the large number of preferences reported in many person-
centered plans. In an attempt to keep staff work expectations at a reasonable level when supplementing person-centered planning with systematic preference assessments, Green and colleagues (2000) developed
a brief, embedded assessment process. In this approach, the assessment
is embedded into the individual's daily routine during the implementation phase of person-centered planning. Items and activities that are
reported in the plan as being preferred are provided during the day, and
a quick assessment of how the person responds to each item and activity is conducted. By observing whether the individual approaches or
avoids the first daily presentation of each item and activity, a valid
assessment of whether the item or activity is truly desired can be completed in only a few minutes.

The embedded assessment process reported by Green and colleagues (2000) represents one way to reduce the time and effort required of support team members to ensure that reported preferences in person-centered plans are accurate. As with other areas of person-centered planning, however, there is insufficient research on the embedded assessment process to definitively determine the utility of this approach. Additional research is warranted to continue to develop and validate more efficient means of supplementing person-centered planning with systematic preference assessments.

IMPLEMENTING PERSON-CENTERED PLANNING IN TYPICAL ENVIRONMENTS

If person-centered planning is to be successful on a large scale basis with people who have severe multiple disabilities, then the process needs to occur within routine environments in which these individuals live, work, and play. Of course, a goal of a person-centered plan may be to support an individual in changing his or her current situation. Nevertheless, initially, person-centered approaches must be successfully incorporated within the environments in which people with severe multiple disabilities typically receive most of their supports and services.

The residential agency is the most common setting in which person-centered planning is attempted with individuals who have severe multiple disabilities. Relative to people who have less serious disabilities, a greater proportion of individuals with severe multiple disabilities reside in large, congregate settings with other individuals who have severe disabilities. An analysis of the residents in state-operated institutions, for example, indicated a much greater percentage of people with severe multiple disabilities residing in the institutions than people with mild or moderate disabilities (Lakin et al., 1999). Considerable numbers of people with severe multiple disabilities also reside in large community settings of a congregate nature (e.g., group homes with as many as six residents). Successfully adopting a person-centered approach in large congregate residences can be a very difficult process.

The difficulty in conducting person-centered planning in large residential settings is primarily due to the system-centered way in which such agencies tend to operate. System-centered supports and services stand in stark contrast to a person-centered way of operating. Actually, part of the impetus for the attention directed to person-centered planning was recognition of the shortcomings of traditional system-centered agencies (Everson & Reid, 1999). In system-centered agencies, supports and services are designed around the needs of the group of consumers served by the agency more than the needs and desires of each individual consumer. Supports and services are likewise designed around existing staff schedules, resources, and agency-wide rules and regulations that tend to treat all consumers in the same way. To illustrate, in large residential units or homes, all consumers are typically expected to get up and go to bed at approximately the same time, eat at the same approximate time, and attend the same day treatment program. In short, system-centered agencies operate in a manner that is essentially the antithesis of person-centered approaches.

Although the adoption of a person-centered approach can be difficult in system-centered agencies such as large residential settings, person-centered planning has become very popular in these settings. On closer examination, however, it is apparent that person-centered planning has not really been adopted in many agencies. Rather, key executive personnel tend to publicly endorse a person-centered approach but do not provide the training or support for agency staff to significantly change how they do business. In many agencies, person-centered planning has been adopted only to the degree that the names of agency forms are changed to reflect person-centered language: *interdisciplinary teams* are renamed *person-centered support teams,* and *program plans* are renamed *person-centered plans.* Such modifications often are not accompanied by significant changes in the lives of agency consumers.

Superficial changes in the name of person-centered planning are not necessarily due to an agency management's lack of sincere efforts to improve services. Again, adopting a person-centered approach in a traditional, system-centered agency is a difficult and time-consuming process. It is beyond the scope of this chapter to adequately describe all of the issues and strategies involved in helping system-centered agencies successfully adopt person-centered approaches (see Everson & Reid, 1999, for in-depth discussion). However, the following section presents information that is relevant to making traditional, system-centered agencies more person centered. The issue of concern here is that because many people with severe multiple disabilities live in large congregate settings and because such settings render person-centered approaches difficult, successful person-centered planning in these agencies must involve more than verbally adopting person-centered values and tools. Successful applications of person-centered planning in congregate settings require major changes in how agencies operate on a day-to-day basis.

ENSURING ADEQUATE STAFF PERFORMANCE FOR ACHIEVING PERSON-CENTERED CONSUMER OUTCOMES

The quality of any agency's services is heavily determined by the adequacy with which the agency's support staff fulfill their job responsibilities. In turn, it is the responsibility of agency management to ensure that staff perform their jobs adequately. Two key issues are involved in effectively managing staff performance for agencies attempting to adopt person-centered approaches. First, agency management must arrange resources to effectively train staff in person-centered values and tools that are specifically applicable to people who have severe cognitive and physical disabilities. Second, management must actively supervise and support the staff's implementation of person-centered plans after the plans have been developed.

Training Staff in Person-Centered Values and Tools

Whenever an agency attempts to change an aspect of how it functions, attention should be directed to ensuring that staff know how to perform duties that coincide with the agency changes. Often, management must arrange for staff to be trained in new work skills. Numerous reports describe research and application of successful means of training work skills to human service personnel (see Jahr, 1998, and Chapter 3 of Reid et al., 1989, for reviews). When an agency serving people with severe multiple disabilities begins to adopt a person-centered approach, however, several key issues warrant attention with staff training.

If management personnel expect staff to successfully participate in person-centered planning, then the staff must know how to conduct person-centered planning. In particular, staff must have the skills to effectively facilitate person-centered planning meetings. The essence of person-centered planning is supporting individuals in achieving their dreams and desires, and those dreams and desires are derived from planning meetings. The importance of training for facilitators of person-centered meetings is discussed elsewhere (Everson & Reid, 1999). Of concern here is *how* agency personnel are trained to facilitate planning meetings.

To effectively facilitate the meetings, facilitators must have knowledge of the values and tools of person-centered planning, as well as the skills to actually facilitate planning meetings. Knowledge and skills regarding expected work responsibilities for facilitating person-centered planning meetings involve two sets of staff competencies. In many cases, training in human service agencies provides staff with the necessary information or knowledge to understand a given work responsibility. In contrast, the training often is ineffective for training the skills to actually apply that knowledge on a routine basis.

Ensuring staff know how to perform a given duty, such as facilitating person-centered planning meetings, usually requires performance-based staff training. Performance-based training requires additional training procedures relative to teaching a knowledge base to staff. Table 8.1 summarizes the key steps of performance-based training for effectively facilitating planning meetings. Of particular relevance here is that typical training programs for preparing facilitators are terminated after the first three or four steps identified in Table 8.1. As a result, there is considerable variability in the skills of facilitators in many human service agencies. If facilitators are to have the skills to effectively facilitate meetings, then staff training programs must include opportunities for staff to practice facilitation skills and receive feedback on their skill application (Step 5 in Table 8.1). Furthermore, these training procedures must be continued until facilitators demonstrate effective use of facilitation skills during actual planning meetings (Step 6).

The importance of observing staff for competency in facilitating planning meetings is particularly relevant for consumers who have severe multiple disabilities. As indicated previously, there are a number of special considerations for identifying preferences of these individuals. Facilitators must be able to determine how and at what level an individual can participate in the planning process. Special consideration is also warranted for obtaining accurate input of support team members regarding their opinions of the individual's most important desires. Likewise, special attention is required to ensure that the opinions are expressed in specific terms so that the resulting plans can be implemented effectively.

Table 8.1. Steps in performance-based training for facilitating person-centered planning meetings

1. Provide a rationale for the target training skills.
2. Provide a written description of the target skills.
3. Verbally describe the target skills.
4. Demonstrate the target skills.
5. Observe trainee practice on target skills and provide supportive and/or corrective feedback.
6. Continue Step 5 until the trainee demonstrates competence with the facilitation skills.

The only way to ensure that facilitators of meetings for people who have severe multiple disabilities effectively address each of these issues is to observe their facilitation of planning meetings (again, see Table 8.1). It should also be noted, however, that although the skills for effectively facilitating person-centered planning meetings have been described in general (e.g., Lyle O'Brien et al., 1997), additional information is needed on how those skills should be refined specifically for people with severe multiple disabilities.

Ensuring Management Support for Implementation of Person-Centered Plans

The second key issue for ensuring adequate staff performance in the person-centered process pertains to providing management support for implementation of person-centered plans. Providing management support is important for all aspects of staff performance in human service settings (Babcock, Fleming, & Oliver, 1998). However, it is particularly important to support implementing person-centered plans for consumers who have severe multiple disabilities. Without such support, plans often are not implemented effectively. To illustrate, in evaluating how person-centered plans were implemented for one group of individuals living in one residential facility, we found that the majority of individuals rarely had access to what their plans identified as their most desired leisure activities. In some cases, there was no difference in an individual's daily life after the development of a person-centered plan, even though the plan identified many desired changes. Significant attention was directed to identifying and transcribing consumer dreams and desires but little attention was directed to supporting consumers in actually realizing those dreams and desires. Consultations with other agencies suggest that this phenomenon is rather common for individuals with severe disabilities; person-centered planning tends to begin and end with the development of the plan.

Problems in implementing person-centered plans for consumers with severe multiple disabilities heighten the need for management oversight for three primary reasons. First, due to communication challenges, these individuals often experience difficulty expressing something that they do not like. For example, if access is not provided for an individual to a certain activity that was identified as important in the individual's person-centered plan, the person may not be able to readily express the desire to gain access to the activity. Rather, support staff usually must provide a specific opportunity for the individual to indicate a desire for the activity. The individual is more dependent on staff support in this type of situation than people with less serious disabilities who can readily express their displeasure. The latter individuals can more easily seek support to gain access to an activity from other team members, advocates, or managers, and sometimes they can resolve the problems themselves. For people with severe multiple disabilities, gaining access to desired activities or resolving problems is more related to how well staff implement aspects of person-centered plans and attend to problem situations. Hence, management attention is often critical for ensuring that staff implement person-centered plans in the way the plans are intended to be implemented.

Second, management attention to staff implementation of person-centered plans is warranted because of where many people with severe multiple disabilities spend their time. As noted previously, most participate in congregate living and day treatment settings, which tend to be system centered and to encounter formidable challenges in adopting person-centered practices. In system-centered organizations, it is inherently difficult for staff to provide sufficiently individualized supports, which are key to the success of person-centered planning. To ensure that staff have sufficient time and resources to interact with and respond to each consumer, considerable management attention usually must focus on staff members' day-to-day functioning.

Third, management attention also should be directed to the staff's implementation of person-centered plans because of the constituency of person-centered support teams. Person-centered support teams should consist of people who know the focus person very well and have a special interest in that person's welfare. This special interest normally serves as a potent motivator for team members to effectively implement a person-centered plan such that an individual experiences the desired lifestyle changes reflected in the plan. In congregate settings, membership on support teams often includes people who do not have special relationships with the focus person. Team members may be mandated to participate on person-centered planning teams because of regulatory guidelines or licensing requirements (e.g., rules that require certain types of professionals to participate on all support teams regardless of their relationship with the individual) or simply because of historical precedent in a given agency. When people participate on support teams solely due to job requirements, their motivation to follow through on implementing person-centered plans can be reduced compared with the motivation of people who have a special relationship with an individual.

These reasons should not be interpreted as reflecting negatively on support staff in human service agencies. Support staff have many duties to fulfill and often are given competing responsibilities from different supervisory personnel that can impede implementation of person-centered plans (Chapter 2 of Reid et al., 1989). The concern here is that because of the significant challenges facing people who have severe multiple disabilities and the types of environments in which they reside, management must provide considerable attention and support to ensure that person-centered plans are well developed and implemented. Precisely how management can oversee the operation of agencies to ensure that the plans serve their intended purpose is beyond the scope of this chapter. Our opinion, however, is that the component procedures of an outcome management approach represent an effective means of managing human service agencies in a person-centered manner. In outcome management, the management process begins with the delineation of desired outcomes of agency consumers (e.g., as derived from person-centered plans) and then specifies necessary staff and supervisory actions to support consumers in attaining the outcomes (Everson & Reid, 1999). Consumer outcome attainment and expected staff actions to support consumers in attaining the outcomes are routinely monitored. Supportive or corrective management actions are then taken depending on how well or poorly the outcomes are observed to occur and on how well or poorly staff are performing, respectively. Following the steps of outcome management, managers can take an active role in ensuring that person-centered plans are effectively implemented.

CONCLUSION

Person-centered planning has had a profound impact on the quality of life of many individuals with disabilities. However, the benefits of this approach to designing and providing supports have been much less pronounced for people who have severe multiple disabilities. Three key issues must be addressed to extend the benefits of person-centered planning to these people. First, caution must be exercised in making sure that preferences identified in person-centered planning meetings represent the focus person's true preferences. Research suggests that the validity of preferences identified through person-centered planning can be enhanced by supplementing the process with systematic preference assessments. However, continued research is needed to develop more efficient preference assessment processes and to find valid ways to identify more life-encompassing preferences.

A second key issue warranting attention if person-centered planning is to expand its benefits to more people with severe multiple disabilities entails demonstrating ways to make congregate settings more person centered. Congregate settings are typically very system-oriented, and they often make only superficial changes under the guise of person-centered planning.

The third issue pertains to effectively training and managing staff performance regarding person-centered planning. More attention is needed on performance-based staff training procedures to adequately equip staff to use the tools of person-centered planning. Management attention also must be directed to ensuring staff adequately implement person-centered plans. If serious attention is directed to these issues, then more people with severe multiple disabilities are likely to realize the benefits of person-centered planning.

REFERENCES

Babcock, R.A., Fleming, R.K., & Oliver, J.R. (1998). OBM and quality improvement systems. *Journal of Organizational Behavior Management, 18*, 33–59.

Browder, D.M., Bambara, L.M., & Belfiore, P.J. (1997). Using a person-centered approach in community-based instruction for adults with developmental disabilities. *Journal of Behavioral Education, 7*, 519–528.

Brown, F., Gothelf, C.R., Guess, D., & Lehr, D. H. (1998). Self-determination for individuals with the most severe disabilities: Moving beyond chimera. *Journal of The Association for Persons with Severe Handicaps, 23*, 17–26.

Everson, J.M. (1996). Using person-centered planning concepts to enhance school-to-adult life transition planning. *Journal of Vocational Rehabilitation, 6*, 7–13.

Everson, J.M., & Reid, D.H. (1997). Using person-centered planning to determine employment preferences among people with the most severe developmental disabilities. *Journal of Vocational Rehabilitation, 9*, 99–108.

Everson, J.M., & Reid, D.H. (1999). *Person-centered planning and outcome management: Maximizing organizational effectiveness in supporting quality lifestyles among people with disabilities.* Morganton, NC: Habilitative Management Consultants.

Favell, J.E., & Cannon, P.R. (1976). Evaluation of entertainment materials for severely retarded persons. *American Journal of Mental Deficiency, 81*, 357–361.

Favell, J.E., Realon, R.E., & Sutton, K.A. (1996). Measuring and increasing the happiness of people with profound mental retardation and physical handicaps. *Behavioral Interventions, 11*, 47–58.

Fisher, W., Piazza, C.C., Bowman, L.G., Hagopian, L.P., Owens, J.C., & Slevin, I. (1992). A comparison of two approaches for identifying reinforcers for persons with severe and profound disabilities. *Journal of Applied Behavior Analysis, 25*, 491–498.

Green, C.W., Gardner, S.M., & Reid, D.H. (1997). Increasing indices of happiness among people with profound multiple disabilities: A program replication and component analysis. *Journal of Applied Behavior Analysis, 30*, 217–228.

Green, C.W., Middleton, S.G., & Reid, D.H. (2000). Embedded evaluation of preferences sampled from person-centered plans for people with profound multiple disabilities. *Journal of Applied Behavior Analysis, 33*, 639–642.

Green, C.W., & Reid, D.H. (1996). Defining, validating and increasing indices of happiness among people with profound multiple disabilities. *Journal of Applied Behavior Analysis, 29*, 67–78.

Green, C.W., Reid, D.H., Canipe, V.S., & Gardner, S.M. (1991). A comprehensive evaluation of reinforcer identification processes for persons with profound multiple handicaps. *Journal of Applied Behavior Analysis, 24*, 537–552.

Green, C.W., Reid, D.H., White, L.K., Halford, R.C., Brittain, D.P., & Gardner, S.M. (1988). Identifying reinforcers for persons with profound handicaps: Staff opinion versus systematic assessment of preferences. *Journal of Applied Behavior Analysis, 21,* 31–43.

Hagner, D., Helm, D.T., & Butterworth, J. (1996). "This is your meeting": A qualitative study of person-centered planning. *Mental Retardation, 34,* 159–171.

Holburn, S. (1997). A renaissance in residential behavior analysis? A historical perspective and a better way to help people with challenging behavior. *The Behavior Analyst, 20,* 61–85.

Ivancic, M.T., Barrett, G.T., Simonow, A., & Kimberly, A. (1997). A replication to increase happiness indices among some people with profound multiple disabilities. *Research in Developmental Disabilities, 18,* 79–89.

Jahr, E. (1998). Current issues in staff training. *Research in Developmental Disabilities, 19,* 73–87.

Kincaid, D. (1996). Person-centered planning. In L.K. Koegel, R.L. Koegel, & G. Dunlap (Eds.), *Positive behavioral support: Including people with difficult behavior in the community* (pp. 439–465). Baltimore: Paul H. Brookes Publishing Co.

Lakin, K.C., Anderson, L., Prouty, R., & Polister, B. (1999). State institution populations less than one third of 1977, residents older with more impairments. *Mental Retardation, 37,* 85–86.

Lyle O'Brien, C., O'Brien, J., & Mount, B. (1997). Person-centered planning has arrived . . . or has it? *Mental Retardation, 35,* 480–484.

Mount, B. (1994). Benefits and limitations of personal futures planning. In V.J. Bradley, J.W. Ashbaugh, & B.C. Blaney (Eds.), *Creating individual supports for people with developmental disabilities: A mandate for change at many levels* (pp. 97–108). Baltimore: Paul H. Brookes Publishing Co.

Mount, B. (1997). *Person-centered planning: Finding directions for change using personal futures planning.* New York: Graphic Futures.

Newton, J.S., Ard, W.R., & Horner, R.H. (1993). Validating predicted activity preferences of individuals with severe disabilities. *Journal of Applied Behavior Analysis, 26,* 239–245.

O'Brien, J. (1987). A guide to life-style planning: Using The Activities Catalog to integrate services and natural support systems. In B. Wilcox & G.T. Bellamy, *A comprehensive guide to The Activities Catalog: An alternative curriculum for youth and adults with severe disabilities* (pp. 175–189). Baltimore: Paul H. Brookes Publishing Co.

Pace, G.M., Ivancic, M.T., Edwards, G.L., Iwata, B.A., & Page, T.J. (1985). Assessment of stimulus preference and reinforcer value with profoundly retarded individuals. *Journal of Applied Behavior Analysis, 18,* 249–255.

Parsons, M.B., & Reid, D.H. (1990). Assessing food preferences among persons with profound mental retardation: Providing opportunities to make choices. *Journal of Applied Behavior Analysis, 23,* 183–195.

Parsons, M.B., Reid, D.H., Reynolds, J., & Bumgarner, M. (1990). Effects of chosen versus assigned jobs on the work performance of persons with severe handicaps. *Journal of Applied Behavior Analysis, 23,* 253–258.

Reid, D.H., Everson, J.M., & Green, C.W. (1999). A systematic evaluation of preferences identified through person-centered planning for people with profound multiple disabilities. *Journal of Applied Behavior Analysis, 32,* 467–477.

Reid, D.H., Parsons, M.B., & Green, C.W. (1989). *Staff management in human services: Behavioral research and application.* Springfield, IL: Charles C Thomas.

Reid, D.H., Phillips, J.F., & Green, C.W. (1991). Teaching persons with profound multiple handicaps: A review of the effects of behavioral research. *Journal of Applied Behavior Analysis, 24,* 319–336.

Ringdahl, J.E., Vollmer, T.R., Marcus, B.A., & Roane, H.S. (1997). An analogue evaluation of environmental enrichment: The role of stimulus preference. *Journal of Applied Behavior Analysis, 30,* 203–216.

Roane, H.S., Vollmer, T.R., Ringdahl, J.E., & Marcus, B.A. (1998). Evaluation of a brief stimulus preference assessment. *Journal of Applied Behavior Analysis, 31,* 605–620.

Roscoe, E.M., Iwata, B.A., & Kahng, S.W. (1999). Relative versus absolute reinforcement effects: Implications for preference assessments. *Journal of Applied Behavior Analysis, 32,* 479–493.

Wehman, P. (1996). Expanding supported employment opportunities. *Journal of Vocational Rehabilitation, 6,* 121–122.

Whitney-Thomas, J., Shaw, D., Honey, K., & Butterworth, J. (1998). Building a future: A study of student participation in person-centered planning. *Journal of The Association for Persons with Severe Handicaps, 23,* 119–133.

Windsor, J., Piché, L.M., & Locke, P.A. (1994). Preference testing: A comparison of two presentation methods. *Research in Developmental Disabilities, 15,* 439–445.

Zhou, L., Goff, G.A., & Iwata, B.A. (2000). Effects of increased response effort on self-injury and object manipulation as competing responses. *Journal of Applied Behavior Analysis, 33,* 29–40.

9

Residential Preferences in Person-Centered Planning

Empowerment Through the Self-Identification of Preferences and Their Availability

Paula Davis and Gerald Faw

Person-centered planning strives to uncover the unique gifts and capacities of a person with a disability, to discover his or her hopes and dreams, and to develop supports that assist the individual in attaining them. One of the core values of person-centered planning is that the preferences of the individual with the disability should be honored and the person should be supported in making choices in all aspects of his or her life.

A national survey of the self-determination of adults with mental retardation revealed that the opportunity to participate in decisions that affect their lives is related to the importance of the decision (Wehmeyer & Metzler, 1995). That is, simple choices of minor consequence, such as what to wear, are likely to be granted. Conversely, the same person is less likely to be involved in decisions about major lifestyle issues such as choosing where to live. In fact, decisions about where to live often reflect the wishes of those who are legally responsible for the individual rather than the preferences of the individual with the disability. In other cases, the person moves to a group home because an opening exists rather than because the home reflects the preferences of the individual who will be living there (Turnbull, Turnbull, Bronicki, Summers, & Roeder-Gordon, 1989). Yet, choosing where to live is one of the most important decisions that adults make and clearly affects overall satisfaction with life in many areas over a long period of time.

The purpose of this chapter is to describe how to include people with mental retardation in the process of selecting a place to live and in the development of a support plan that accompanies that selection. Systematic procedures for identifying an individual's community living preferences are explained. Also described is a program to teach individuals to determine whether their preferences are available and, thus, whether a home or an apartment would be a good place to live. That section of the chapter examines the discrepancy between preferences and their availability in traditional group living arrangements. Finally, a method for teaching consumers to play a more active role in planning meetings is recommended. Our suggestions are derived from projects that we conducted to assist individuals in moving from large, congregate care settings to smaller, group home living arrangements. The procedures described in this chapter have been modified to illustrate how they can be used within the context of more individualized supported living arrangements and person-centered planning.

METHOD FOR IDENTIFYING COMMUNITY LIVING PREFERENCES

Many factors should be considered when moving from one living arrangement to another. For one person, a critical consideration may be whether he or she will have a private bedroom; for another, it may be whether the home or apartment is near a favorite restaurant or shopping center; and for still another, it may be whether the yard has room for a garden. Unfortunately, many people with mental retardation have a difficult time identifying critical home characteristics if asked that question in an open-ended fashion. Furthermore, if the person has limited life experiences, as is often the case for many individuals with mental retardation, the person may not even know which options exist with respect to home features. Therefore, the first step in helping a person select a home in the community is to develop a systematic assessment procedure that makes the identification of preferences reliable and valid. The assessment procedures recommended in this section are based on work done by Faw, Davis, and Peck (1996) and Foxx, Faw, Taylor, Davis, and Fulia (1993).

Based on a review of the literature and an examination of existing questionnaires, we developed a 30-item preference assessment. Because the individuals in our study were moving into group living arrangements rather than into individually supported homes or apartments, the items focused on issues having to do with privacy (e.g., sharing a bedroom), house rules (e.g., curfew, use of the telephone), and other service issues (e.g., having opportunities to cook, handling one's own money). Table 9.1 lists the items that we used in the study. For people moving into more individualized arrangements, other home characteristics may be crucial. Choices regarding concerns such as location of the home (e.g., proximity to public transportation, restau-

Table 9.1. Lifestyle items and contrasting options

Lifestyle item	Contrasting options
Bedroom	You have your own bedroom.
	You share a bedroom.
Bathroom	You have your own bathroom.
	You share a bathroom.
Pets	Pets are allowed.
	Pets are not allowed.
Neighbors	Neighbors live near the home.
	Neighbors live far away from the home.
Work	You have a job.
	You do not have a job.
Pay	You receive real money as payment for your job.
	You do not receive real money as payment for your job.
Handling money	You handle your own money.
	Staff handle your money for you.
Classes	You take training classes.
	You do not take training classes.
Visitors	Family and friends can visit whenever they want.
	Family and friends can only visit during visiting hours or on certain days.
Smoking	Cigarette smoking is allowed in the home.
	Cigarette smoking is not allowed inside the home.

(continued)

Table 9.1. *(continued)*

Lifestyle item	Contrasting options
Number of residents	Many other people live in the home.
	Only a few other people live in the home.
Curfew	The home has a curfew.
	The home does not have a curfew.
Getting up in the morning	Staff wake you up in the morning.
	You wake up in the morning on your own.
Sleeping late	You get up at the same time every day.
	You can sleep late some days.
Meals with staff	Staff eat meals with you.
	Staff do not eat meals with you.
Permission to leave the home	You can come and go as you please.
	You must have staff permission to leave the home.
Counselor	A counselor is available.
	A counselor is not available.
Keys	You have a key to your bedroom and/or locker.
	Only staff members have keys.
Telephone	You can talk on the telephone whenever you want.
	You must have permission to talk on the telephone.
Public transportation	Public transportation is available.
	Public transportation is not available.
Staff gender	The majority of staff are male.
	The majority of staff are female.
	Approximately the same number of male and female staff work at the home.

Staff turnover rate	There is a low staff turnover rate.
	There is a high staff turnover rate.
Grocery shopping	You shop for your own groceries.
	Staff shop for your groceries.
Cleaning	Staff clean the home.
	You and the other residents clean the home.
Laundry	You do your own laundry.
	Staff members do your laundry for you.
Serving meals	Staff fill your plate and serve your meals.
	You and the other residents eat family style and fill your own plates.
Fast-food restaurants	The home is near fast-food restaurants.
	The home is far away from fast-food restaurants.
Doctor appointments	Staff make doctor appointments for you.
	You make your own doctor appointments.
Familiar residents	You knew some of the residents before moving into the home.
	You did not know any of the residents before moving into the home.
Noise level	The home is usually noisy.
	The home is usually quiet.

rants, church, shopping centers, work) and physical characteristics of the home (e.g., number of bedrooms, number of stories, size of yard, type of heat) should be included. One way to identify which items should be included in the assessment is to examine the preferences identified by other individuals who have already participated in person-centered planning. The home-related items that are noted on the preference list would be a good starting point for developing a comprehensive list of items to include on the preference assessment.

To determine a person's preferences for each assessment item, contrasting items are developed. The questions should reflect the home characteristics most relevant to the type of living arrangement being considered (e.g., renting an apartment, buying a home, having a roommate, living alone). For instance, for a person buying a home, the type of heat available might be important, so the contrasting items would be "Do you want a house with electric heat or gas heat?" For an individual sharing a home or an apartment, one important question might be "Do you want your own bathroom, or do you want to share a bathroom?" Each item on the assessment has two (or perhaps more) contrasting options.

To identify each individual's preferences and then to determine which of those preferences are most important, a two-step assessment procedure is recommended. Table 9.2 provides a task analysis for conducting the assessment. The purpose of the first portion of the assessment procedure, within-item task tests, is to determine which of two contrasting options represents the person's preference. For example, does the person prefer a home in which he or she has a private bathroom or one in which the bathroom is shared? After completing this first portion of the assessment, each individual's preferences are identified.

The second portion of the assessment procedure, across-item tests, is designed to determine which of the identified within-item preferences are most important to the individual. This is accomplished by randomly pairing items selected in the within-item tests and "forcing" a choice between the two. For example, the question might be, "Which is more important—being near a grocery store or having your own bathroom?" Repeated random pairings across three trials identifies the consumer's strongest preferences. The items identified through this systematic procedure reflect valued, reliable indicators of the person's preferences regarding the type of home in which he or she wants to live.

Although some individuals may be able to identify their preferences when asked in a typical interview format, others may not. For those individuals, a visual representation of the choices may be helpful. Photographs that represent the options are shown side by side as the questions are asked. For example, for the item regarding sharing a

Table 9.2. Preference assessment procedures

Type of assessment	Procedures
Within-item tests	1. Display photographs of preference items that depict two contrasting options (e.g., a bedroom with one bed, a bedroom with two beds).
	2. Label the options for the consumer.
	3. Have the consumer label the options.
	4. Point to one option and say, "In some homes, people [e.g., have their own bedrooms]." Point to the other option and say, "In other homes, people [e.g., share a bedroom]."
	5. Cue a choice by saying, "In which home would you rather live?"
	6. Have the consumer describe or label the option that he or she chooses.
	7. Record the option choice.
	8. Repeat Steps 1–7 for all preference items.
	9. Conduct three of these tests with several days between each assessment. On each test, reverse the position of the photographs.
Across-item tests	1. Display photographs of two of the consumer's chosen options from the within-item test (e.g., a person with a pet, a bedroom with one bed).
	2. Remind the consumer of previous choices by saying, "Remember, you told us that you want [e.g., to live where you can have a pet] and that you also want to [e.g., have your own room]."
	3. Cue a choice between the consumer's selections by pointing to the respective photographs and saying, "Which is more important to you, being able to [e.g., have a pet] or being able to [e.g., have your own room]?"
	4. Have the consumer describe the choice that he or she selected.
	5. Record the consumer's preference.
	6. Randomly pair the consumer's remaining preferences from the within-item test, and repeat Steps 1–5 for all pairings, ensuring that each item is paired against a different item on every trial.
	7. Conduct three of these tests, making sure to use a different pairing each time.
	8. Create a "Top 10" list for the consumer by first including options that the consumer selected three times.
	9. To complete the Top 10 list, ask the consumer to choose the most important options that he or she selected on two of three tests.

209

bedroom, the person is shown a picture of a bedroom with one bed and told, "In this home, you would have your own bedroom." At the same time, the person is shown a picture of a bedroom with two beds and told, "In this home, you would share a bedroom." The person is then asked which home he or she prefers. The same photographs are used in the forced choice questions as well. Using either/or questions and photographs facilitates responding and minimizes the errors associated with a traditional interview format.

The critical issue is to ensure that the items represent the important characteristics of homes and that individual preferences are determined in a systematic fashion that ensures that the answers are reliable. Our studies show test–retest agreement scores between 70% and 93% with a mean of 87% (Foxx et al., 1993) and 67% and 100% with a mean of 86% (Faw et al., 1996). The procedures that we used provide guidance on how to develop systematic preference assessments.

It is often assumed that living in the community, by definition, provides individuals with access to a desired lifestyle. To determine the accuracy of that assumption, we conducted a survey to see what preferences were available in the supervised community homes in our area. Therefore, the residential choices for the individuals surveyed in our studies were limited to traditional supervised group living options. Individualized arrangements that are consistent with the philosophy and values of person-centered planning were not available. We then compared that information yielded by our study with the consumer preferences identified in the studies described previously (Davis, O'Guin, & Faw, 1994). The data collected in the studies on what people want and the availability of those preferences in traditional group living arrangements underscore why more individualized residential options are important.

The left-hand column in Table 9.3 shows the lifestyle options that frequently are selected by consumers as being top priorities (e.g., having a job, living near fast-food restaurants, being able to have visitors anytime). The right-hand column reveals the availability of those options in 14 homes. As an example, the results show that 63% of the consumers identified working and receiving money as pay as one of their strongest preferences, but only 7% of the homes reported that the people who lived in them would have a community job in which they received real money as pay. In contrast, 43% of the homes responded that the people living in them would work in and be paid by sheltered work or training programs. Half reported that the individuals would attend programs in which they would do simulated work and may or may not receive money as pay. As another example, 53% of the consumers

Table 9.3.   Availability of top preferences

Top lifestyle preference	Percentage of homes in which available	
Job with money as pay	7	Community job, real pay
	43	Sheltered or training, real pay
	50	Simulated work, may or may not receive real money as pay
Fast-food restaurant nearby	57	Yes
	43	No
Handle own money	43	All money, all decisions
	57	Some money, some decisions
	0	No access to own money
Come and go as please (into town)	29	Anytime
	21	Certain hours
	50	With permission
(into own yard)	79	Anytime
	7	Certain hours
	14	With permission
Wake up on own	36	Independently every day
	36	Independently on weekends only
	28	Never
Have own keys	14	To bedroom
	36	To locker or closet
	50	No keys to either
Visitors	64	Anytime
	29	Specified hours or days
	7	With permission
Buy own groceries	14	All groceries
	43	Snack foods only
	43	No groceries

selected living near a fast-food restaurant as a priority, but that option was available at only 57% of the homes.

These data underscore the fact that simply living in the community does not necessarily result in access to the items that are most important to an individual. For individuals who need ongoing support to live in the community, such as those individuals with whom we worked, the supports provided should reflect the concerns and preferences of the individuals living in the home so that they have access to their chosen lifestyles. Human services agencies that provide support services could use the same preference assessment procedures described in this section to ensure that the supports that they are providing reflect the preferences of the individuals whom they are serving.

METHOD FOR DETERMINING PREFERENCE AVAILABILITY AND THE CHOICE BETWEEN A HOME OR AN APARTMENT

Knowing a consumer's preferences does not ensure that he or she plays an active role in selecting where to live or identifying desired supports. Person-centered planning requires meaningful involvement from the individual with a disability. One way to involve consumers is to have them visit homes before deciding where to live. Yet, visits alone may be insufficient if the person does not ask about preference availability. Our research shows that consumers rarely ask questions about their preferences when taken on tours of group homes, even when they are asked if they have any questions (Foxx et al., 1993). There is no reason to expect that they are any more likely to ask questions when taken to visit more individualized options.

One way to ensure that consumers' preferences are considered is to teach them to ask questions about the availability of their preferences when touring houses that they might purchase or rent and then to evaluate the home based on that information. The procedures suggested next are based on the previously described studies (Faw et al., 1996; Foxx et al., 1993). Although those studies were conducted within the context of teaching people to identify whether various group homes possessed their preferences, the following procedures are applicable to assisting individuals to evaluate more individualized living arrangements.

The first step is to ensure that the person remembers to ask questions about his or her preferences. This can be accomplished by developing an individualized booklet that lists the person's strongest preferences (identified using the procedures described in the previous section). For individuals with limited or no reading skills, small photograph albums are recommended, with a photograph of each of the individual's strongest preferences on its own page. Below each photograph is a question regarding the preference item (e.g., "Would I have my own bedroom if I picked this home?" "Would I be able to walk to McDonald's if I lived here?") and three boxes labeled "yes," "no," and "maybe." "Maybe" is an option because the availability of a certain preference may not be known immediately. For example, it may be necessary to check with the owner of an apartment building to determine whether pets are allowed or permitted only in certain circumstances. The person can then record the answer by using a grease pencil to circle "yes," "no," or "maybe." A sample page from an album is shown in Figure 9.1. Using the booklet, a person can be taught to determine preference availability when touring homes to be rented or purchased. Similarly, the booklet can be used to determine supports available in the case of an individual who is moving to a supervised home or apartment.

After obtaining information about preference availability, the person can use the evaluation sheet shown in Figure 9.2 to determine

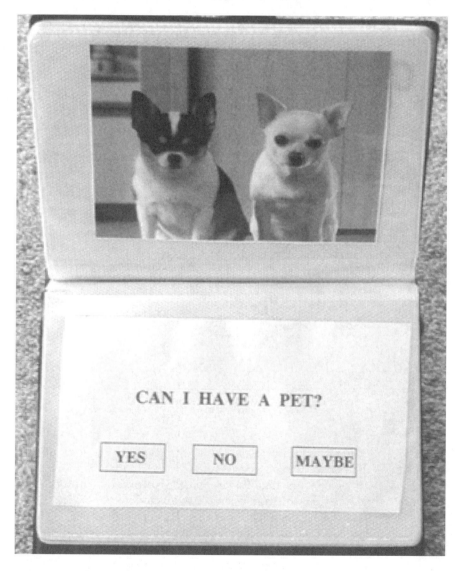

Figure 9.1.   Sample photograph album page.

PREFERENCES	**ANSWERS**

1. Can I have a pet?	YES= [X] [X] NO= [ ] MAYBE= [X]
2. Are there two bedrooms?	YES= [X] [X] NO= [ ] MAYBE= [X]
3. Are there two bathrooms?	YES= [X] [X] NO= [ ] MAYBE= [X]
4. Is there a screened-in porch?	YES= [X] [X] NO= [ ] MAYBE= [X]
5. Is it near my church?	YES= [X] [X] NO= [ ] MAYBE= [X]
6. Is it near my family?	YES= [X] [X] NO= [ ] MAYBE= [X]
7. Is it near a fast food restaurant?	YES= [X] [X] NO= [ ] MAYBE= [X]
8. Is it near a park?	YES= [X] [X] NO= [ ] MAYBE= [X]
9. Is it on the bus line?	YES= [X] [X] NO= [ ] MAYBE= [X]
10. Is it near a grocery store?	YES= [X] [X] NO= [ ] MAYBE= [X]

Come in

Home Sweet Home

BASED ON THIS INFOMATION, IS THIS A GOOD PLACE FOR YOU TO LIVE?

YES   NO

START HERE

Figure 9.2. Evaluation worksheet for the fit between a home and a consumer's top preferences.

whether the home would be a good place to live. The top half of the worksheet lists the person's strongest preferences in question form. By referring to the answers that the individual recorded in his or her album while touring the home, he or she circles "yes," "no," or "maybe" next to each question on the evaluation worksheet. If needed, a family member, friend, or staff member can read the questions on the evaluation sheet. The bottom half of the worksheet is used to determine whether the toured home might be a good place to live. For each "yes," "maybe," and "no" answer that is marked on the top half of the sheet, two, one, or zero squares, respectively, are crossed off on the sidewalk in front of the house, as shown by the boxes next to the words. Reaching the shaded squares on the sidewalk indicates that "yes" or "maybe" was scored for at least half of the preference questions. If any of the shaded squares are crossed off after the worksheet is completed, then the person answers that the home would be a good place to live.

Table 9.4 presents the task analysis for teaching individuals to determine whether their preferences are available and to evaluate the home. Role-play training (using individually determined prompts), feedback, and reinforcers are recommended to teach the skills. Our instructional methods were successful in teaching individuals who previously did not have the skills to obtain information about their preferences and to make decisions about the suitability of the homes that they toured.

Table 9.4.   Training task analysis

Ask preference questions	1. Bring the necessary materials on the tour (e.g., the individual's preference booklet).
	2. Initiate preference questioning (e.g., "I have some questions that I would like to ask.").
	3. Suggest sitting at a table.
	4. Ask the first question from the booklet.
	5. Ask for clarification (e.g., "Is that a 'yes,' 'no,' or 'maybe'?") when the person does not answer with a simple "yes," "no," or "maybe."
	6. Record the answer in the book.
	7. Repeats Steps 4–6 for the remaining questions.
	8. Terminate the interaction politely.
Evaluate the home	1. Open the booklet to the first preference question and transcribe the answer at the corresponding space on the evaluation worksheet.
	2. Mark the appropriate number of boxes on the sidewalk leading to the home.
	3. Complete transcribing and marking boxes for the remaining questions in the order that they appear in the preference book.
	4. State whether the marks on the sidewalk reach the shaded area.
	5. Answer decision box correctly (i.e., "yes" if the marks reached shaded area or "no" if the marks fell short).
	6. Show and state decision.

The results of our studies illustrate that individuals with mental retardation can play an active role in making decisions about where to live. They were shown how to make decisions based on the availability of at least half of their preferences. The number of top preferences considered (10) and the percentage that should be available (50%) were arbitrarily selected. No consideration was given to weighting the importance of any of the preferences. If certain preferences are known to be critical to an individual, then additional questions can be added to the evaluation form. For example, any characteristic that an individual or his or her circle of support deems nonnegotiable can be listed on the evaluation sheet along with the words "yes" and "no." If any nonnegotiable item is not available at a particular home, then that home would not be a choice regardless of the score received. As this variation illustrates, the procedures can be modified to include even more individualization while still ensuring that the process is systematic and reliable.

In most cases, it is not possible for an individual to look at every home that is available for rent or purchase. In much the same way as a realtor works with a potential home buyer, the individuals supporting the person with the disability might assist him or her in screening homes to identify those that most closely mirror individual preferences. The person would then tour those homes and evaluate them using the previously described procedures. This screening process would be efficient for both the consumer and his or her support network.

Figure 9.3 shows how a quick visual analysis can be made regarding the fit between an individual's preferences and the availability of those preferences at several homes. Lynn's top 10 preferences are listed under the figure. The graph shows that for five houses or apartments (named A, B, C, D, and E), the number of Lynn's preferences that are available ranges from one (at A and D) to five (at C and E). Based on this analysis, Lynn would find at least half of her preferences available in two houses or apartments and nearly half available in one. Therefore, Lynn might want to visit C and E and maybe also home B. Because homes A and D have few of the important home characteristics that Lynn desires, neither is a good match, and tours of those houses or apartments are unnecessary.

Honoring the preferences of individuals may result in their being more satisfied with their living arrangements. Likewise, people who participate in decision making about where to live and have access to their preferences may have fewer behavior problems. In addition, their return to a restrictive environment may be less likely. Future research that examines these variables is warranted.

Name: Lynn

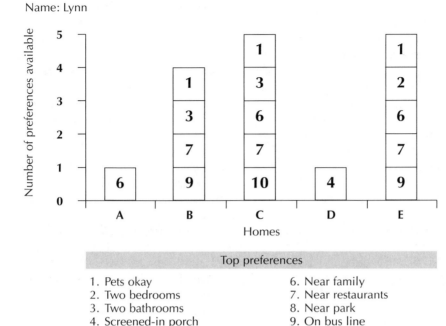

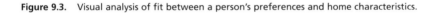

	Top preferences
1. Pets okay	6. Near family
2. Two bedrooms	7. Near restaurants
3. Two bathrooms	8. Near park
4. Screened-in porch	9. On bus line
5. Near church	10. Near grocery store

Figure 9.3.   Visual analysis of fit between a person's preferences and home characteristics.

METHOD TO INCREASE CONSUMER PARTICIPATION IN MEETINGS

Supporting an individual in identifying and moving into a preferred living arrangement is only one aspect of person-centered planning. In many cases, the person will need ongoing support and assistance to be as successful as possible in the home and to accomplish additional dreams. This support is often provided by human service agencies (Everson & Reid, 1999). Some type of plan (e.g., habilitation plan, support plan), written in a person-centered manner, is usually employed to identify the supports that an individual needs (Everson & Reid, 1999). Traditional habilitation or support planning meetings often emphasize identifying treatment goals that address an individual's deficits (McDonnell, Mathot-Buckner, & Ferguson, 1996). In contrast, person-centered planning focuses on the focus person's goals and desires and dictates that the individual plays a key role in expressing those preferences and discussing intervention goals. Research on person-centered planning has shown, however, that consumers are not as active in these meetings as desired and expected (Hagner, Helm, & Butterworth, 1996). Part of the reason may be that individuals do not know how to advocate for themselves. Yet, learning to self-advocate is probably no different than learning any other skill.

Using materials and procedures similar to those described previously in this chapter, we taught individuals with developmental disabilities to play a more active role in their planning meetings (Faw et al., 1997). As a result, those meetings became more person centered and outcome oriented. Specifically, the top 10 preferences of each individual were identified, and corresponding picture albums were developed. Using a task analysis nearly identical to the one shown in Table 9.4, individuals were shown how to make statements regarding individually determined preferences during the meetings (e.g., "I would like to come and go as I please") and how to determine whether they had access to those preferences as part of their plans. Instead of deciding whether a home was a good place to live, individuals were taught to decide whether they were happy with the answers that they received in their meeting by using a form similar to the one shown in Figure 9.2. If the individual is already living where he or she chooses to live, then the preferences may focus on supports, services, and requested community access (e.g., being able to handle one's own money, being able to come and go as one pleases).

To evaluate the impact of individuals being more active in their planning meetings, interactions between the person with the disability and the planning team should be recorded. We observed meetings in which consumers had not been taught to ask questions about their preferences and meetings in which consumers had received the training. Results revealed that when consumers were not trained, 17% of the interactions occurred between the team and the consumer, whereas the remainder of the interactions occurred among team members. In contrast, in meetings in which consumers had been trained to self-advocate, 57% of the interactions were between the team and the consumer. These results suggest that people with disabilities can be active participants in their planning meetings when provided with the right support and training.

It is important to recognize that this study is a preliminary investigation. Although the results appear promising because they show that teaching individuals to self-advocate can result in increased interactions in meetings, we do not know whether the individuals gained access to their preferences more often as a result. Additional studies should examine whether the goals and objectives included on plans that are developed at the meetings reflect consumer preferences or whether the plans continue to reflect the desires of others (i.e., the planning team). It should be noted that the desires of the consumer can be incorporated easily into the recommendations of the team. For example, if an individual expresses a desire to handle his or her own money, not only should the team find some way to address this issue because it is a preference, but also money management should be included as an objective on the plan.

From a service delivery perspective, it is important to recognize that some preferences may not be immediately available or may not be fully available. In those cases, a mutually negotiated alternative may be appropriate. Say that a person expresses a desire to have a pet. If this is not possible in the current (or future) living arrangement, then maybe that desire can be fulfilled in another way. For example, the person could volunteer at the local humane society or walk the neighbor's dog daily. In other cases, the expressed preference may not be an accurate description of the person's real desire, which may become clear upon further discussion. For instance, after talking with the individual, the desire to "live in the country" may reflect a desire to go hiking in the woods regularly. In that case, perhaps the preference originally identified as "living in the country" can be achieved by providing the person with support to go on a weekly hike. In other words, each identified preference should be discussed with the individual to ensure that the true desire is understood.

By choosing objectives that include consumer preferences, it seems likely that a more meaningful plan will be developed than one that only addresses skill deficits. In addition, when planning meetings to develop objectives focus on the individual's preferences, it seems that consumers will be more likely to report satisfaction with their meetings and plans. Finally, such an approach is consistent with the tenets of person-centered planning with respect to the values of honoring consumer preferences and dreams; assisting consumers in becoming more skilled and, therefore, more independent; and, ultimately, leading a more inclusive community life. Including individually determined preferences and having the focus person play an active role in plan development should result in a person-centered process, content, and outcome. Future research is needed to examine whether that in fact occurs.

CONCLUSION

The purpose of person-centered planning is to support individuals with disabilities in achieving the lives that they desire. To attain this goal, it is essential to understand each person's unique hopes and dreams in areas including—but not limited to—where the person wants to live. The studies that have been described in this chapter were conducted with individuals who were moving from large, congregate care settings to smaller, group living arrangements in a traditional continuum model of community living. This chapter has suggested modifications to these procedures that are consistent with the more individualized arrangements emphasized by the supported living philosophy (i.e., people living where they choose with the supports necessary to assist them in achieving that goal).

Using the systematic assessment procedures described in this chapter will not detract from the individualized nature of person-centered planning. Yet, their use should permit the person's circle of support to feel more confident that the hopes, dreams, and preferences identified are reliable, accurate indicators of his or her true wishes. In addition, by teaching a consumer to determine whether his or her preferences are available and whether a particular home is a good place to live permits that consumer to play a more central role in decisions about his or her life, a critical tenet of person-centered planning. Finally, when a consumer is able to express his or her wishes in person-centered planning meetings, the resulting support plans are more likely to reflect the consumer's preferences than his or her deficits. Future research is needed to evaluate the changes in support plans, outcomes, and consumer satisfaction that occur when a person's preferences are systematically identified and honored.

REFERENCES

Davis, P.K., O'Guin, D., & Faw, G.D. (1994). *Development of an assessment instrument to evaluate the availability of lifestyle preferences in homes serving individuals with developmental disabilities.* Unpublished manuscript, Southern Illinois University at Carbondale.

Everson, J.M., & Reid, D.H. (1999). *Person-centered planning and outcome management: Maximizing organizational effectiveness in supporting quality lifestyles among people with disabilities.* Morganton, NC: Habilitative Management Consultants.

Faw, G.D., Davis, P.K., McCord, B., Troutman, L., Holden, M., & Livesay, J. (1997, May). *Teaching people with mental retardation to self-direct their habilitation planning meetings.* Poster presented at the meeting of the Association for Behavior Analysis, Chicago.

Faw, G.D., Davis, P.K., & Peck, C. (1996). Increasing self-determination: Teaching people with mental retardation to evaluate residential options. *Journal of Applied Behavior Analysis, 29,* 173–188.

Foxx, R.M., Faw, G.D., Taylor, S., Davis, P.K., & Fulia, R. (1993). "Would I be able to . . .?" Teaching clients to assess the availability of their community living life style preferences. *American Journal of Mental Retardation, 98,* 235–248.

Hagner, D., Helm, D.T., & Butterworth, J. (1996). "This is your meeting": A qualitative study of person-centered planning. *Mental Retardation, 34,* 159–171.

McDonnell, J., Mathot-Buckner, C., & Ferguson, B. (1996). *Transition programs for students with moderate/severe disabilities.* Pacific Grove: CA: Brooks/Cole Thomson Learning.

Turnbull, H.R., Turnbull, A.P., Bronicki, G.J., Summers, J.A., & Roeder-Gordon, C. (1989). *Disability and the family: A guide to decisions for adulthood.* Baltimore: Paul H. Brookes Publishing Co.

Wehmeyer, M.L., & Metzler, C.A. (1995). How self-determined are people with mental retardation? The National Consumer Survey. *Mental Retardation, 33,* 111–119.

10

"I Don't Know How They Made it Happen, but They Did"

Efficacy Perceptions in Using a Person-Centered Planning Process

Shelley Dumas, Denise De La Garza, Penny Seay, and Heather Becker

[My plan] helped me to be my own person, take care of my family . . . and you learn a whole lot about yourself you don't even know about, like what you can do on your own . . . they still help me out but not a whole lot . . . they have more other people that need their help worser than I do . . . but I still contact them, though, ever now and then.
—Ethel, study participant with developmental disabilities

If individuals with developmental disabilities are to develop more independence and to operationalize the self-determination principles of freedom, support, authority, and responsibility (Nerney & Shumway, 1996), then they must be intrinsically involved in the shaping of their lives (Bradley, 1990). It is possible that a life based on these principles of self-determination can be achieved through a person-centered planning process, and a more effective person-centered planning process can be achieved when people and their families believe in their self-efficacy in the planning process (Bandura, 1998). An integral part of believing that person-centered planning has value in meeting needs and expectations is believing in personal agency in the process. At the heart of person-centered planning are people's beliefs, not only in the efficacy of the process, but also in their own abilities to participate in developing and carrying out activities in a plan. Without a perception of efficacious performance in an activity, people will typically abandon efforts to continue that activity (Bandura, 1998). If individuals do not believe that the process will work for them, then they are less likely to participate fully in the person-centered planning process. If they are not participating fully in the process, then it can become more agency driven than person centered or directed. Thus, self-efficacy can become part of a reciprocal process for the design of person-centered plans and the implementation of those plans.

There is little information about self-efficacy and individuals with developmental disabilities. Investigation of beliefs in self-efficacy may reveal what motivates people to initiate and continue participating in the person-centered planning process. People who are confident of their skills for participating in a person-centered planning process may expect successful outcomes and want to continue the process; people who doubt their ability to participate might have little expectation of achieving outcomes they want. It is possible that without perceptions of efficacious results, individuals with disabilities and their families will not seek to be a part of their person-centered planning process. Diminished person-centered planning participation may result in fewer opportunities for achieving freedom, support, authority, and responsibility for people with disabilities (Nerney & Shumway, 1996).

This chapter is based on a qualitative research study, designed and conducted by the first author, that examined the role of self-efficacy in the person-centered planning process of individuals with developmental disabilities. A discussion of Bandura's (1997) theory of self-efficacy, focusing specifically on personal self-efficacy and proxy self-efficacy, provides a theoretical framework. The qualitative methods used in the study are explained, along with the findings, which are based on the perceptions and experiences of the individuals interviewed. Finally, the implications of this study are considered as well as recommendations for the future efforts in person-centered planning.

THEORY OF SELF-EFFICACY

Bandura's concept of self-efficacy expectations is one of the most theoretically and practically useful concepts formulated in modern psychology in that practical applications of the theory have been shown to improve people's capacity to have a positive impact on their lives (Betz & Hackett, 1998; Pajares, 2000). Bandura (1997) defined *self-efficacy* as people's beliefs in their capacity to organize, create, and manage the circumstances that affect the course of their lives. This self-efficacy theory has been widely studied and applied in the areas of aging, education, employment, health, organizational management, psychology, social culture, sports, and technology (Pajares, 2000). Studies on practical applications of the theory have shown, for example, that people can develop capacities to deal more positively with the effects of illness or aging or that students can improve in their academic studies

(Betz & Hackett, 1998; Pajares, 2000). According to Bandura's theory, individuals have a range of self-efficacy expectations, or beliefs, in their capabilities to successfully perform a given behavior or set of behaviors. These expectations or beliefs will influence their choices, performance, and persistence in any activity (Betz & Hackett, 1998). Self-efficacy can be evident in both personal and/or proxy forms of efficacy (Bandura, 1997).

Application of the self-efficacy theory (Bandura, 1997) can provide a framework for understanding and promoting intrinsic involvement in person-centered planning by individuals with developmental disabilities and their family members. In addition, self-efficacy may influence initiation and maintenance of the person-centered planning process, and it may increase the quality of their person-centered planning participation.

Personal Efficacy

Personal efficacy theory states that a person's behavior is the result of two expectations: efficacy expectations and outcome expectations. *Efficacy expectations* are defined as perceptions or judgments about one's capability to accomplish a certain level of performance (Bandura, 1986). Efficacy expectations are the belief that one's actions make a difference. These beliefs are influenced by the following experiences: mastery experiences in which a person successfully performs a skill or behavior; vicarious experiences through which there is an opportunity to observe other people performing a skill or behavior; social persuasions in which a person receives verbal judgment or feedback about performance; and emotional and physiological states, such as stress in performing the behaviors. This information can be applied to person-centered planning to enhance the self-efficacy strategies of the process (see Table 10.1).

Outcome expectations, both immediate and distant, are important constructs of the self-efficacy theory. Bandura (1997) believed that the outcomes people expect depend on their perception of their adequate performance, or their efficacy expectations, in a given situation. People must believe, therefore, that their behavior influences outcomes. For example, a person must believe that he or she is capable of completing the person-centered plan's successive steps that are necessary to become employed (the perceived adequate behavior performance) in a job that provides more money to spend (the expected outcome). If people believe they can effectively participate in the person-centered planning process, then it is more likely that they will achieve the outcomes they expect and will continue to be involved in ongoing person-centered planning, which is a critical requirement for the success of person-centered planning (Bradley, 1990, 1994; Smull & Bellamy, 1991).

Table 10.1. Self-efficacy and person-centered planning

Strategies for developing self-efficacy	Implications for person-centered planning
Does a person have opportunity for mastery experiences? Does the person successfully perform a skill or behavior?	Does the person experience personal success in completing person-centered planning action steps toward a goal?
Does the person have vicarious experiences?	Does the person have the opportunity to observe other people with disabilities using person-centered planning to complete action steps toward a goal?
Does the person have exposure to verbal judgments of others, or social persuasions?	Does the person experience positive verbal reinforcement to be involved in a person-centered planning process?
Are the person's emotional and physiological states noted in connection with an activity?	How do the emotional or physiological states of a person (in connection with person-centered planning) affect that process?
Does the person recognize that behavior in a process influences outcomes?	Does the person recognize a connection between behavior and achieving outcomes? That is, does the person believe that he or she is capable of completing each successive action step necessary to become employed in a job that provides money to spend?

Few people are completely independent in their actions, however; most operate more from a position of interdependence. According to Bandura, human action is more appropriately described as a "product of a dynamic interplay of personal and situational influences" (1999, p. 155). This stance is most compatible with the use of person-centered planning in service delivery to people with disabilities, and it is found in the proxy form of self-efficacy.

Proxy Efficacy

According to Bandura (1997), proxy efficacy results in an individual's giving up direct control to other people to perform the activities necessary to attain outcomes. This type of efficacy behavior is often found in people who do not have control over social conditions and institutional practices. They try to get those who have expertise or who are influential to intercede on their behalf to get the desired outcomes. It can be difficult to build skills and competencies that lead to outcomes and to accept the responsibility for those outcomes. Bandura believed the underlying reason for assigning proxy efficacy is that people do not want to or cannot take on the stress that having control produces.

These reasons, plus the lack of control over social conditions and institutional practices, cause many people with cognitive disabilities to turn to advocates or people within the system to support them to get what they want (Wehmeyer, 1993). Yet, unless they have a high sense of personal efficacy to influence the actions taken on their behalf, they are vulnerable to the competency and power wielded by their advocate (Bandura, 1997).

In person-centered planning, people with cognitive disabilities may use proxy efficacy, but personal efficacy is still required to achieve a desired outcome. Similar to the concept of task analysis or Gold's (1982) concept of "try another way," individuals proximally build skills in person-centered planning if skill acquisition in the process is difficult. With experience, more responsibility is accepted, and the ability to deal with the stressors continues to develop as more control is assumed (Bandura, 1998). If planning processes are to remain person centered or directed, then it is important to know what motivates someone to be an intrinsic part of them, both initially and throughout the planning process.

METHOD

Because there is little literature about the effectiveness of using person-centered planning to direct support and service delivery, a qualitative study of perceptions of people with disabilities and their family members in using person-centered planning was used to gather information. This description of lived experiences forms a realistic body of knowledge from which the field can begin to understand the subjective aspects of person-centered planning. The following sections describe the participants, procedure, and data analysis techniques used in this study.

Participants

Thirteen individuals with developmental disabilities were interviewed for this study. In addition, five mothers of these participants agreed to take part in the study. All participants had been involved in a person-centered planning process from 6 months to 2 years, for an average of 14.8 months per family unit. The average age of the participants with developmental disabilities was 33.5 years, and the average length of time receiving services was 17 years. Twelve participants were Anglo American and one was African American. Participants had a range of support needs, from infrequent to total, as determined by the Inventory for Client and Agency Planning (ICAP; Bruininks, Hill, Weatherman, & Woodcock, 1986). The ICAP is a functional assessment tool used to determine the level of support needs of individuals served by an agency. It measures motor, social, communication, personal living, and community living skills. ICAP levels of need are extensive personal care and/or constant supervision, regular personal care and/or close supervision, limited personal care and/or regular supervision, and infrequent or no assistance for daily living.

Each participant had functional verbal communication and had participated in at least two person-centered planning meetings. Table 10.2 displays specific participant information.

Procedure

Data were collected from three different sources. Individual interviews and follow-up meetings with participants and/or family members were conducted. In addition, person-centered plans were reviewed, as well as the actual agency service plans.

Interviews   At least one face-to-face interview with each participant was conducted and audiotaped. When necessary, follow-up interviews were also scheduled. Five of the participants were unable to complete an interview because of language or communication difficulties. In these instances, close family members were identified and interviewed.

All participants were currently involved in a person-centered planning process, and each had a person-centered service plan that was facilitated by a service coordinator. All of the individuals had participated in an initial profile meeting and then in 90-day follow-up meetings, during which plans were reviewed, evaluated, or updated to meet newly identified support needs.

Based on Seidman's (1991) qualitative research interview format, the Participant Interview Guide had three separate sections and generally took approximately 1½ hours to conduct. Section One consisted of participant background information, such as living arrangement, daytime activities, services, and supports received. Section Two elicited experiences in person-centered planning. For example, participants answered questions about who participates in their person-centered planning meetings and what happens in a meeting. Section Three built on Sections One and Two and asked participants to reflect on the meaning and outcomes of their experiences with person-centered planning. Table 10.3 displays selected questions from the Participant Interview Guide.

Document Review   Two documents were reviewed for each participant. First, the person-centered plan was reviewed to determine how well it documented participants' lifestyle preferences. According to Smull (personal communication, July 28, 2000), although the person-

Table 10.2.   Participants in the study

Name	Support need	Lives with	Supported in interview by	Years in services	Time involved in person-centered planning
Brett	Infrequent	Mother	Mother	4	1 year
Ethel	Infrequent	No one	No one	22	2 years
Helen	Infrequent	Husband	No one	15	1 year
Johnny	Infrequent	No one	No one	35	1 year
Kitty	Infrequent	No one	No one	16	6 months
Sarah	Infrequent	No one	No one	14	2 years
George	Extensive	Mother	Mother	4	1 year
Coleman	Limited	Mother	Mother	3	1 year
Eugene	Limited	Girlfriend	No one	30	6 months
Scott	Limited	Parents	No one	25	1 year
Clayton	Extensive	Mother	Mother	3	1 year
Bunny	Total	Group home	No one	30	2 years
Jeffrey	Total	Parents	Mother	20	2 years

centered plan format may vary for individuals, at a minimum, each plan should reflect participant preferences throughout the six basic areas of the Essential Lifestyle Planning process (Smull, Sanderson, & Burke Harrison, 1996) that was used with participants in this study. These six areas include 1) the individual's perspective on what is

Table 10.3.   Selected questions from the Participant Interview Guide

Background Information

- Tell me about the services and supports that you have always received from the (Mental Health/Mental Retardation) agency.
- What is your living arrangement? Do you live with your family, in a group home, in a foster family home, with a roommate, or alone?
- When did you first learn about person-centered planning?
- How often do you have person-centered planning meetings?

Experience with Person-Centered Planning

- Who participates in your person-centered planning process?
- What is successful person-centered planning for you? What does a good person-centered planning meeting look like?
- Have you ever wanted something different than what your family/friends wanted for you? What happened?
- Did you get what you wanted?
- Did you feel people were listening to you?

Meaning of the Person-Centered Planning Experience

- In what way is your life different because of person-centered planning?
- Do you have more choices in your life now that you have used person-centered planning?
- Has person-centered planning helped you to identify what's important? What do you need?
- Describe an outcome for me. What is your understanding of outcomes?

important to have in life, 2) family members' or others' perspectives on what is important for the person, 3) information on how to support the person to obtain what is important in his or her life, 4) what already works in the individual's life, 5) what specific desirable activities need to be added to the person's life, and 6) what undesirable activities need to be changed or deleted. Second, the agency plan of service was reviewed to determine whether the plan's goals and objectives related to the person's stated desired outcomes.

The three data sources were compared: interview transcripts, person-centered plans, and the service agency's individual service delivery plan. The comparison provided information about what was learned from the person directly and how that learning was ultimately incorporated into a plan of action, or a service delivery plan. It was also used to assess the consistency of information in the plans (see Table 10.4).

Data Analysis

An interactive model described by Miles and Huberman (1994) was used to analyze this data. This is a process of selecting, focusing, simplifying, abstracting, and transforming the data that appear within and

Table 10.4. Participant identification and achievement status of important goals

Participant	Agency providing service (A, B, or C)	Important goal identified in interview	How goal was noted in Essential Lifestyle Planning	How goal was noted in service agency plan	Goal achieved? (yes, no, or proximal)
Coleman	Agency A	Have friends	Find social activities with other teenagers	Not noted in plan	No
Eugene	Agency A	Get a house and a dog	Prefers to live in a house and not an apartment; wants a pet	Needs assistance in determining a place to move; needs money to move	No
Helen	Agency A	Having a job in a restaurant or a pet store	Indicated job development in working with animals	Tour an animal shelter; identify 2–3 jobsites; with Helen, develop a list of interests in a pet care career	No—was placed in a job as a janitor at a Mental Health Mental/Retardation center
Johnny	Agency A	Get a vacuum cleaner	Needs support in getting a vacuum cleaner	Not noted in plan	Proximal—obtained a vacuum cleaner but no vacuum cleaner bags
Clayton	Agency B	Be included in school	Be included in general education classes and after-school care	Has direct staff funding for after-school support and service coordinator attends individualized education program meetings to advocate for inclusion	Yes
Ethel	Agency B	Get an apartment	Find a new place to live	Not noted in plan—she found a place before the agency plan was written	Yes

(continued)

231

Table 10.4. (continued)

Participant	Agency providing service (A, B, or C)	Important goal identified in interview	How goal was noted in Essential Lifestyle Planning	How goal was noted in service agency plan	Goal achieved? (yes, no, or proximal)
Scott	Agency B	Live alone in apartment	Move to his own place	Get training in independent living skills	No
Jeffrey	Agency C	Keep him at home, not in an institution	Remodel garage into a room for Jeffrey	Remodel garage with money from the agency and labor by church volunteers	Yes—remodeled the garage into his room
Brett	Agency C	Learn to play the guitar	Include this as an addendum to his original Essential Lifestyle Plan	Receive a guitar to use; arrange lessons	Proximal—began lessons
Bunny	Agency C	Have a home	Having her own home	Check with the Home of Your Own program	Proximal—moved into an apartment of her own
George	Agency C	Take sign language lessons	Needs sign language lessons	Enroll in sign language lessons	Yes
Kitty	Agency C	Get new things for her apartment	Needs wallpaper and bathroom decorations	Save money for her apartment decorations (make a budget)	Proximal—not achieved yet because she was still saving money
Sarah	Agency C	Be able to leave a job that she does not like	Is in a boring job that she dislikes	Received support to find her a new job	Proximal—moved from disliked job to another job that was also disliked, so she was looking for another job

between transcripts in an attempt to identify themes and patterns. Final conclusions were verified by rechecking transcriptions, field notes, and memos, as well as by peer review.

For a qualitative inquiry to be credible, study participants must agree that the constructed realities understood and reported by the researcher are representative of their own viewpoints. Three activities were employed to further strengthen credibility: member checks, triangulation, and peer review and debriefing (LeCompte & Preissle, 1993; Lincoln & Guba, 1985).

Member Check   The member check requires reviewing data, interpretations, and conclusions with those participants from whom the data were collected. It is often difficult to understand the perceptions of a person with a cognitive disability because of a tendency to want to please the interviewer by agreeing, accepting, or complying (Biklen & Moseley, 1988). Thus, interviewees were encouraged to give responses that reflected their true beliefs and perceptions. This was accomplished by the interviewer's use of open-ended questions, audiotaping, and a comfortable interview site for the participant. Ongoing member checks were employed to verify that the recorded responses accurately represented participants' thinking or perceptions. These checks with participants happened during the interviews and periodically throughout the data analysis process.

Triangulation   Triangulation is a procedure of checking multiple sources of information for consistency in what is being learned about the participant's constructions (Lincoln & Guba, 1985). In this study, the document review, which was a part of the data collection, was used to triangulate data gathered from the interviews. As information was gathered in an interview about what was important to an individual, that information was validated against the Essential Lifestyle Plan; the agency individual service plan; and additional field notes from interactions with other people such as family members, agency staff, or friends. Discrepancies were noted and clarified, which also helped alleviate the problem of interviewee overcompliance.

Peer Review and Debriefing   Reviewers were asked to give written suggestions for directions that the study was taking, and to comment on emerging categories, themes, and hypotheses. The peer reviewers for this study were familiar with similar qualitative research methods, disability issues, and the population of people with disabilities. One reviewer had an extensive background in person-centered planning training and individual plan development, whereas the other had participated as a member of one person's person-centered plan. The peer review included written reactions to and feedback on field notes, observer comments, and memos. Debriefing sessions with the reviewers were scheduled throughout the study and focused on identifying possible biases, exploring meanings, and clarifying interpretations and findings.

FINDINGS

In analyzing the participants' reflective comments of their experiences in the person-centered planning process, five findings, or themes, emerged from the data. These were interpreted as descriptions of the presence or absence of elements of self-efficacy. The themes were organized into the categories of personal efficacy and proxy efficacy. Three of the themes were related to personal efficacy, and two themes were related to proxy efficacy. The themes, described and illustrated in the following sections, are formative, not exhaustive. They provide a basis to begin thinking more broadly about the meaning and experience of self-efficacy for individuals with developmental disabilities.

Personal Efficacy

Efficacy is not simply about the knowledge and skill that one might have in an activity; rather, it is the belief about successfully using whatever skills and resources one has to get what is wanted (Bandura, 1997). Therefore, to begin to perceive personal efficacy in the person-centered planning process, people must have some degree of knowledge and skills in that process. More important, they must believe that successful participation in that process is possible and will have positive outcomes. Emerging themes relating to personal efficacy in the person-centered planning process included 1) an understanding of the planning process, 2) opportunities for plan implementation, and 3) control in planning services.

An Understanding of the Planning Process   Most participants in this study, as well as their family members, expressed little understanding of the person-centered planning process that was being used. Lack of understanding significantly limits the development of a sense of personal efficacy in the process. Participants' knowledge of the planning format ranged on a continuum from minimal (e.g., an awareness that there is a process but no understanding of the steps of the process) to more understanding (e.g., having knowledge of the process steps).

For example Scott expressed a minimal level of understanding of the process when he described it as follows:

> [We] talk about different things, that's all. . . . You get a couple of people and sit down. . . . I don't know, just talk, this and that, that's all I know. . . . I just hope it works out, that's what I'm hoping.

This example indicates he was aware that something was going on (the process) and that there was a meeting to share information, but he did not identify the action planning, implementation activities, and assessment of the process.

To determine whether Eugene knew the steps of the process, he was asked what kind of instructions he would give a new service coordinator on how to conduct person-centered planning. He answered, "I don't know . . . I'd just ask her . . . for help and all that, that I need help with my things and other things." Although Eugene was vague, he knew the purpose of the meetings was help and also knew he could ask.

Bunny said that her person-centered planning meetings took place with her service coordinator and that they "talk about the things that we've done and the things that we want to do . . . you've got to tell people what you want, and if you change your mind, that's okay." She, too, was minimally aware of the information sharing part of the planning process. Yet she had some recognition of assessment of the process in that she knew it was okay to change her mind if she did not like the outcomes.

Ethel indicated more understanding. She had been to a 3-day person-centered planning training session, and she described her person-centered planning meetings as follows:

> Well, I go up and see Gloria when I need something. . . . Then, we do some planning. Gloria kinda goes through that up at her office, and we keep on doing that 'til everything is done . . . what we was supposed to get done. . . . That's about it.

Ethel demonstrated a fairly clear understanding of the process. In her first plan, she indicated that she wanted to move from foster care into her own apartment. She had mastery experiences in self-efficacy expectations when she shared information with her service coordinator, reviewed the plan, and participated in plan action steps that resulted in her moving to her own rent-subsidized apartment. Ethel had knowledge and skill, as well as the belief that a plan could work for her.

Opportunities for Plan Implementation   As seen in Bunny's case, the person-centered planning process was sometimes limited because of lack of opportunities available to the participants. Although needs and desires were identified, many times plans were not implemented because of a lack of viable service or support solutions. Sometimes, outcomes could not be created because of a lack of creative support ideas generated within the existing agency rules and regulations.

Bunny had clearly identified a desire to move from a group home, where she had roommates, into a home of her own. Speaking of her roommates, she said,

> That's why I want to move. . . . I want to get to move. I want to pick. I want to get out of here. . . . my roommate makes noise and she hollers and the [staff] that lives here gets up at 4 A.M. and they are so loud, so rowdy . . . and [my roommate] won't let me have a puppy.

Written into her plan was beginning the process to find a home. In a follow-up interview, Bunny was asked how the plan to move into her own home was progressing. She responded, "It's at a standstill now. It's at a standstill. Strangely enough we don't have any money to fund a house." Asked whether she would consider moving to an apartment, Bunny refused, saying,

> There's too much killing going on in an apartment. In a house you got time to move, but in [an apartment] they sneak up on you . . . and the landlord sneaks up on you. . . . They've got a pass key and you never know when they're going to come in. So I don't want no apartment for myself . . . and you can't have a puppy in an apartment.

Obviously, creative support ideas around safety in the apartment complex environment could have been generated as well as other actions to work toward pet ownership.

When asked if things were better now that a person-centered planning process was in place, Eugene answered, "Not really . . . 'cause I don't like living where I'm at." Eugene had asked for supports to move because his apartment had no hot water for almost a month. In a follow-up interview a month later, Eugene was asked if he had hot water yet. He informed the interviewer that the building still had no hot water and that "they use the water in the swimming pool. . . . That's why I want to get out of there as soon as I can." Moving to a new apartment was not an option because of his bad credit history with the local apartment association, and no creative or alternative living arrangements were being explored.

Control in Planning Services   Like Sarah, most participants seemed to believe that they were prisoners of program models of service delivery rather than free agents in gaining access to individualized services and supports. An important factor in developing self-efficacy expectations is having perceptions of control in one's life, the idea that one is not totally helpless to have an impact on his or her environment (Wehmeyer, 1994, 1995). To have a sense of self-efficacy in a person-centered planning process, people must believe they have some possibility of control in gaining access to services and supports. Certainly in the realm of human services, and especially for people with developmental disabilities and their family members, a lack of perceived personal control is often pervasive throughout the service delivery system (Wehmeyer, 1995). In this study, many participants' and their family members' perceptions of control were more external than internal. Instead of believing that they could use person-centered planning to have supports structured to meet their individual needs, most participants believed their only choice was to go along with choosing from an existing array of services. Little real personal efficacy was observed.

When Sarah was asked whether person-centered planning helped her determine what was important, she responded, "Yes . . . it's easier to know what you want to do . . . but I felt pressured into having to find a job . . . and I have been kind of forced to make decisions which I'm not ready for." Her plan revealed that she wanted to work but only part time because of her husband's disability. Instead, a full-time job was developed for her, and she believed that she had no option but to take the job.

Johnny left a large state institution to live in his own apartment in the community. He was very proud of his home and was a fastidious housekeeper. In his first person-centered plan, he identified that he needed a vacuum cleaner to keep his apartment clean. Six months later, he still had not gotten a vacuum, but he believed that there was still a possibility of getting one. He said, "Gonna get one [a vacuum] pretty soon . . . [my service coordinator] is gonna give me the money . . . it's in my plan." At some point in the next 3 months, a new service coordinator found a funding source for the purchase of a vacuum that arrived with extra bags. Within a few months, Johnny had used all of the bags and asked his service coordinator for a supply of new bags. Two weeks after the request, he still had no bags; the service coordinator said that the requisition had been made but approval to buy the bags still had not been granted.

It took almost 9 months for Johnny to get his vacuum cleaner. He had little belief that he could direct his service plan so that he could receive vacuum cleaner bags on a regular basis. After many years of institutionalization, Johnny believed that he just had to wait for something to happen; circumstances with his plan continued to support that belief. Johnny had the skills—that is, he could have picked up a telephone and called for bags—but he had no perception of himself as having the control or power to do that.

Many of the participants believed that person-centered planning gave them more control, albeit limited, because they also still believed that they had to accept whatever services and supports were offered to

them. Although service providers were listening better, many participants' plans were still shackled by inflexible rules and regulations.
They appeared to have no perception that they could use the person-
centered planning process to develop more creative means of support
and service delivery.

Summary   Although these interviews and plan reviews indicate
little understanding of the planning process, few fully realized outcomes, and little sense of control, an interesting undercurrent runs
through these snapshots: hope. This study focused on self-efficacy;
however, the value of a qualitative study is that unexpected phenomena can often emerge from the data. It was surprising to see the degree
of optimism and hope expressed by participants even when outcomes
were delayed or nonexistent. This hopefulness certainly could be considered as much an aspect of ongoing person-centered planning's success as the concrete outcomes.

Participants were achieving some immediate goals, such as obtaining an apartment, but not distant goals, such as home ownership or
having a puppy. Even having no realistic expectations of achieving outcomes, which is a critical concept in developing self-efficacy, most participants continued to be optimistic that their lives would get better
because they believed that their service coordinators would make it
happen. This outlook is consistent with another category of efficacy:
proxy efficacy.

Proxy Efficacy

According to Bandura (1999), people often turn to proxy efficacy even
when situations allow them to be in some degree of control. This may
occur because they do not know what to do, they believe that others
can do it better, or they do not want to take on the complexities of direct
control. The participants' service agencies were attempting to become
more responsive to individual needs and to offer more individual
choice and control in services, yet most of the participants appeared to
primarily use proxy efficacy. Service coordinators were trained to be
the facilitators of the plans. As a result, most participants believed that
the service coordinators were the major factors that either facilitated or
inhibited the person-centered planning process. Two final themes
emerged in the study relating to the category of proxy efficacy: service
coordinators as agents of success in achieving plan outcomes and service coordinators as agents of failure in achieving plan outcomes. In the
first case, the proxy or service coordinator was personally responsible
for positive plan outcomes; in the second, the service coordinator was
personally responsible for plan failure.

Service Coordinators as Agents of Success   Scott's statement, "I wouldn't get nothing at all if I didn't have her," captures that belief of the service coordinator as the change agent, not the plan itself. Participants believed that they could expect outcomes because they asked service coordinators do things for them. These perceptions are an excellent example of Bandura's (1999) description of proxy efficacy. Proxy efficacy, or relying on the efforts of others, occurs most often when people do not have direct control over conditions and institutional practices that affect their lives. Many of this study's participants had long histories of institutionalization and learned helplessness. It was natural for them to rely almost completely on service coordinators to use the person-centered planning process to attain outcomes. Family members also relied heavily on service coordinators, although not as much as the participants.

George's mother was asked what caused an increase in services, such as sign language and assistive technology, for her son. There was a magical quality in her description of what the service provider did:

> It was important for George to have [sign language and assistive technology]. . . . It's amazing how much [sign language] changed his whole attitude toward life. He's communicating and people listen. . . . and they made it happen. I don't know how they made it happen, but they did.

Eugene had the experience of changing service coordinators and found the new person, who now facilitated his person-centered plan, to be a significant improvement. He commented, "Well . . . I just like doing a lot of things with [my service coordinator]. I think she's nice." When asked how the new service coordinator was an improvement, Eugene said, "Well, things changed on me. . . . She's trying to help me now. . . . She's trying to help me make better things in life . . . like, being independent and all that."

Bunny believed that her service coordinator was what made her person-centered plan work. When asked how she could make the person-centered planning process work if her service coordinator left, she responded, "They would have to hire someone to take his place. That's all. That would be rather hard because [he] is really special."

Service Coordinators as Agents of Failure   In this study, the assignees—that is, the participants' service coordinators and person-centered planning facilitators—were also seen as possible inhibitors or reasons for failure in facilitating outcomes. In Scott's case, proxy efficacy was only as useful as the assignee's degree of ability to achieve outcomes for the assignor (Bandura, 1997).

Scott's hope that his service coordinator (Tricia) was getting him an apartment is a good example of proxy efficacy with little personal and assignee efficacy. Scott's personal efficacy was "wheedling"—that is, continuing to ask his service coordinator to get him an apartment. He asked, and asked, and asked again. As Scott said, "I try . . . I try, all I can do is try." However, he lived at home with his parents, who were strongly against his moving out; Tricia was having difficulty in facilitating Scott's desired outcome because she did not believe that she could resolve the conflict with his parents. Tricia stated in a follow-up planning meeting for Scott that she did not know what to do because his parents would not discuss Scott's wish to move. Not only was she unable to resolve the family conflict, but she also apparently could not generate creative viable solutions to the problem.

As an individual with disabilities, Helen evidenced considerable personal efficacy in combination with proxy efficacy. Although she depended on the service coordinator for arranging the details of one of her goals (home ownership), she also participated to some extent by going out on her own to look for houses that would meet her criteria. She filled out the paperwork and met with a lender. When asked what had happened since the first person-centered planning meeting, she said, "Well, I got a job . . . and I am working on trying to arrange to get enough money for the house . . . [I've] looked at houses and they're expensive." At the time of this study, however, the process had fallen apart because the service coordinator did not believe that she could overcome the mortgage lender's objections to the home purchase, and she was not seeking the support of outside organizations (e.g., Home of Your Own) to support Helen in the process. Helen's use of proxy efficacy was only as good as the efficacy of her service coordinator, who was having difficulty in overcoming barriers to support Helen's achieving her goal.

In addition, Helen's service coordinator had assistance in obtaining a job for Helen; yet, it was not the type of work that Helen had requested in her plan. Helen had hoped to work in a restaurant or in a pet store (she loved animals and could not have one of her own). Instead she was working as a janitor at the provider agency. Helen said, "I'd rather work as a janitor than stay home . . . I had to get the janitor work." Although the service coordinator and job development staff had listened to what was important to Helen, they had placed her in a type of job that Helen did not request.

Summary   In this study, most participants were still giving control to their service coordinators. Nonetheless, there was evidence of participants beginning to display potential for self-efficacy in a process that was beginning to provide preferred outcomes. Perceptions of what facilitated or inhibited the process, as well as what parts of the person-centered planning process worked and did not work, were beginning to surface in the participants' awareness of the process.

It is logical that individuals who have experienced extensive institutionalization more easily relinquish control to professionals. In many cases, individuals with disabilities are unable to negotiate complex social service systems and they need help. There is a difference between help and control, and the service coordinators in this study often seemed unable to differentiate them or to recognize the ways that they assumed control.

IMPLICATIONS

The findings indicate both positive and negative aspects of the person-centered planning process for these participants. We hope that this information provides a basis to facilitate the development of more effective and efficacious person-centered planning processes, with resulting increased self-determination, for people with developmental disabilities and their family members.

An important aspect of these findings is the lack of understanding many participants had about their own person-centered planning process. For many participants, the plan seemed capricious and out of their control. Institutional behaviors that prevented individuals from taking action, and control seemed pervasive. Most participants understood the process to be dependent on the service coordinator, a single person affiliated with an agency, and not on the plan. Participants did not seem to connect their actions in the planning process with achieving outcomes. Therefore, person-centered planning processes need to include assistance for people to increase their own self-efficacy, however limited or complex, in developing and implementing ongoing plans.

Another striking aspect of the data was the simplicity of many requests, such as a vacuum cleaner. Those unique requests can only be known by close, consistent, and long-term interactions that are possible in the person-centered planning process. It was also interesting to note the consistency of the big goals. Many participants wanted a job, a house, and a dog. The undercurrent of those requests is the emotional need for security and relationships—basic human longings that must be appreciated and respected in individuals with developmental disabilities.

It can be easy to focus on what did not happen for participants and to lament that what did happen occurred slowly, as part of this chapter's purpose is to highlight what can be improved and expanded in the person-centered planning process. However, it is essential to appreciate that some things did change for the participants: jobs were found, living arrangements were changed, vacuum cleaners were purchased. The participants, individuals with developmental disabilities, were actually asked what they wanted and what they preferred. Even when those preferences were not what the service provider might have chosen, they were often honored. The result, sometimes even without concrete outcomes, was the participants' hope and belief that life would get better. The optimism expressed by most of the participants may simply have been a result of the attention and communication, but hope and belief combined with skills and knowledge can be a powerful force for self-efficacy and change.

Limitations

Limitations of this study included interviewing a small number of people involved in a specific person-centered planning process, interviewing people who needed interpretive supports, and having only one face-to-face interview with many participants. In this study, the single interview with participants limited the researcher's ability to investigate changes over time. If multiple interviews had been conducted with each participant, then the outcome might have been a fuller picture of their journeys through the person-centered planning process. The snapshots from this study lend support for further research with more interviews over time per participant. Even with these limitations, the study provided a basis for developing strategies that create supportive environments for individuals, agencies, and communities to build self-efficacy for person-centered planning.

Recommendations

If the heart of person-centered planning is the full involvement of individuals with disabilities, then an emphasis on self-efficacy is a logical addition to training in the planning process. This training and technical assistance should be comprehensive and include people with disabilities and their families, service agency staff, and community members. The training is self-fulfilling in that any training in the planning process enhances self-efficacy, and training specifically in self-efficacy enhances participation in the person-centered planning process.

Training agendas for individuals should include opportunities for learning with structured practice of self-efficacy concepts. Helping to increase a person's self-efficacy may be a general way to increase life satisfaction, and it would most immediately help with involvement in the person-centered planning process. In fact, increasing self-efficacy in the context of person-centered planning can provide the first steps to developing self-efficacy in other life skills areas. People with developmental disabilities and their families need training in the person-centered planning process, self-advocacy, and negotiation skills (Smull & Bellamy, 1991). Individuals receiving training should also have opportunities to see other people successfully engaged in the steps of the planning process.

Training alone is not adequate, however; mentoring or technical assistance should always be factored into any training endeavor. All people benefit by having opportunities for practicing what they have learned, receiving feedback, and then practicing the learning again. For people with disabilities, having a mentor is necessary, in much the same way as having a job coach.

The marriage of self-efficacy training with information on person-centered planning would be useful for all parties involved in person-centered planning. Agency staff, community members, and family members should receive background knowledge of person-centered planning process steps, mediation and negotiation skills, and mentoring skills. Effective training to increase self-efficacy within the person-centered planning process should also include failure training: how to help individuals rebound when impediments or barriers occur or strategies to use when a person fails. With repeated failures, people gain or regain self-efficacy with graduated steps in the process (Bandura, 1998). Agency staff and community and family members often need support in learning to develop a tolerance for allowing people with disabilities to fail and to learn from those failures.

The concept of self-efficacy is not limited to an individual level. Another important area of self-efficacy training includes the concept of collective efficacy and how that type of advocacy results in systems change. Bandura (1997) defined *collective efficacy* as a group's shared belief in its capabilities as a group to organize and implement the actions needed to produce outcomes; group members work together to achieve what they cannot accomplish alone. Although group collaboration is an implicit assumption of person-centered planning processes, techniques in collaborative and collective planning might be further promoted and enhanced. Helping people with disabilities and families to develop collective efficacy as they move toward fully realized self-efficacy could be a key factor in training success. A person-centered planning team is an example of a group using collective efficacy; the group attainments are products of team members' shared knowledge and/or the skills of individual members (Bandura, 1997). A person with developmental disabilities contributes knowledge of what is important and what is desirable to attain, whereas other group members (e.g., family, friends, agency staff, community members) apply their knowledge and skills to make possible the attainment of those goals. Working collaboratively in groups to initiate, develop, implement, assess, and maintain person-centered plans may be a more effective way to change systems than to use personal efficacy alone

(Bandura, 1998). Including a broad perspective in training would be beneficial in achieving greater outcomes in the planning process.

If you are an administrator or practitioner, then it is hoped that this chapter has given you a framework for assessing the self-efficacy strategies that are built into your own person-centered planning process. The continuous evaluation of your person-centered planning program to include strategies that support and enhance the self-efficacy of participants will ensure the empowerment and genuine choice making of the individuals with disabilities whom the plan is designed to support. Does your planning process include opportunities for mastery, opportunities to see others' planning processes, and feedback experiences for individuals having plans? Routinely ask yourself whether your plans reflect a balance between what is important to the person and what is important for the person, such as health and safety issues. Are those plans flexible enough to allow consumers to explore and to change their minds? Does consumer preference exploration include the awareness of the individual's need to please or comply? Do you work toward outcomes even when the ultimate goals feel impossible, or do you ignore a person's preference when the barriers seem insurmountable? Is there an organizational system in place so that resources can be shared, ideas brainstormed, and problems creatively solved? Is there an organizational culture of trust, respect, and partnership, which must be present for real person-centered planning to take hold and take place? Continuous evaluation will result in a person-centered planning process that is empowering and focused on what is important to the individual.

CONCLUSION: LOOKING TO THE FUTURE

The importance of person-centered planning in the lives of individuals with developmental disabilities cannot be overstated. In the study described in this chapter, individuals received operational support and achieved some self-identified outcomes. It is easy as a professional to look at what the individuals did not obtain and ask why, but one also must focus on what was gained. As noted, one of the most significant gains for the individuals in this study may have been hope. Many of these individuals lived in state institutions for several years of their lives and, by many standards, would have little reason to hope that anything could change for the better. The fact that the ongoing person-centered planning process gave them a reason to hope and dream—to imagine themselves in a home with a puppy—is reason enough to say this process is valuable. If we believe that the lives and perspectives of individuals with disabilities have value, then we believe that this process has value and should be continued, expanded, and implemented as well and as completely as possible.

Those in the field always need to know more. This study was the first to examine self-efficacy beliefs of people with developmental disabilities and their family members in the person-centered planning process. It illuminated a need for further research on personal, proxy, and collective efficacy of people with developmental disabilities and their families, as well as agency staff, as they navigate the human service system. If training programs are implemented that incorporate self-efficacy concepts, then they should be thoroughly evaluated in terms of individual and program outcomes.

Bandura's theory indicated that people's beliefs in their efficacy affect almost everything they do (i.e., how they think, motivate themselves, feel, and behave). Thus, it is reasonable to assume that an individual's capacity to effectively participate in person-centered planning is compromised by low expectations; lack of control, solutions, and opportunities; and the exclusive use of proxy efficacy. This study demonstrated that people with developmental disabilities and their families have the capacity to be personally and collectively efficacious in the person-centered planning process, and they want the planning process to continue. If person-centered planning is to continue being widely used, then the field must support people to move beyond accepting the service delivery status quo to expecting the achievement of their desired outcomes.

REFERENCES

Bandura, A. (1986). *Social foundations of thought and action: A social cognitive theory.* Upper Saddle River, NJ: Prentice Hall.

Bandura, A. (1997). *Self-efficacy: The exercise of control.* New York: W.H. Freeman.

Bandura, A. (1998, March). *Health promotion through self-efficacy.* Paper presented at the Thirteenth Annual LaVerne Gallman Distinguished Lecture in Nursing, Austin, TX.

Bandura, A. (1999). Social cognitive theory of personality. In L. Pervin & O. John (Eds.), *Handbook of personality* (2nd ed., p. 155). New York: The Guilford Press.

Betz, N., & Hackett, G. (1998). *Manual for the Occupational Self-Efficacy Scale* [Online]. Available: http://seamonkey.ed.asu.edu/~gail/occse1.htm.

Biklen, S.K., & Moseley, C.R. (1988). "Are you retarded?" "No, I'm Catholic": Qualitative methods in the study of people with severe handicaps. *Journal of The Association for Persons with Severe Handicaps, 13*(3), 155–162.

Bradley, V.J. (1990). Conceptual issues in quality assurance. In V.J. Bradley & H.A. Bersani (Eds.), *Quality assurance for individuals with developmental disabilities: It's everybody's business* (pp. 3–15). Baltimore: Paul H. Brookes Publishing Co.

Bradley, V.J. (1994). Evolution of a new service paradigm. In V.J. Bradley, J.W. Ashbaugh, & B.C. Blaney (Eds.), *Creating individual supports for people with developmental disabilities: A mandate for change at many levels* (pp. 11–32). Baltimore: Paul H. Brookes Publishing Co.

Bruininks, R.H., Hill, B.K., Weatherman, R.F., & Woodcock, R.W. (1986). *Inventory for Client and Agency Planning.* Itasca, IL: The Riverside Publishing Co.

Gold, M.W. (1982). *A look at values with Dr. Marc Gold* [Video]. Ocean Springs, MS: Marc Gold & Associates.

LeCompte, M.D., & Preissle, J. (1993). *Ethnography and qualitative design in educational research.* San Diego: Academic Press.

Lincoln, Y.S., & Guba, E.G. (1985). *Naturalistic inquiry.* Thousand Oaks, CA: Sage Publications.

Miles, M.B., & Huberman, A.M. (1994). *Qualitative data analysis: An expanded sourcebook.* Thousand Oaks, CA: Sage Publications.

Nerney, T., & Shumway, D. (1996). *Beyond managed care: Self-determination for people with disabilities.* Concord, NH: The Self-Determination National Program Office.

Pajares, F. (2000). *Information on self-efficacy* [On-line]. Available: http://www.emory.edu/EDUCATION/mfp/effpage.html.

Seidman, I.E. (1991). *Interviewing as qualitative research: A guide for researchers in education and the social sciences.* New York: Teachers College Press.

Smull, M.W., & Bellamy, G.T. (1991). Community services for adults with disabilities: Policy challenges in the emerging support paradigm. In L.H. Meyer, C.A. Peck, & L. Brown (Eds.), *Critical issues in the lives of people with severe disabilities* (pp. 527–536). Baltimore: Paul H. Brookes Publishing Co.

Smull, M.W., Sanderson, H., & Burke Harrison, S. (1996). *Reviewing essential lifestyle plans: Criteria for best plans.* Unpublished manuscript.

Wehmeyer, M.L. (1993). Sounding a certain trumpet: Case management as a catalyst for the empowerment of people with developmental disabilities. *Journal of Case Management, 2,* 14–18.

Wehmeyer, M.L. (1994). Employment status and perceptions of control of adults with cognitive and developmental disabilities. *Research in Developmental Disabilities, 15,* 119–131.

Wehmeyer, M.L. (1995). How self-determined are people with mental retardation? *Mental Retardation, 33,* 111–119.

11

Active Support

Planning Daily Activities and Support for People with Severe Mental Retardation

David Felce, Edwin Jones, and Kathy Lowe

Mount defined *person-centered planning* as "an approach for learning about people with disabilities and creating a lifestyle that can help people contribute in community life" (1998, p. 55). It is a means to an end; it is not advocated for its own sake but as a mechanism to improve a person's quality of life. According to Routledge and Sanderson, the objective of person-centered planning is "to support the person to have the lifestyle that they choose in their local community," with "self-determination, relationships and valued social roles" being given the highest priority (2000, p. 10). The selected priorities have a restricted breadth compared to most definitions of quality of life. However, this restriction is probably not intended to deny the importance of other aspects of the human condition, such as health, self-image, income, employment, or activity interests. Accordingly, one might consider that an understanding of quality of life as experienced by citizens in general, as well as by people with mental retardation, would be central to implementing person-centered planning.

Typically, quality of life refers to the breadth of lived experience. Most commentators agree that it is a multidimensional construct that must reflect the essential aspects of human existence. Therefore, a concern for a person's quality of life provides a potentially broad agenda encompassing such diverse areas as

- Physical well-being
- Emotional well-being
- Interpersonal relationships

The research reported in this chapter was supported by two grants from the Wales Office of Research and Development for Health and Social Care.

- Social inclusion and belonging
- Material circumstances and security
- Personal development and identity
- Self-determination
- Rights
- Occupation, contribution, or role at home or in school, the work-place, or the community (e.g., Cummins, 1997; Felce, 1997; Schalock, 1996)

In common parlance, the word *quality* suggests excellence. The focus of interest is to establish whether life is experienced as good and whether circumstances that constrain quality of life can be altered to allow life experiences to improve.

People differ in their preferences and interests and what they want from life. There is not a uniform standard for quality of life. Having personal values and self-determination in line with preferences is crit-ical at an individual level in the pursuit of a fulfilling day-to-day lifestyle and longer-term accomplishments. Hence, a structure is required to allow individuals to set the direction for their lives and to decide arrangements that affect them. Person-centered planning pro-vides such a structure. However, the emphasis on individual determi-nation should not prevent recognition that people with substantial dis-abilities may be at a general disadvantage in conducting their lives within environments and social structures or processes that are de-signed for and maintained by people without such disabilities.

There is now considerable evidence that objective indicators of many quality of life domains among people with mental retardation are significantly correlated with personal ability as assessed by a stan-dardized adaptive behavior scale. Stancliffe and Lakin reported that "a striking feature of the analyses of individual outcomes was the consis-tently strong positive relation with adaptive behavior" (1998, p. 565). Higher ability was related to greater variety of community environ-ments used, more social activities, better community inclusion, more contact with family members, and greater choice. Emerson and col-leagues found that personal ability "was the single most powerful pre-dictor of variation in the quality of outcomes experienced" (1999, p. xi). Higher ability was associated with greater use of leisure and commu-nity facilities, greater social inclusion, greater choice, and a more active lifestyle. Associations between higher ability and both more frequent social and community activities and greater participation in activity have also been found by Felce, Jones, and Lowe (in press); Felce, Lowe, Beecham, and Hallam (2000); Hatton, Emerson, Robertson, Henderson, and Cooper (1996); and Perry, Felce, and Lowe (2000). Perry and colleagues (2000) and Felce and colleagues (2000) also found that higher ability was associated with greater choice and autonomy.

The consistency of these findings across different groups of research participants suggests that severity of developmental disability constrains the achievement of a variety of common life experiences. The associations found between individual ability and lifestyle outcome can be ascribed to personal preference only if people with more severe mental retardation actually want lower self-determination, less social and community participation, and less constructive occupation than their counterparts with less severe disabilities and, by extension, citizens in general. However, there is no evidence in support of this proposition. A much more reasonable assumption would be that people with severe mental retardation are no different than others in the nature and diversity of their personal lifestyle preferences. In other words, one would hypothesize that all things being equal, lifestyle would be independent of measured personal characteristics such as adaptive ability. The fact that an association is so clearly evident between adaptive ability and a range of quality of life indicators suggests that not all things are equal. People with more severe mental retardation appear to experience significant disadvantage. The way that societal arenas (e.g., homes, workplaces, community amenities) function discriminates against people with mental retardation in leading typical lifestyles.

This analysis is consistent with the redefinition of level of disability in terms of intensity of needed support arrangements (Schalock et al., 1994). It highlights the imperative to enhance typical environmental conditions for people with significant disabilities by providing a sufficient "bridge," which enables them to achieve a quality of life that is within the normative range and reflects their personality, values, and aspirations. Active Support is designed to provide a bridge to participation in everyday activities for people who lack the skills to participate independent of assistance. In brief, Active Support is a way of training staff in small community residences to plan and monitor activities in consultation with or on behalf of residents with severe mental retardation, as well as to interact with them in a way that supports and encourages their participation in the activity. (Active Support is described more fully later in this chapter.)

The remainder of this chapter considers 1) the importance of participation in activity as an indicator of quality of life, 2) the need for Active Support among people with severe or profound mental retardation, 3) implementing Active Support—that is, staff training and its relationship to supporting choice, 4) our research on the impact of

Active Support, and 5) our conclusions about the wider implications of this research.

IMPORTANCE OF PARTICIPATION IN ACTIVITY

As illustrated by the foregoing discussion, people with severe mental retardation have restricted experience in many aspects of life. Our work on Active Support has proceeded from a concern that such people are usually not given the support required to participate in the activities which typify daily life. Rather, activities are frequently done for them. As a result, people are not given the opportunity to occupy the multiplicity of valued social roles that characterize the way that society is organized. In thinking only about home life, for example, one can be a cook; a cleaner; a good neighbor; a shopper; a gardener; an activity partner; or the person who does the laundry, decorating, or household maintenance. Participation and contribution are valued; passivity and dependence are not. Our view is that the commonly observed passivity and dependency of people with severe mental retardation (even when apparently "doing" an activity with a supporter) is greater than it should be.

Although some commentators do refer to the importance of daily rituals and the ordinary nature of what most people want (e.g., Smull, 1998a, 1998b), we are conscious that making participation in everyday activities a priority is out of step with the common appeal to bigger-sounding themes found in the language surrounding person-centered planning. Whereas others talk of empowerment, self-determination, relationships, visions, and dreams, we appear to be interested in promoting the mundane. One hardly wants to dream about getting the laundry done. So, why have we persisted with this emphasis when others have not?

Our first reason is based in the fact that participation in activity refers to the process of everyday living. People interact with their social and physical environments, second by second, minute by minute, hour by hour, day by day, conducting their affairs. "I was bored; there wasn't enough to do," "It's been a good day; I achieved a lot," and "Life is crazy at the moment; I haven't stopped all day" are familiar and meaningful commentaries on life. Whether people are satisfied with what they have done during the day plays a large part in how they sum up the day and, successively over time, what they might think about their quality of life.

Second, many of the grander-sounding quality of life abstractions are what Gilbert (1978), Gilbert and Gilbert (1992), and O'Brien (1987) term *accomplishments*. Accomplishments are states of existence that endure beyond the transient ebb and flow of moment-to-moment behavior. O'Brien (1987), for example, listed five accomplishments that ordinary citizens have or acquire: community presence, community participation, competence, status and respect, and choice and rights. However, neither Gilbert nor O'Brien suggest that gaining accomplishment can be divorced from participation in everyday activities. Accomplishments cannot be attained in a vacuum. They are gained or conferred as a result of engaging in life. Therefore, we believe that it is impossible to achieve the accomplishments set out by O'Brien unless steps are taken to support people with severe mental retardation to be participants in, rather than observers of, life. Unfortunately, supporting such people to participate in conducting their own affairs rather than doing activities for them appears to be a skill that is not naturally taught to ordinary community members. Instilling such an approach, therefore, becomes a matter for staff training, which is detailed later in this chapter.

THE NEED FOR ACTIVE SUPPORT

The often gross understimulation and lack of constructive activity experienced in institutional services was a familiar and depressing problem. The move to small-scale community housing carried the expectation that access to more normative environments and opportunities would set the occasion for a radically improved pattern of existence. Yet, there is evidence that low participation in activity, at least among people with severe mental retardation, is an enduring problem, even in decent homelike environments with high staffing levels and apparent adherence to contemporary service philosophies (Emerson & Hatton, 1996; Emerson et al., 2000; Felce & Perry, 1995). Moreover, in critical ways, how staff do their jobs has not been sufficiently altered. If patterns of support were related to need, then one would have expected people with lower assessed adaptive behavior to receive more attention and, in particular, more practical assistance to do activities than their colleagues who have more skills. However, research has found that neither attention nor assistance is differentiated in favor of people with greater support needs (Felce & Perry, 1995; Felce et al., 1998; Felce et al. 1999; Hewson & Walker, 1992). The great majority of staff attention given to people supported in community homes is in the form of conversation, which contributes little to enabling participation in activity.

A housing development project in Britain for adults with severe and profound mental retardation provided a rare example of staff–resident interaction patterns relating to service users' needs for support

(Felce, de Kock, & Repp, 1986). People with lower assessed adaptive behavior received more attention than people with higher assessed adaptive behavior, and approximately 75% of the attention received was in the form of assistance to do activities. As a result, people with more severe disabilities had higher levels of engagement in activity than have been found in other small-scale community housing (Felce, 1996). These findings were interpreted as dependent on the organizational approach followed by staff. Staff were trained to 1) plan opportunities for service user activity proactively; 2) plan their own division of responsibility for supporting that activity; 3) support people's participation by supplementing verbal instruction with gestural or physical prompting, demonstration, or physical guidance as necessary and increasing the help provided until the person was able to participate in the activity successfully; 4) give the majority of their attention to people when people were constructively occupied; and 5) monitor the opportunities provided to individuals each day.

This approach has come to be called Active Support. The following subsection describes Active Support in more detail. Subsequent sections discuss staff training for Active Support and our work in evaluating the experimental introduction of Active Support within community residences.

Active Support Defined

The previously outlined five components of Active Support involve three organizational elements: 1) staff use a paper-based system for planning activities and the use of their time on a daily basis, 2) staff interact with those whom they support in a way that encourages participation in these activities, and 3) staff use a paper-based system for recording and summarizing the activities that individuals have been given the opportunity to do.

In terms of planning daily life, it appears that most people tread a path somewhere between the two extremes of having no shape to their days or weeks and having a rigid and unchanging routine. Most people have a sense of routine, which may reflect their personal interests and their roles and responsibilities within the family or household in which they live. Often, it is the busy nature of life and the richness of opportunity and social interdependency that necessitate planning and organization. Yet, people also appreciate change and spontaneity and want to be in control of their lives. Plans and routine should be sufficiently flexible to serve the best interests of people, not to overrule them.

The planning within Active Support attempts to strike a balance between flexibility and rigidity by recognizing the following:

- There may be an implicit weekly routine of major household tasks (e.g., preparing breakfast Monday through Friday at a regular time, doing most of the laundry or shopping on particular days).

- Individuals may have activity interests that are arranged or occur at routine times (e.g., talking to a friend who tends to call on a particular evening, attending a club at a regular time, following a television series that has a regular time).

- Some activities are regularly done by individuals and others are done either by taking turns or out of choice.

- A need exists for times that are free to do irregular, new, or unusual activities to add variety and interest to life.

Decision-making about who is going to do what and when needs to allow for spontaneity; therefore, it should be possible to change plans as circumstances dictate. An example of an Activity and Support Plan is given in Figure 11.1. It covers part of one day. In practice, meals are good times to discuss what everyone wants to do the next morning, afternoon, or evening. In this example, time unfolds down the left-hand axis and the columns refer to people's activities (one column per person), household activities, and other activity options. It is important to stress that we have only implemented Active Support within small community residences, where the idea of having individualized activity schedules is realistic.

A basic weekly timetable is first devised by listing all regular activities—that is, all domestic, gardening, and maintenance activities that are done to keep up household standards; each person's personal and self-care activities; and each person's regular leisure, vocational, and social activities—and the typical times at which they are done. These are then transferred to the various Activity and Support Plans spanning the week. All activities that are particular to an individual are located in that individual's activity column. These may form personal preferences or agreed-on contributions to household tasks. Otherwise, regular household tasks that are usually done at that time but not necessarily by a particular individual are listed in the "Household" column. In addition, episodic activities or other possible activity options are listed in the "Options" column.

Planning on the day achieves two things: 1) activities from the undesignated household and options lists are distributed among people to ensure that people have the opportunity of reasonably full occupation and 2) staff assign themselves to support particular individuals and activities. Both of these objectives are indicated on Figure 11.1 by entries made in bold script. The reverse side of the planning grid can

Activity and Support Plan

Support worker (SW) shift times   *Monday morning*

SW: *Anne Jones*   Time: *7:00-1:30*   SW: *Helen Ingram* Time: *1:15-5:15*
SW: *Colin Edwards* Time: *7:00-1:30*   SW: *Janet Davies* Time: *2:00-10:00*

Time	Olive	SW	Roger	SW	Diane	SW	Household	Options
7:00	Get up, wash, dress **Put trash out**	AJ	Get up, wash, dress Prepare breakfast	CE	Get up, wash, dress (on own) **Set table**	AJ	Put trash out Set table	
8:00	Eat breakfast	AJ	Eat breakfast	CE	Eat breakfast	CE		
8:30	**Clear breakfast dishes**	AJ	Wash up/load dishwasher	AJ	**Start laundry**	CE	Clear breakfast dishes Wash up/load dishwasher Start laundry	
9:00	Shopping	CE	Clean bedroom and bathroom	AJ	Go shopping and to the post office— collect benefit and pay bills	CE		Take a good walk Water the plants
10:00			Start laundry	AJ				
	Unpack groceries	CE	Have coffee with mother	Mrs. F	Finish laundry	AJ	Unload dishwasher and stack coffee cups	Do gardening Cut the grass
11:00	Have coffee with Diane **Do gardening Cut grass**	CE	Have physiotherapy session **Unload dishwasher and stack cups**	FG AJ	Have coffee with Olive Prepare lunch	AJ		Polish wooden furniture Clean windows
12:00								
12:30	Lunch	AJ	Lunch	CE	Lunch	CE		Have lunch in town or at the pub
1:00	Watch TV		Clear lunch dishes Clean up kitchen	CE HI	Wash up/load dishwasher	CE HI	Clear lunch dishes Wash up/load dishwasher Clean up kitchen	

Figure 11.1. Sample Activity and Support Plan.

be used to reinforce effective communication between staff working at different times. For example, it might be relevant to communicate 1) a planned activity that was not done (e.g., there was no time for Olive to do her laundry this morning; can she wash her clothes this evening?), 2) the occurrence of something unexpected (e.g., Roger's father has invited him to dinner this evening; please ask Roger what he wants to do when he comes in), or 3) reminders about what must be done now so that something can be achieved later (e.g., someone needs to buy steak this afternoon so Diane can marinade it before cooking tomorrow evening).

The second organizational element is for staff to give individuals sufficient assistance to facilitate their participation in activity and then to motivate continued participation by showing interest. Repp, Barton, and Brulle (1981) found that nonverbal instruction, with or without physical assistance, was the form of instruction most likely to help people with severe mental retardation respond correctly. Active Support therefore seeks to train staff to supplement verbal instruction with gestural or physical prompting, as well as demonstration or physical guidance, depending on how much help the person needs to complete a particular activity. In addition, staff are trained to give people attention when they are constructively occupied. Provision of attention contingent on engagement has been shown experimentally to increase activity levels (Mansell, Felce, de Kock, & Jenkins, 1982; Porterfield, Blunden, & Blewitt, 1980).

The third organizational element is monitoring and review of the activity opportunities that have been extended to each person. Each individual has a personalized record of participation (see Figure 11.2 for a typical example). At the end of each period at work, staff check off the activities in which the person has been involved. These activities can be arranged in categories as indicated; indeed, which activities are listed and how they are categorized can be personalized. The frequency of participation in activities within a category can be totaled for the week. Totals can be transferred to a summary record, which can be used to monitor at a glance the balance of opportunities offered a person and the increase, decrease, or maintenance of opportunities over time (see Figure 11.3).

ACTIVE SUPPORT TRAINING

Active Support training comprises two stages: a workshop related to the planning and monitoring elements, followed by practical training in the workplace on how to interact to assist and encourage participation. The workshop is a 2-day event attended by the entire staff of the

Figure 11.2 Participation Record

Name: _Olive Carpenter_   Date: _Week ending August 25_

Meals/laid table	Sun	Mon	Tues	Wed	Thurs	Fri	Sat	Total
Prepared breakfast/lunch/dinner/tea	✓✓	✓✓	✓✓	✓	✓	✓✓	✓✓	10
Prepared snack/drink	✓✓✓	✓✓		✓✓	✓	✓	✓✓	12
Laid table	✓					✓✓	✓	7
Other: _Made picnic_	✓							1
							Total	30

Cleaning up after meals	Sun	Mon	Tues	Wed	Thurs	Fri	Sat	Total
Wiped table, put away mats, etc., and cleaned dining room	✓		✓✓	✓	✓	✓✓		6
Washed up/used dishwasher	✓			✓	✓	✓	✓	4
Dried up/emptied dishwasher		✓		✓			✓	3
Put dishes/cutlery away	✓	✓		✓✓			✓	5
Other								–
							Total	18

Tidying and cleaning	Sun	Mon	Tues	Wed	Thurs	Fri	Sat	Total
Daily dusting and tidying	✓	✓✓	✓	✓	✓✓	✓✓	✓	9
Cleaned kitchen	✓			✓	✓	✓	✓	5
Housework downstairs	✓		✓		✓		✓	4
Cleaned bathroom/toilet			✓			✓		2
Did upstairs housework		✓		✓		✓	✓	4
Other: _Polished furniture_				✓				1
							Total	25

Laundry	Sun	Mon	Tues	Wed	Thurs	Fri	Sat	Total
Did handwashing								–
Used washing machine		✓			✓			2
Hung out clothes		✓						1
Used tumble dryer				✓		✓	✓	3
Ironed clothes		✓		✓				2
Put clothes away						✓	✓	2
Other								–
							Total	10

Shopping	Sun	Mon	Tues	Wed	Thurs	Fri	Sat	Total
Did personal or small local shopping	✓	✓				✓	✓	3
Did big supermarket shopping		✓	✓					2
Put groceries away		✓	✓			✓		3
Other								–
							Total	8

Gardening/maintenance	Sun	Mon	Tues	Wed	Thurs	Fri	Sat	Total
Worked in the garden	✓	✓			✓		✓	4
Cleaned windows, car, etc.							✓	1
Did house maintenance				✓				1
Other: _Hung picture_	✓							1
							Total	7

Hobbies at home	Sun	Mon	Tues	Wed	Thurs	Fri	Sat	Total
Watched TV	✓				✓		✓	3
Listened to radio or music							✓	1
Looked at magazines or books								–
Collected things								–
Made things				✓				1
Other								–
							Total	5

Social life	Sun	Mon	Tues	Wed	Thurs	Fri	Sat	Total
Had visitors	✓	✓			✓		✓	3
Visited other people's homes						✓		1
Went out with people other than staff	✓			✓				2
Other								–
							Total	6

Hobbies in the community	Sun	Mon	Tues	Wed	Thurs	Fri	Sat	Total
Played sports								–
Watched sports or other event				✓				1
Attended church, club, or society	✓							1
Attended an education class					✓			1
Other								–
							Total	3

Other community use	Sun	Mon	Tues	Wed	Thurs	Fri	Sat	Total
Had a drink or meal at pub or restaurant								–
Went to cinema/theatre/museum/gallery				✓				1
Went to library/bank/post office						✓		1
Went for a good walk								–
Other								–
							Total	2

Participation Summary

Name: _Olive Carpenter_ Date: _Week ending 9/22_

Week ending	Activity										Totals
	Meals	After meal chores	Tidying and cleaning	Laundry	Shopping	Garden main-tenance	Hobby at home	Social life	Hobby in the community	Other community activity	
8/25	30	18	25	10	8	7	5	6	3	2	114
9/1	28	17	20	12	10	6	9	10	5	4	121
9/8	31	18	22	8	8	6	6	8	4	5	116
9/15	27	22	16	8	7	6	8	8	5	2	109
9/22	30	18	18	10	8	6	9	10	3	3	125
											etc.
Total											

Figure 11.3. Sample Participation Summary.

residence and its manager. It consists of presentations, group work sessions, and exercises in which staff do the following:

- Consider individuals' activity preferences, the household routine and other domestic requirements, and the breadth of other activities which might be offered.
- Draw up preliminary Activity and Support Plans for each day of the week based on these considerations.
- Consider the monitoring component and the layout of the Participation Record.
- Discuss practical arrangements, administrative issues, and quality maintenance.
- Receive instruction, supported by a videotape illustrating desired practice, on providing different levels of assistance to match a person's need for help and attention to reinforce participation in activity.

The content of the workshop is reinforced in short guidance booklets written for staff.

Immediately following the workshop, the interaction training phase begins. A trainer works with each staff member in the residence to teach him or her how to give assistance and attend to people in practice. This involves working directly with staff and the people whom they support by using an iterative process of demonstrating recommended performance, observing staff practice, and giving feedback. The goal is to teach staff 1) to adjust the level of assistance that they give according to each person's need for support (to accomplish successive steps of activities and successive activities) by appropriately combining verbal instruction, gestural or physical prompting, demonstration, or physical guidance and 2) to sustain that participation by giving appropriate attention and further assistance when necessary. Each staff member receives 1–2 hours of training. This stage of training takes approximately 3 days to complete per residence.

Regular weekly staff meetings are recommended so that staff can monitor progress and introduce whatever changes are judged to be required. Staff are encouraged to implement Active Support in the week following the interaction training. Staff check and finalize the Activity and Support Plans that were prepared in the workshop, in consultation with the people whom they support, to ensure sufficient opportunity for each person to be occupied constructively throughout each day. Staff are encouraged to update Activity and Support Plans regularly. Activity and Support Plan and Participation Record forms are provided on disk to facilitate their revision.

Active Support and Choice

The emphasis on supporting people to participate in activities—particularly the emphasis on the activities of routine daily life—may appear incompatible with self-determination and its primary component: choice. However, the intention is not to be coercive. Rather, it is to offer people who may be disengaged through no choice of their own genuine opportunities to participate in typical, constructive pursuits. For people with more severe or profound mental retardation—thus, who have extremely limited independent skills—three factors appear necessary if opportunities to participate are to exist: 1) availability of activity, 2) availability of staff support, and 3) matching the level of assistance given by support staff to that which is required to participate successfully. The planning element within Active Support should increase the occasions when the first two factors are present. The practical training should increase staff skills to achieve the third.

Self-determination is also encouraged by emphasizing that staff should involve the people they support as much as possible in the construction of their activity plans and take account of the individuals' activity preferences and aspirations. Typically, planning is more about filling available time than choosing between competing activity opportunities. Therefore, there is not usually a problem in accommodating personal activity preferences. However, difficulties in understanding and using language and other symbolic means of communication exist among a proportion of the people for whom Active Support appears relevant. This means that staff effectively make many decisions about the opportunities and support that are offered to individuals. The assumption underlying Active Support in these circumstances is that people would prefer to be occupied in a similar range of activities that occupy other people than not to be.

RESEARCH ON THE IMPACT OF ACTIVE SUPPORT

We have undertaken two evaluations of the impact of Active Support. The first study aimed to train staff in five community residences for adults with severe mental retardation to test the hypotheses that implementing Active Support would result in residents 1) receiving more assistance and 2) engaging in more activity (Jones et al., 1999). A total of 19 people lived in these houses and participated in the research, four in each of four houses and three in one. Their ages ranged from 30 to 67 years. The great majority of participants had severe mental retardation. Participants' scores on Part One of the AAMR Adaptive Behavior

Scales, Second Edition (ABS-2; Nihira, Leland, & Lambert, 1993), averaged 115. Participants living in Houses 1–5 had mean ABS-2 scores of 108, 97, 135, 131, and 98 respectively. Overall, the ABS-2 score range was wide, from 12 to 236, reflecting a policy of heterogeneous groupings within some environments. However, only three people had domain scores that consistently ranked them in the higher two quartiles of the domain profiles. Additional physical disabilities, sensory impairments, severe challenging behavior, and mental health problems were present among 8, 5, 4, and 3 individuals out of 19 respectively. Although most could walk independently and feed themselves, the majority needed help to dress and wash and had very limited speech.

All five houses were managed by the same voluntary sector provider. They had been open for 3–6 years and had 42.5 full-time equivalent staff among them. Most staff had prior experience working with people with mental retardation, and 70% had been in their current post for 2 years or longer, but only 12% had a professional qualification that was relevant to supporting people with mental retardation.

Houses 1, 2, and 3 were reported as having systems of individual planning already in operation, which set and reviewed goals with and on behalf of the people living in the houses. Houses 4 and 5 held ad hoc case review meetings but did not operate a regular individual planning system. House 2 was reported to use a system for deciding teaching priorities and setting teaching programs, which were recorded and reviewed. Teaching was also conducted in an ad hoc way in House 4, but no regular behavioral assessment or system for setting teaching programs was reported in the other three houses. All houses had underdeveloped ways for ensuring that residents had adequate opportunities for participation in activities. Any activity timetables that did exist were incomplete, accounting for less than half of residents' available time. In all of the houses, the staff role was broadly defined in terms of giving residents support, but staff were left to their own initiative as to how to put this into practice. All settings provided their own in-house orientation training, with other training opportunities provided in response to staff requests. Normalization was a priority in the agency's mission statement and training.

Experimental Design

The intervention was staggered across the five houses at monthly intervals following a multiple-baseline design with 10 data points in each phase. Two further data points were collected at follow-up 6 months after the last post-baseline observation and 8–12 months after intervention. Control for the passage of time and other extraneous variables potentially affecting all environments was strengthened by the fact that all houses were drawn from the same agency. This provided a basis for assuming that one house could be a control for another in relation to introducing general organizational, management, or training changes during the study. There were no trends in a therapeutic direction during baseline.

Measurement

Participants were directly observed for a similar 2-hour period on each occasion just before the evening meal. Their activity and the attention that they received from staff were recorded using a handheld computer. Observation distinguished 1) receiving assistance (instruction, prompting, demonstration, guidance) from receipt of other attention (other conversation, other physical touch) and 2) engagement (doing a social, leisure, domestic, self-care, or other activity) from disengagement (exhibiting challenging behavior or being unoccupied). Interobserver reliability was satisfactory. Readers are referred to Jones and colleagues (1999) for further details of observation procedures and measurement definitions.

Results

Figure 11.4 provides a summary of the results. Following the introduction of Active Support, all houses had statistically significant increases in the level of assistance that participants received (from a mean level overall in baseline of 5.9% of time to 23.3%) and in their engagement in domestic activities (from a mean level overall in baseline of 12.8% of time to 32.2%). The total level of participant engagement in activity increased in all of the houses, from a mean level overall in baseline of 33.1% of time to 53.4% (increases in Houses 1, 2, 3, and 5 were statistically significant). Increased levels of assistance and engagement in activity were observed immediately on implementation of Active Support. At the point that Active Support was successively introduced in each house, no change in a therapeutic direction was observed in houses remaining in baseline.

Across individuals, proportional changes in assistance and engagement in activity between baseline and postintervention were significantly and positively associated (Spearman rank correlation, $rho = .84$, $N = 19$, $p < .001$). Moreover, before Active Support was introduced, staff gave more attention and assistance to people with higher ABS-2 scores ($rho = .67$ and .58 respectively, both $N = 19$, both $p < .01$). Afterward, receipt of attention was unrelated to ability, and participants with lower ABS-2 scores tended to receive more assistance ($rho = -.26$, $N = 19$, $p = .288$). As a result, the disparity in activity between people

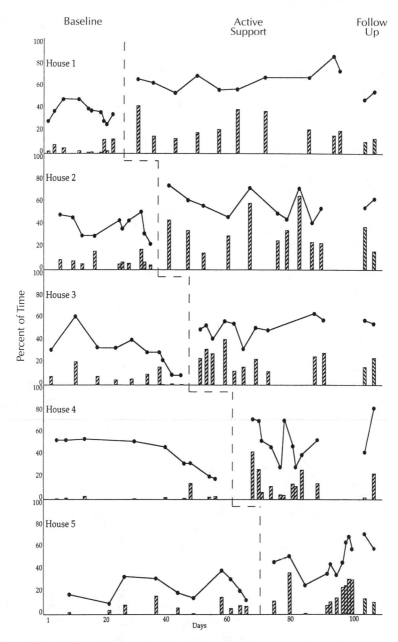

Figure 11.4. Staff assistance and resident engagement in five community residences before and after the implementation of Active Support. (*Key:* ▨ = staff assistance, ● = resident engagement.) (From Jones, E., Perry, J., Lowe, K., Felce, D., Toogood, S., Dunstan, F., Allen, D., & Pagler, J. [1999]. Opportunity and the promotion of activity among adults with severe intellectual disability living in community residences: The impact of training staff in Active Support. *Journal of Intellectual Disability Research, 43,* 173; published by Blackwell Science Ltd.; reprinted by permission.)

with more and less severe disabilities was reduced. The eight participants with ABS-2 scores greater than the mean of 115 received assistance for 7.9% of the time in baseline and for 18.1% of the time after intervention. Their total engagement levels increased from 52.7% to 67.5%. The 11 participants with ABS-2 scores below the mean received assistance for 4.8% of the time in baseline and for 24.2% after intervention. Their total engagement levels increased from 20.2% to 41.8%.

Gains were fully maintained at follow-up in Houses 2, 3, and 5 and partially maintained in House 1. Results were variable in House 4 after training and at follow-up. Across the five houses, participants received assistance from staff at follow-up for 16.0% of time, engaged in domestic activities for 32.3% of time, and were engaged in activity overall for 57.2% of time. Variability and loss of performance over time coincided with senior staff turnover or absence through sickness and use of untrained relief staff.

Dissemination of Active Support

The aim of the second study was to conduct a widespread replication of Active Support training in similar community residences run by three Welsh nonprofit agencies. One of the agencies had participated in the previous study, and the other two agencies had similar service philosophies (Jones et al., 2001). The study was conducted in 38 staffed houses that accommodated 106 people in mean groups of 2.8 (range 1–4). Fifty-four percent of the participants were male and their mean age was 43 years (range 22–76 years). The mean score on Part One of the ABS-2 was 144 (range 20–293). There were 303 full- or part-time staff working in the houses, giving a mean of 7.2 full-time equivalent staff per house and 2.6 per participant. Their mean age was 40.4 years (range 20–64 years) and 32.8% were male. Their mean length of service was 3.9 years (range birth–12 years). A minority (8.5%) had a professional nursing or social care qualification that was relevant to supporting people with mental retardation. Slightly more than a quarter (26.5%) had prior experience working with people with mental retardation before taking their current jobs.

Most settings had preexisting arrangements for individual or person-centered planning, but procedures for conducting behavioral assessments or systematic teaching were underdeveloped. Plans for participant activity were generally confined to social or leisure activities outside the home. Little attention was given to planning daily household tasks. None of the environments had a system for organizing staff availability to support participant activity throughout the day. Any planning of staff availability that did exist focused on activities outside the home.

A simple pre-post evaluation design used observational measurement similar to the first study. In addition, three staff report measures were administered before and after the introduction of Active Support: 1) an assessment of the extent of planned activities between 9:00 A.M. and midnight each day for a typical week for each participant, 2) the Index of Participation in Domestic Life (IPDL; Raynes, Wright, Shiell, & Pettipher, 1994), and 3) the Index of Community Involvement (ICI; Raynes et al., 1994) as modified by Felce and colleagues (1998).

Reported activity for participants in a typical week indicated a 35% increase in planned activity for participants following the implementation of Active Support. The main increase was in activities occurring within the houses, which rose from a combined baseline level of 3.7 to 11.0 hours per week per person. There were statistically significant increases in observed receipt of assistance (from 7.5% to 14.6% of time), engagement in domestic activities (from 18.4% to 24.0% of time), and total engagement in activity (from 46.7% to 54.6% of time). Similar patterns of association were found between individual ABS-2 scores and changes in assistance and engagement before and after the implementation of Active Support. Before the introduction of Active Support, people with higher ABS-2 scores received more attention than those with lower scores ($rho = .26, N = 106, p < .01$). Afterward, receipt of attention was not associated with ability and people with lower ABS-2 scores received more assistance ($rho = -.45, N = 106, p < .001$). Change in engagement at an individual level was positively associated with change in assistance ($rho = .40, N = 106, p < .001$). A descriptive analysis was undertaken to explore how mean changes in total and domestic engagement levels varied among participants according to their ABS-2 scores. Increased engagement in activity overall was experienced by people with ABS-2 scores in the 0–180 range. Increased engagement in domestic activity was experienced by people with ABS-2 scores in the 0–210 range. Active Support did not have a positive effect among people with higher ABS-2 scores.

Increased engagement in domestic activities was also reflected in significant IPDL score increases. In addition, the range and frequency of social and community activities as measured by the ICI increased. Participants undertook a greater range of social activities after Active Support (1.6 types out of a possible 5 categories assessed, compared with 1.2) at a higher frequency (4.1 events per month, compared with 2.9). They undertook more types of community activities after Active Support (6.7 out of a possible 10 categories assessed, compared with 6.0) at a higher frequency (20.2 events per month compared with 18.1). However, these latter results should be viewed with caution, as staff informants were not blind to the experimental conditions and no interrespondent reliability data were collected. This lack of rigor allows for biased reporting to indicate improvement in response to training where none such existed.

CONCLUSION

The consistency of results between the two studies described in this chapter—a small, well-controlled experimental demonstration and a larger, uncontrolled dissemination study—demonstrates that Active Support training has a significant impact on the level of assistance received by people with more severe mental retardation and on their engagement in household and other activities. Active Support, there-fore, appears to provide a means of meeting the goal of supporting people with few independent skills to participate in daily, typical activ-ities. The prime focus of Active Support is creating the conditions that make homes places where people with severe mental retardation can *live* as opposed to be accommodated. In this respect, it has much in common with the Supported Routines approach advocated by Saunders and Spradlin (1991). Saunders and Spradlin drew attention to the low or episodic staff involvement with individuals and a lack of constructive activity found among people living in residential services. They observed that these features of staff and resident activity may coexist with or even arise from the preoccupation with individual needs assessment, objective setting, and skills teaching that stems from widely held notions of active treatment. In emphasizing the prime function of a home as a place to live daily life, Saunders and Spradlin argued that it is

> The responsibility of the facility to assist the individual in adopting and performing a daily routine that is enjoyable and functional. The facility must support that routine by creating the necessary environmental and social conditions within which it can occur and be sustained. The facility must also ensure that the routines are similar to the types and purposes of the routines evidenced by persons without handicaps in the general com-munity. (1991, p. 24)

As already stated, we assume that people prefer to have the same level of occupation and to experience the same range of activities as other people. Evidence from service user participation events and sur-veys in Britain (Audit Commission/Social Services Inspectorate Wales, n.d.) shows that self advocates want responsibility, opportunities to do things for themselves, and help when they need it. A focus group con-sultation with a sample of residents capable of giving their views about Active Support, which was undertaken by independent consultants who support the tenants associations of two of the three agencies involved in the second study, confirmed this general impression. Despite the indication that Active Support had less impact among people with higher adaptive behavior, 80% of those surveyed said that Active Support helped them and only one person said that it did not. One of the independent consultants commented that all respondents appeared to find Active Support meaningful and enjoyable, almost speaking about it with affection. Respondents described Active Support as "doing things for yourself," "making sure the staff care for you properly," and "something to think about and it helps you remember things."

Respondents viewed doing things for themselves, learning new skills and being involved as positive experiences. Their comments on the changes accompanying Active Support included the following:

- "It was boring before; now I do lots of things in the house."
- "We do so much more now that we've got plans."
- "It's important we know when things are going to happen. I just have to look at my chart."
- "It's good to see the men doing housework in our house."
- "We get a chance to do things a lot of the time now."
- "I do ironing now—I never used to. I don't mind it."

When asked to comment on activities that they do now but had not done previously, respondents highlighted participation in domestic tasks—such as cooking, cleaning, doing the laundry, and shopping—and personal care. They also mentioned participating in more hobbies and going to the town center more often. When asked about negative changes, most people said that there were none. A quarter of those surveyed said that doing housework was tiring and that there was too much housework to do. When asked whether they thought that the training had changed staff, responses were positive and revealed a good understanding of Active Support. Comments included

- "It gives staff an idea of what they are meant to be doing."
- "I didn't know staff could teach me so well! They are good teachers."
- "It's good for us. Staff should help us as much as they can and they do."
- "They give us more attention now in our house."

One independent consultant commented that people believed that relationships with staff had improved since the introduction of Active

Support and that staff were more attentive to the needs and wishes of the people whom they supported.

That Active Support is not an effective approach for people with moderate or mild mental retardation would seem consistent with the research of Stancliffe (1997) and Stancliffe and Keane (2000). These studies demonstrated that semi-independent living was associated with equivalent or better outcomes than fully staffed accommodation for people within this ability range. The service effectiveness issue at this end of the ability spectrum appears not to be about how to train available staff to promote activity better but, rather, about how to reduce staff presence so that people become more autonomous and still receive the episodic help, skills teaching, and supervision that they require. In contrast, the benefit of Active Support is experienced by those people whose severe mental retardation necessitates continuous staffing. Where there is a general concern about low activity levels in community homes or when person-centered planning sets goals for increasing the range of activities or experiences for one or more individuals within a home, Active Support is an effective intervention system.

REFERENCES

Audit Commission/Social Services Inspectorate Wales. (n.d.). *Learning disabilities, quality and the All Wales Strategy: Enabling service users to set the agenda.* Cardiff, United Kingdom: Welsh Office.

Cummins, R.A. (1997). Assessing quality of life. In R. Brown (Ed.), *Quality of life for people with disabilities: Models, research and practice* (pp. 116–150). Cheltenham, United Kingdom: Stanley Thorne.

Emerson, E., & Hatton, C. (1996). Deinstitutionalization in the UK and Ireland: Outcomes for service users. *Journal of Intellectual and Developmental Disability, 21,* 17–37.

Emerson, E., Robertson, J., Gregory, N., Hatton, C., Kessissoglou, S., Hallam, A., Knapp, M., Järbrink, K., Netten, A., Walsh, P., Linehan, C., Hillery, J., & Durkan, J. (1999). *Quality and costs of residential supports for people with learning disabilities: Summary report.* Manchester, United Kingdom: University of Manchester, Hester Adrian Research Centre.

Emerson, E., Robertson, J., Gregory, N., Kessissoglou, S., Hatton, C., Hallam, A., Järbrink, K., Knapp, M., Netten, A., & Linehan, C. (2000). The quality and costs of community-based residential supports and residential campuses for people with severe and complex disabilities. *Journal of Intellectual and Developmental Disabilities, 25,* 265–281.

Felce, D. (1996). Quality of support for ordinary living. In J. Mansell & K. Ericcson (Eds.), *Deinstitutionalization and community living: Intellectual disability services in Britain, Scandinavia and the USA* (pp. 117–133). London: Chapman and Hall.

Felce, D. (1997). Defining and applying the concept of quality of life. *Journal of Intellectual Disability Research, 41,* 126–143.

Felce, D., de Kock, U., & Repp, A. (1986). An eco-behavioural analysis of small community-based houses and traditional large hospitals for severely and profoundly mentally handicapped adults. *Applied Research in Mental Retardation, 7*, 393–408.

Felce, D., Lowe, K., Beecham, J., & Hallam, A. (2000). Exploring the relationships between costs and quality of services for adults with severe intellectual disabilities and the most severe challenging behaviours in Wales: A multivariate regression analysis. *Journal of Intellectual and Developmental Disability, 25*, 307–326.

Felce, D., Lowe, K., & Jones, E. (in press). Association between the provision characteristics and operation of supported housing services and resident outcomes. *Journal of Applied Research in Intellectual Disability.*

Felce, D., Lowe, K., Perry, J., Baxter, H., Jones, E., Hallam, A., & Beecham, J. (1998). Service support to people with severe intellectual disabilities and the most severe challenging behaviours in Wales: Processes, outcomes and costs. *Journal of Intellectual Disability Research, 42*, 390–408.

Felce, D., Lowe, K., Perry, J., Jones, E., Baxter, H., & Bowley, C. (1999). The quality of residential and day services for adults with learning disabilities in eight local authorities in England: Objective data gained in support of a Social Services Inspectorate inspection. *Journal of Applied Research in Intellectual Disabilities, 12*, 273–293.

Felce, D., & Perry, J. (1995). The extent of support for ordinary living provided in staffed housing: The relationship between staffing levels, resident dependency, staff:resident interactions and resident activity patterns. *Social Science and Medicine, 40*, 799–810.

Gilbert, T.F. (1978). *Engineering worthy performance.* New York: McGraw-Hill.

Gilbert, T.F., & Gilbert, M. B. (1992). Potential contributions of performance science to education. *Journal of Applied Behavior Analysis, 25*, 43–49.

Hatton, C., Emerson, E., Robertson, J., Henderson, D., & Cooper, J. (1996). Factors associated with staff support and user lifestyle in services for people with multiple disabilities: A path analytic approach. *Journal of Intellectual Disability Research, 40*, 466–477.

Hewson, S., & Walker, J. (1992). The use of evaluation in the development of a staffed residential service for adults with mental handicap. *Mental Handicap Research, 5*, 188–203.

Jones, E., Felce, D., Lowe, K., Bowley, C., Pagler, J., Gallagher, B., & Roper, A. (2001). Evaluation of the dissemination of Active Support training in staffed community residences. *American Journal on Mental Retardation, 106*, 344–358.

Jones, E., Perry, J., Lowe, K., Felce, D., Toogood, S., Dunstan, F., Allen, D., & Pagler, J. (1999). Opportunity and the promotion of activity among adults with severe intellectual disability living in community residences: The impact of training staff in Active Support. *Journal of Intellectual Disability Research, 43*, 164–178.

Mansell, J., Felce, D., de Kock, U., & Jenkins, J. (1982). Increasing purposeful activity of severely and profoundly mentally handicapped adults. *Behaviour Research and Therapy, 20*, 593–604.

Mount, B. (1998). More than a meeting: Benefits and limitations of personal futures planning. In J. O'Brien & C. Lyle O'Brien (Eds.), *A little book about person-centered planning* (pp. 55–68). Toronto: Inclusion Press.

Nihira, K., Leland, H., & Lambert, N. (1993). *AAMR Adaptive Behavior Scales–Residential and Community (ABS-RC:2)* (2nd ed.). Austin, TX: PRO-ED.

O'Brien, J. (1987). A guide to life-style planning: Using The Activities Catalog to integrate services and natural support systems. In B. Wilcox & G.T. Bellamy, *A comprehensive guide to The Activities Catalog: An alternative curriculum for youth and adults with severe disabilities* (pp. 175–189). Baltimore: Paul H. Brookes Publishing Co.

Perry, J., Felce, D., & Lowe, K. (2000). *Subjective and objective quality of life assessment: Their interrelationship and determinants.* Cardiff, United Kingdom: Welsh Centre for Learning Disabilities, University of Wales College of Medicine.

Porterfield, J., Blunden, R., & Blewitt, E. (1980). Improving environments for profoundly handicapped adults: Using prompts and social attention to maintain high group engagement. *Behavior Modification, 4,* 225–241.

Raynes, N., Wright, K., Shiell, A., & Pettipher, C. (1994). *The cost and quality of community residential care.* London: David Fulton Publishers.

Repp, A.C., Barton, L.E., & Brulle, A.R. (1981). Correspondence between effectiveness and staff use of instructions for severely retarded persons. *Applied Research in Mental Retardation, 2,* 237–245.

Routledge, M., & Sanderson, H. (2000). *Work in progress: Implementing person centred planning in Oldham.* Whalley, United Kingdom: North West Training and Development Team.

Saunders, R.R., & Spradlin, J.E. (1991). A supported routines approach to active treatment for enhancing independence, competence, and self-worth. *Behavioral Residential Treatment, 6,* 11–37.

Schalock, R.L. (1996). Reconsidering the conceptualization and measurement of quality of life. In R.L. Schalock (Ed.), *Quality of life: Vol. 1. Conceptualization and measurement* (pp. 123–139). Washington, DC: American Association on Mental Retardation.

Schalock, R.L., Stark, J.A., Snell, M.E., Coulter, D.L., Polloway, E. A., Luckasson, R., Reiss, S., & Spitalnik, D.M. (1994). The changing conception of mental retardation: Implications for the field. *Mental Retardation, 32,* 181–193.

Smull, M.W. (1998a). Positive rituals and quality of life. In J. O'Brien & C. Lyle O'Brien (Eds.), *A little book about person-centered planning* (pp. 51–54). Toronto: Inclusion Press.

Smull, M.W. (1998b). Revisiting choice. In J. O'Brien & C. Lyle O'Brien (Eds.), *A little book about person-centered planning* (pp. 37–49). Toronto: Inclusion Press.

Stancliffe, R.J. (1997). Community living: Unit size, staff presence, and residents' choice-making. *Mental Retardation, 35*(1), 1–9.

Stancliffe, R.J., & Keane, S. (2000). Outcomes and costs of community living: A matched comparison of group homes and semi-independent living. *Journal of Intellectual and Developmental Disability, 25,* 281–305.

Stancliffe, R.J., & Lakin, K.C. (1998). Analysis of expenditures and outcomes of residential alternatives for persons with developmental disabilities. *American Journal on Mental Retardation, 102,* 552–568.

IV

Challenging Behavior

12

Person-Centered Planning from a Behavioral Perspective

Gregory A. Wagner

Starting in the 1960s, procedures derived from the experimental and applied analyses of behavior have had dramatic impacts on the lives of people with developmental disabilities. These procedures have effectively reduced challenging behavior and provided the tools for teaching functional life skills. Indeed, these techniques made possible the shift from the medical model to a developmental, habilitative model of service delivery (Anderson & Freeman, 2000). Since the late 1980s, further changes have occurred within the service system for people with developmental disabilities. These changes reflect the shift from program-centered to person-centered services, with a focus on consumer choice (e.g., Mount, 1992; O'Brien, 1987). This transformation and related events have affected the provision of behavioral services both philosophically and technologically. The values on which person-centered approaches are based—self-determination (consumer choice), dignity and respect, community inclusion—have resulted in widespread adoption of these approaches. These values are relatively noncontroversial. However, a paucity of research and related empirical support for person-centered planning has generated controversy, at least among behavioral researchers and clinicians. This book is the first concerted attempt to address this controversy by examining the existing empirical evidence and related issues for person-centered planning.

Although the book focuses principally on current research and practice in person-centered planning, this chapter is a conceptual analysis of person-centered planning. It consists of three major components: 1) the historical events that led to the current emphases on positive behavioral supports and person-centered planning, 2) a behavioral conceptual analysis and comparison of some person-centered

The opinions expressed in this chapter do not necessarily reflect those of the California Department of Developmental Services.

planning processes and outcomes, and 3) a discussion of issues regarding empirical support and experimental analysis of person-centered planning.

EARLY HISTORY

Early behavioral efforts to treat challenging behavior frequently consisted of some combination of reinforcement for not engaging in the target behavior (or for engaging in some prespecified appropriate behavior) and a punishing consequence delivered contingent on the occurrence of the challenging behavior. These procedures were typically used without regard for the function served by the behavior (Bates & Wehman, 1977; Lennox, Miltenberger, Spengler, & Erfanian, 1988). In fact, a pretreatment assessment of the function served by the target behavior (i.e., a functional assessment) was rarely conducted (Scotti, Evans, Meyer, & Walker, 1991). These early efforts were often initially effective in reducing the targeted challenging behavior; however, maintenance and generalization of response reduction were often absent, and other challenging behaviors often emerged. In addition, the relative intrusiveness or restrictiveness of interventions was not matched with the relative severity of behavior (i.e., the most intrusive interventions were not reserved for the most severe behavior).

Starting in the late 1970s, a number of events led to improvements of these early behavioral approaches. First, the excessive use of restrictive or aversive procedures resulted in mounting pressure from advocates to reduce their use. In response to this pressure, human services agencies promulgated policies and regulations to reduce the use of these procedures and to ensure the clinical appropriateness of their use. Second, behavioral practitioners began to acknowledge the importance of social validity (e.g., Wolf, 1978) and intervention acceptability (e.g., Morgan, 1989). The primary focus of these topics is the extent to which primary consumers, intervention providers, and society in general find particular procedures and outcomes acceptable. These issues are particularly salient in community environments, in which procedures such as restraint are subject to public observation and may be stigmatizing for consumers. Third, and directly related to social validity and treatment acceptability, is a growing emphasis on community-referenced procedures (e.g., Koegel & Koegel, 1989). Again, these are procedures considered to be culturally or socially normative for the problem. They frequently involve avoiding or modifying the situations that cause or increase the likelihood of challenging behavior (i.e., antecedent or ecological events). Fourth, procedures for identifying the causes or functions of challenging behavior—that is, functional assessment and analysis—have been dramatically improved (e.g., Iwata, Dorsey, Slifer, Bauman, & Richman, 1982/1994). This change allows people to treat the actual conditions that are responsible for challenging behavior. This is a major improvement over the earlier practice of arranging reinforcing and/or punishing consequences for a behavior without regard to the function that the behavior served. Fifth and finally, as an outcome of the previously noted events, a technology of positive behavioral support has emerged. According to Carr and colleagues, this approach to challenging behavior "focuses on the remediation of deficient contexts (i.e., environmental conditions and/or behavioral repertoires) that by functional assessment are documented to be the source of the problem" (1999, p. 1). Furthermore, instead of simply reducing targeted challenging behavior, effective outcomes should include increases in appropriate behavior and an overall improvement in quality of life. Person-centered planning is often considered a positive behavioral approach (Wagner, 1999).

The transition to a person-centered service model reflected broad, humanistic efforts toward consumer self-determination and empowerment by allowing consumers to choose their own individualized services and supports, rather than imposing preexisting menus of services and decisions made primarily by professionals. This shift also reflected a growing antibehavioral sentiment by some segments of the developmental disabilities field. The sentiment was based on semantic confusion, misconception, and ideological predisposition. An example of semantic confusion and misconception involved the inconsistent, vague, and ambiguous use of terms such as *aversive, restrictive,* and *intrusive.* Ideological predisposition includes the perception that purposely arranging or altering the environment to change behavior (as in behavioral programming) is dehumanizing. Indeed, behavioral approaches, including relatively benign procedures such as planned positive reinforcement, came to be viewed as simplistic, narrow, and mechanistic control procedures (Holburn, 1997; Wagner, 1999). Similar criticisms were raised when behavioral procedures were initially applied to human behavior in the 1960s. In this context, Holburn noted, "Ironically, these criticisms of behaviorism helped to promote person-centered planning" (p. 73; see also Holburn & Vietze, 2000). On a similar note, some authors suggested that person-centered planning arose in response to "people whose behaviors or needs for personal assistance severely challenged existing programs" (Lyle O'Brien, O'Brien, & Mount, 1997, p. 481) and "as a countermeasure to conventional approaches and interventions that were not working very well" (Holburn & Vietze, 1998, p. 487). At the same time, many person-centered planners were reporting reductions in challenging behavior as a result of implementing person-centered planning, thus obviating the need for formal behavioral techniques in these cases (e.g., Smull & Burke Harrison, 1992). As person-centered planning gained acceptance in the field of developmental disabilities, however, some behaviorists came to view person-centered planning as just another fad that was couched in nonbehavioral (or antibehavioral) terms and based largely on anecdotal stories with a corresponding lack of data (e.g., Osborne, 1999).

Controversy notwithstanding, Holburn (2001) showed that person-centered planning is compatible with several basic dimensions of applied behavior analysis. Furthermore, the typical processes and reported outcomes of person-centered planning can be easily interpreted and understood from a behavioral perspective. Indeed, from the context of a behavioral conceptual framework, changes in a person's behavior as an outcome of person-centered planning appear lawful and systematic. Behavioral procedures and person-centered planning may also complement and benefit each other in a number of ways (Kincaid, 1996; Reid, Everson, & Green, 1999; Risley, 1996; Wagner, 1996, 1999; Wagner & Martin, 1995). When viewed from the same perspective, both approaches have useful roles in the provision of contemporary services and supports.

RELATIONSHIPS BETWEEN BEHAVIORAL AND PERSON-CENTERED APPROACHES

Years of behavioral research and application have repeatedly demonstrated that behavior operates under a set of laws and can often be explained by various environmentally based principles of behavior. If person-centered planning causes reductions in challenging behavior, then these behavioral principles can readily explain the reductions. For example, in describing person-centered planning, Holburn observed that "for the most part, its [person-centered planning's] philosophy and practices are consistent with radical behaviorism" and that person-centered planning is essentially "environmentalistic in strategy" (1997, pp. 73, 77). In fact, the person-centered emphasis on changing the environment rather than the person is thoroughly consistent with behavior analysis: The fundamental discourse of behavior analysis involves the study of behavior–environment interactions, and the hallmark of the field involves the identification of environmental events of which behavior is a function. Changing the environment changes behavior. On an applied level, the emerging area of positive behavioral support (of which some would consider person-centered planning to be a part) involves remediating environments that are deficient "to the extent that they involve lack of choice, inadequate teaching strategies, minimal access to engaging materials and activities, poorly selected daily routines, and a host of other proximal and distal antecedent stimuli" (Carr et al., 1999, p. 4). When person-centered planning results in reduction in challenging behavior, most of the reduction can be parsimoniously explained by two broad behavioral principles: 1) the person-centered planning process minimizes or eliminates the aversive events (e.g., people, places, tasks) that the person has historically escaped or avoided through challenging behavior or 2) the process provides the person with ready access to reinforcers (e.g., attention, preferred items) that the challenging behavior has produced in the past. Thus, in either case, person-centered planning can render the challenging behavior unnecessary (Wagner, 1999).

An initial strategy of person-centered planning consists of minimizing, eliminating, or otherwise modifying aversive events. Challenging behavior often allows a person to escape or avoid such events. These types of events occur before (antecedent to) or as part of the overall environmental context (ecological conditions) surrounding the challenging behavior. By eliminating or altering these events, challenging behavior can be reduced or eliminated. Holburn noted that these types of manipulations "can result in immediate reductions in challenging behavior, largely in part by the sweeping modifications in establishing operations and occasioning stimuli" (1997, p. 74). Such antecedent or ecological manipulations are increasingly characteristic of many current behavioral interventions (see Carr et al., 1999). These strategies may include altering events that closely precede challenging behavior, such as eliminating unnecessary demands that evoke the behavior; altering events that are relatively distant (in time) from the occurrence of challenging behavior, such as ensuring adequate sleep or alleviating hunger (Horner, Vaughn, Day, & Ard, 1996); or altering ecological events such as noise, crowding, or a lack of stimulating materials.

A second strategy of person-centered planning consists of providing ready access to reinforcers (Osborne, 1999; see also Holburn & Vietze, 1999, for a good example contrasting behavioral and person-centered approaches to providing access to preferred activities). In addition to allowing escape from or avoidance of aversive events, challenging behavior may provide access to reinforcers (e.g., social attention, preferred items or activities). The person-centered process of providing ready access to these reinforcers is very similar to a current behavioral approach to treating some challenging behavior. That is,

many behavioral studies conducted during the 1980s and 1990s identified social attention or access to preferred activities as the reinforcer
that maintains a person's challenging behavior. The researchers conducting these studies then provided the same or other high-preference
reinforcers on an ongoing basis, independently of the person's behavior (i.e., noncontingently). The challenging behavior was thereby
reduced (e.g., Fischer, Iwata, & Mazeleski, 1997; Fisher, O'Connor,
Kurtz, DeLeon, & Gotjen, 2000; Hagopian, Fisher, & Legacy, 1994;
Vollmer, Iwata, Zarcone, Smith, & Mazeleski, 1993).

Functional Assessment and Analysis

Person-centered planning strives to minimize aversive events in a person's life—and, conversely, to maximize positive events—through the
identification of preferences, choices, and dislikes. This process is very
similar to the behavioral procedures of functional assessment and
analysis. These behavioral assessment procedures identify the func-
tion(s) that challenging behavior serves. Holburn (1997) described the
person-centered planning process in behavioral terms as clarifying
past and present reinforcement contingencies by identifying relevant
antecedents and consequences. Both the person-centered planning
and behavioral assessment processes often include structured interviews, observations or trials in real-life situations, and, ultimately, the
identification of events that the person chooses to maximize or to
avoid and escape. Kincaid described these events as "situations, people, places, capacities, and activities that create motivation, interest
and engagement" versus "strategies, conditions, people, places, and
activities that create frustration, anxiety, or other problems" (1996,
p. 452).

    Person-centered planning and behavioral assessment processes
are not simply similar in concept. Functional assessment and analysis
methodologies offer procedures that may complement and contribute
to person-centered planning processes by identifying important events
in a person's life (Kincaid, 1996; Risley, 1996; Wagner, 1999). Given the
extensive developments in functional assessment methodologies since
the 1980s, their inclusion in the person-centered planning process
would provide important additional information and help ensure the
accuracy of the information gathered. Indeed, the accuracy of the information regarding a person's reinforcers (positive and negative) is a prerequisite for developing strategies that make sense or otherwise match
the identified function(s) served by challenging behavior. (For excellent
discussions of functional assessment and analysis research, issues, and
directions, see Carr, 1994; Horner, 1994; and Mace, 1994.)

Choice

Person-centered planners often report that when a person is allowed to make informed choices such as where to live, with whom to spend time, and what to do, challenging behavior decreases. This emphasis on choice is not foreign to behavior analysis. Choice has long been an area of behavioral research and application (see Fisher & Mazur, 1997, for an excellent review of the basic and applied literature on choice). Holburn similarly observed, "One particularly behavioristic rule of person-centered planning is that people should make more choices for themselves " (1997, p. 76). Similar to person-centered planners, behaviorists have described reductions in challenging behavior and increases in adaptive skills as a function of choice (cf. Dunlap, 1990; LaVigna, Willis, & Donnellan, 1989). In addition, behavioral procedures are useful for teaching informed choice making (e.g., Foxx, Faw, Taylor, Davis, & Fulia, 1993) and accurately assessing preferences (Green, Reid, Canipe, & Gardner, 1991; Lohrmann-O'Rourke & Browder, 1998). Research in the late 1990s has emphasized the importance of accurately assessing preferences. For example, Reid and colleagues (1999)—and subsequently Green, Middleton, and Reid (2000)—demonstrated that participants in person-centered planning meetings may not accurately identify consumer leisure preferences when speaking for consumers with limited verbal skills. This finding is not surprising given research indicating that caregiver opinions of consumer reinforcers may not coincide with the results of preference assessments conducted with those consumers (Fisher, Piazza, Bowman, & Amari, 1996; Green et al., 1988). Rather than relying solely on caregiver opinions, conducting formal behavioral preference assessments helps ensure that consumer preferences are accurately identified (Everson & Reid, 1999; Green et al., 2000; Reid et al., 1999).

In addition to assessing preferences for leisure and other activities, behavioral research has included assessment of consumer preference for behavioral interventions (Hanley, Piazza, Fisher, Contrucci, & Maglieri, 1997). In the Hanley and colleagues study, two consumers indicated their choice of two intervention procedures. One procedure involved teaching a communication response as an alternative to the challenging behavior. This communication response served the same function as the challenging behavior. The second procedure involved providing the reinforcer that was maintaining the challenging behavior (e.g., social attention) on a frequent, ongoing basis that was not contingent on behavior. Both consumers chose the communication training procedure over the noncontingent reinforcement procedure. This creative study could be viewed within the context of behavioral social validation procedures, which are described later in this chapter. Finally, providing choices may be an effective tactic for a number of reasons. For instance, providing choices may be reinforcing in and of itself. Alternatively, providing choices may allow people to choose options that maximize reinforcement for them. By determining which of these characteristics of choice are important, behavioral researchers may help increase the effectiveness of choice in the context of behavioral or person-centered planning procedures (e.g., Fisher, Thompson, Piazza, Crosland, & Gotjen, 1997).

The person-centered focus on allowing consumers to choose their own goals and the means for reaching those goals is similar to behavioral social validation procedures (Wagner, 1999). Wolf (1978) originally articulated social validity within the field of behavior analysis by emphasizing the importance of assessing consumer satisfaction with program procedures and outcomes. Schwartz and Baer further summarized the focus of social validation: "1. Are the goals of the procedures important and relevant to the desired life-style changes? 2. Are the techniques used acceptable to the consumers and the community . . . ? 3. Are the consumers satisfied with the outcome . . . ?" (1991, pp. 192–193). In this context of social validity, Carr and colleagues (1999) later observed that one goal of positive behavioral support is met when consumers find the intervention and outcomes worthwhile. These foci seem remarkably similar to and consistent with those of person-centered planning.

EMPIRICAL SUPPORT AND RELATED ISSUES

In the spirit of scientific inquiry, this book presents research on person-centered planning. Given the history of fads in the field of developmental disabilities and the paucity of research in the area of person-centered planning, this is a much needed and important effort. However, proponents of person-centered planning such as Lyle O'Brien and colleagues lament, "Researchers call for studies to quantify its effects," and further state, "Now some people want to evaluate the effectiveness of person-centered planning by counting its outcomes, sometimes in predefined categories; for them people's stories are anecdotes" (1997, pp. 480, 483). Holburn and Vietze countered, "The position that person-centered planning outcomes should not be evaluated quantitatively is unsupportable" (1998, p. 487). Again, fads in the field of developmental disabilities are all too common. Indeed, the potential negative consequences of adopting ineffective fads include diverting time and scarce resources from otherwise effective approaches and, in some cases, causing actual harm (Osborne, 1999).

The primary research question is, "Does person-centered planning really work?" (Holburn, 1997; Holburn & Vietze, 1998). Given an affirmative answer, subsequent questions might include

- "Does person-centered planning work better than conventional approaches?"
- "What are the effective components?"
- "What are the optimal parameters for those components?"

These questions have been approached both qualitatively and quantitatively. Selecting one approach over the other often depends on the type of information sought or the amount of control that researchers have over the relevant variables. Ultimately, however, quantification of both process and outcomes is necessary for an empirical, experimental analysis (Holburn, Jacobson, Vietze, Schwartz, & Sersen, 2000). That is, to establish a functional, quantitative relationship between person-centered planning and its outcomes with a high degree of certainty, the independent variable (person-centered planning procedures) and dependent variables (outcomes) must first be operationalized; then, appropriate experimental procedures are employed. Such rigor is difficult to achieve in person-centered planning endeavors. Positive behavioral support researchers struggle with the same issues. For instance, Carr and colleagues (1999) noted that questions about the overall effectiveness of positive behavioral support and its components can only be answered by engaging in an experimental analysis. However, the difficulties of conducting controlled research, under naturalistic conditions, with multicomponent interventions, present challenges "tantamount to developing a new applied science" (Carr et al., p. 59). These issues also apply to conducting research in person-centered planning. Indeed, in describing the problem of overlap in independent and dependent variables in person-centered planning, Holburn and Vietze (1998) observed that the most difficult part of evaluating person-centered planning lies in conceptually differentiating the process from its outcomes (see also Osborne, 1999).

As of 2002, virtually no published studies meet these rigorous experimental requirements. A notable exception is a study by Holburn and colleagues (2000). The researchers used a rational-empirical method to construct three instruments for measuring both the person-centered process (and its integrity) and associated outcomes. Although quantitative studies on person-centered planning are lacking, some anecdotal case reports and other qualitative, descriptive studies have been published (e.g., Hagner, Helm, & Butterworth, 1996; Malette et al., 1992; see also Rowe & Rudkin, 1999 and Rudkin & Rowe, 1999). Unfortunately, these studies permit limited conclusions regarding any

functional relationship between person-centered planning and its outcomes. Hagner and colleagues reflected on this problem by describing
"an indirect, tenuous relationship between planning and outcomes"
(1996, p. 168). These authors further describe vague outcomes that
participants "felt" could have or "seemed to result" from the process
(p. 167). Such conclusions offer little for answering the previously
noted research questions.

Quantitative research is necessary to answer questions of cause
and effect in a definitive way. Qualitative research, however, can suggest possible relationships between process and outcome. Qualitative
approaches may also help identify outcomes that are not included in
predefined measures or are otherwise not known ahead of time. Typical qualitative approaches include open-ended interviews and observations. The resulting information may then be analyzed for overall
trends, generalities, or themes, ostensibly without any preexisting conceptual framework (Hagner et al., 1996, p. 161). The resulting studies
are generally anecdotal or case study in nature.

With respect to independent variables (person-centered planning
process), person-centered planning consists of a variety of approaches.
This variety has caused difficulties in operationally defining the overall approach (Schwartz, Jacobson, & Holburn, 2000). Holburn and
Vietze (1998) emphasized these definitional problems by describing
person-centered planning as "a multifaceted approach" that "is artful,
unique, personal, complex, and extended" (p. 486). Mount (1994) further suggested that efforts to standardize this approach result in frag-
mentation and breakdown in the process, as well as concomitant
decreased effectiveness. These realities present a challenge with regard
to operationalizing the approach as an independent variable. In this
context, Holburn (1997) suggested that community involvement and
honoring consumers' preferences and choices are essential elements of
person-centered planning. Researchers have begun to objectively
define the primary characteristics of a person-centered approach
(Schwartz et al., 2000). This type of operational definition is a prerequisite for reliable measurement of the integrity of person-centered
implementation and its outcomes (Holburn et al., 2000).

The dependent variables (i.e., outcomes) associated with person-
centered planning pose similar challenges. Purportedly, "multiple and
profound effects" may occur as a function of person-centered planning, although these may not be known a priori (Holburn, 1997, p. 80).
Some researchers note that person-centered planning outcomes may be
unforeseeable but suggest using predefined categories for dependent
variables (Holburn & Vietze, 1998; Rudkin & Rowe, 1999). For example, Holburn (1997) reported administering a battery of instruments

every 6 months to two groups of 20 people each: one group receiving person-centered planning and the other matched contrast group receiving traditional planning services. This battery apparently measured both the integrity of the independent variable and predefined dependent variables. In a later study, Holburn and colleagues (2000) described instruments that were developed to measure process and outcomes. Risley (1996) also proposed specific outcomes that include whether the person is happy, safe, more independent and productive, and included in community environments. These outcomes can be easily operationalized and measured. In fact, Green and Reid (1996) provided a good example of operationally defining happiness. Others have proposed similar quality of life outcomes (e.g., Holburn, 1997; Kincaid, 1996). Most researchers agree on a general level about the types of outcomes that should occur a priori as a function of person-centered planning. The task at hand, however, is defining these outcomes in sufficiently operationalized terms to permit the reliable measurement that is necessary for quantitative analysis.

When research is conducted under controlled, laboratory conditions, independent variables can be precisely defined and systematically manipulated. Their corresponding effects on specified dependent variables can be measured, and functional relationships between the two sets of variables can be determined. Conducting research in uncontrolled natural environments, however, presents a range of challenges. With regard to conducting research in positive behavioral procedures, Risley succinctly stated, "The recommendation for multicomponent interventions, individually adapted to circumstances and revised over time, is contrary to the [behavioral research] goals of specifiable treatment 'packages,'" and "recommendations for larger interventions, goals, and measures cannot be met while adhering to high requirements of experimental manipulation" (1999, p. xii). Carr and colleagues (1999) further suggested that the standards for rigor for these naturalistic studies must differ from those for tightly controlled experimental, analog research. The difficulties involved in conducting naturalistic research on positive behavioral support also apply to research efforts in person-centered planning. In response to these difficulties, researchers such as Holburn and Vietze (1998) have proposed using multiple research methods, including both quantitative and qualitative approaches. Clearly, both approaches have potential merit for evaluating person-centered planning. Quantitative, experimental and quasi-experimental approaches are necessary to answer basic questions regarding effectiveness and to conduct related component analyses. Holburn (1997), Schwartz and colleagues (2000), and others have appropriately developed for this purpose measures of independent variable integrity and predefined dependent variables. Alternatively, given the difficulties in a priori specification of outcomes, qualitative approaches may initially point to possible idiosyncratic outcomes that researchers would likely miss in the customary practice of predefining targeted outcomes. In addition, the time is right for new experimental approaches that fit the realities of complex interventions under real-world ecological conditions. Finally, in contrast to group designs, single-subject designs such as multiple baseline across subjects should be considered by future researchers. Regardless of experimental tactics, "In order to move practice on in a constructive way, it could be argued that we need more evidence and less ideology" (Rowe & Rudkin, 1999, p. 154).

CONCLUSION

Since the early 1990s, services for people with developmental disabilities have increasingly reflected a shift from program-centered to person-centered approaches. This chapter has 1) described how the field of developmental disabilities arrived at person-centered planning and positive behavioral supports, 2) analyzed person-centered planning from a behavioral conceptual framework, and 3) raised issues regarding research and empirical support. The rise of person-centered planning was fueled by an antibehavioral backlash by some members of the field who came to view behavioral techniques as inappropriate control procedures. However, person-centered planning is essentially environmental in approach, consistent with the focus of behaviorism. In addition, person-centered planning and behavioral procedures may complement each other in many ways. Despite the widespread adoption of person-centered planning, little research exists regarding the effectiveness of this approach or its components. This book is an important step in addressing this paucity.

Behavioral technology provided tools to dramatically increase functional life skills and reduce challenging behavior for people with developmental disabilities. Early efforts to reduce challenging behavior typically involved arranging reinforcers for not engaging in the target behavior and punishers for engaging in the behavior. These punishers were often used indiscriminately. That is, they were not always reserved for the most severe behavior. This frequent, often indiscriminate use resulted in pressure to reduce or eliminate the use of punishers and to replace them with socially valid procedures. In addition, some segments of the developmental disabilities field came to view any behavioral programming as ideologically undesirable. Behavioral procedures were viewed as being incompatible with choice and self-determination. Also, desirable outcomes for people with challenging behavior began to reflect broad quality of life improvements, rather than to simply reduce challenging behavior. Person-centered planning and other positive behavioral approaches arose in this context.

Although many professionals have viewed behavioral and person-centered approaches as incompatible, both are environmental in nature. For example, both frequently involve changing antecedent or ecological conditions, and both may involve providing reinforcers independently of behavior. Risley (1996) provided an especially pragmatic, environmental description of the relationship between behavioral and person-centered approaches. At one end of a hierarchy are precise, behavior analytic procedures; these procedures are followed by less-technical contingency management approaches and, finally, by molar, ecological "life arrangement" interventions. As Risley noted, the latter focuses on identifying and maximizing those things (e.g., people, places) that a person prefers and minimizing those things that a person dislikes.

These approaches require relatively little technical expertise or training, and they should be tried first. According to Risley (1996), the level of intervention necessary for a person is inextricably bound to the flexibility of the environment:

> The wider the latitude available for modifying the life arrangements for a person with challenging behaviors, the less precise and technical the behavior programming needs to be. The opposite is also true in that the less flexible a person's life arrangements are, the more technically precise the behavior programming must be. (p. 429)

This conceptualization is thoroughly environmental and parsimonious.

In addition to sharing an environmental focus, person-centered planning and behavioral approaches may complement each other. For instance, behavioral functional assessment procedures and person-centered planning strive to identify reinforcers and punishers in a person's life. Functional assessment procedures can clarify and enhance the information gathered through the person-centered planning process. Behavioral research on choice can also contribute to person-centered planning. For example, rather than solely rely on caregiver opinions of consumer preference, behavioral preference assessments can directly assess preferences. Finally, the person-centered emphasis on consumer choice of goals and the means for achieving those goals resembles behavioral social validation procedures.

Person-centered planning remains more art than science, but investigators have begun to evaluate person-centered planning and establish an empirical base. It is hoped that the issues raised in this chapter encourage additional research toward this end. The majority of research conducted thus far is qualitative. However, researchers have begun to operationally define independent and dependent variables and to conduct quantitative studies. Both types of research are potentially useful.

Person-centered approaches have helped establish a values base for behavioral science with respect to broader quality of life goals and outcomes. This focus has also set the stage for relatively simple, socially acceptable approaches for addressing challenging behavior. Nonetheless, person-centered planning is not a panacea. Sometimes person-centered planning is feasible for reducing challenging behavior; sometimes it is not. Sometimes it is effective; sometimes it is not. Traditional behavior analytic approaches will continue to be necessary in environments or situations in which person-centered planning alone is ineffective or not particularly feasible. Both approaches, however, will continue to improve the lives of people with developmental disabilities.

REFERENCES

Anderson, C.M., & Freeman, K.A. (2000). Positive behavior support: Expanding the application of applied behavior analysis. *The Behavior Analyst, 23,* 9–14.

Bates, P., & Wehman, P. (1977). Behavior management with the mentally retarded: An empirical analysis of the research. *Mental Retardation, 15,* 9–14.

Carr, E.G. (1994). Emerging themes in the functional analysis of problem behavior. *Journal of Applied Behavior Analysis, 27,* 393–399.

Carr, E.G., Horner, R.H., Turnbull, A.P., Marquis, J.G., Magito-McLaughlin, D., McAtee, M.L., Smith, C.E., Ryan, K.A., Ruef, M.B., & Doolabh, A. (1999). *Positive behavior support for people with developmental disabilities.* Washington, DC: American Association on Mental Retardation.

Dunlap, G. (1990, November/December). Choice-making as a management strategy. *AAMR News and Notes, 6,* 3, 8.

Everson, J.M., & Reid, D.H. (1999). *Person-centered planning and outcome management.* Morganton, NC: Habilitative Management Consultants.

Fischer, S.M., Iwata, B.A., & Mazeleski, J.L. (1997). Noncontingent delivery of arbitrary reinforcers as treatment for self-injurious behavior. *Journal of Applied Behavior Analysis, 30,* 239–249.

Fisher, W.W., & Mazur, J.E. (1997). Basic and applied research on choice responding. *Journal of Applied Behavior Analysis, 30,* 387–410.

Fisher, W.W., O'Connor, J.T., Kurtz, P.F., DeLeon, I.G., & Gotjen, D.L. (2000). The effects of noncontingent delivery of high- and low-preference stimuli on attention-maintained destructive behavior. *Journal of Applied Behavior Analysis, 33,* 79–83.

Fisher, W.W., Piazza, C.C., Bowman, L.G., & Amari, A. (1996). Integrating caregiver report with a systematic choice assessment to enhance reinforcer identification. *American Journal on Mental Retardation, 101,* 15–25.

Fisher, W.W., Thompson, R.H., Piazza, C.C., Crosland, K., & Gotjen, D. (1997). On the relative reinforcing effects of choice and differential consequences. *Journal of Applied Behavior Analysis, 30,* 423–438.

Foxx, R.M., Faw, G.D., Taylor, S., Davis, P.K., & Fulia, R. (1993). "Would I be able to . . .?" Teaching clients to assess the availability of their community living life style preferences. *American Journal on Mental Retardation, 93,* 235–248.

Green, C.W., Middleton, S.G., & Reid, D.H. (2000). Embedded evaluation of preferences sampled from person-centered plans for people with profound multiple disabilities. *Journal of Applied Behavior Analysis, 33,* 639–642.

Green, C.W., & Reid, D.H. (1996). Defining, validating, and increasing indices of happiness among people with profound multiple disabilities. *Journal of Applied Behavior Analysis, 29,* 67–78.

Green, C.W., Reid, D.H., Canipe, V.S., & Gardner, S.M. (1991). A comprehensive evaluation of reinforcer identification processes for persons with profound multiple handicaps. *Journal of Applied Behavior Analysis, 24,* 537–552.

Green, C.W., Reid, D.H., White, L.K., Halford, R.C., Brittain, D.P., & Gardner, S.M. (1988). Identifying reinforcers for persons with profound handicaps: Staff opinion versus systematic assessment of preferences. *Journal of Applied Behavior Analysis, 21,* 31–43.

Hagner, D., Helm, D.T., & Butterworth, J. (1996). "This is your meeting": A qualitative study of person-centered planning. *Mental Retardation, 34,* 159–171.

Hagopian, L.P., Fisher, W.W., & Legacy, S.M. (1994). Schedule effects of non-contingent reinforcement on attention-maintained destructive behavior in identical quadruplets. *Journal of Applied Behavior Analysis, 27,* 317–325.

Hanley, G.P., Piazza, C.C., Fisher, W.W., Contrucci, S.A., & Maglieri, K.A. (1997). Evaluation of client preference for function-based treatment packages. *Journal of Applied Behavior Analysis, 30,* 459–473.

Holburn, S. (1997). A renaissance in residential behavior analysis? A historical perspective and a better way to help people with challenging behavior. *The Behavior Analyst, 20,* 61–85.

Holburn, S. (2001). Compatibility of person-centered planning and applied behavior analysis. *The Behavior Analyst, 24,* 271–281.

Holburn, S., Jacobson, J.W., Vietze, P.M., Schwartz, A.A., & Sersen, E. (2000). Quantifying the process and outcomes of person-centered planning. *American Journal on Mental Retardation, 105,* 402–416.

Holburn, S., & Vietze, P. (1998). Has person-centered planning become the alchemy of developmental disabilities? A response to O'Brien, O'Brien, and Mount. *Mental Retardation, 36,* 485–488.

Holburn, S., & Vietze, P. (1999). Acknowledging barriers in adopting person-centered planning. *Mental Retardation, 37,* 117–124.

Holburn, S., & Vietze, P. (2000). Person-centered planning and cultural inertia in applied behavior analysis. *Behavior and Social Issues, 10,* 39–70.

Horner, R.H. (1994). Functional assessment: Contributions and future directions. *Journal of Applied Behavior Analysis, 27,* 401–404.

Horner, R.H., Vaughn, B.J., Day, H.M., & Ard, W.R. (1996). The relationship between setting events and problem behavior: Expanding our understanding of behavioral support. In L.K. Koegel, R.L. Koegel, & G. Dunlap (Eds.), *Positive behavioral support: Including people with difficult behavior in the community* (pp. 381–402). Baltimore: Paul H. Brookes Publishing Co.

Iwata, B.A., Dorsey, M.F., Slifer, K.J., Bauman, K.E., & Richman, G.S. (1994). Toward a functional analysis of self-injury. *Journal of Applied Behavior*

Analysis, 27, 197–209. (Reprinted from *Analysis and Intervention in Developmental Disabilities, 2,* 3–20, 1982)

Kincaid, D. (1996). Person-centered planning. In L.K. Koegel, R.L. Koegel, & G. Dunlap (Eds.), *Positive behavioral support: Including people with difficult behavior in the community* (pp. 439–465). Baltimore: Paul H. Brookes Publishing Co.

Koegel, R.L., & Koegel, L.K. (1989). Community-referenced research on self-stimulation. In E. Cipani (Ed.), *The treatment of severe behavior disorders* (pp. 129–150). Washington, DC: American Association on Mental Retardation.

LaVigna, G.W., Willis, T.J., & Donnellan, A.M. (1989). The role of positive programming in behavioral treatment. In E. Cipani (Ed.), *The treatment of severe behavior disorders* (pp. 59–83). Washington, DC: American Association on Mental Retardation.

Lennox, D.B., Miltenberger, R.G., Spengler, P., & Erfanian, N. (1988). Decelerative treatment practices with persons who have mental retardation: A review of five years of the literature. *American Journal on Mental Retardation, 92,* 492–501.

Lohrmann-O'Rourke, S., & Browder, D.M. (1998). Empirically based methods to assess the preferences of individuals with severe disabilities. *American Journal on Mental Retardation, 103,* 146–161.

Lyle O'Brien, C., O'Brien, J., & Mount, B. (1997). Person-centered planning has arrived . . . or has it? *Mental Retardation, 35,* 480–484.

Mace, F.C. (1994). The significance and future of functional analysis methodologies. *Journal of Applied Behavior Analysis, 27,* 385–392.

Malette, P., Mirenda, P., Kandborg, T., Jones, P., Bunz, P., & Rogow, S. (1992). Application of a lifestyle development process for persons with severe intellectual disabilities: A case study report. *Journal of The Association for Persons with Severe Handicaps, 17,* 179–191.

Morgan, R.L. (1989). Judgments of restrictiveness, social acceptability, and usage: Review of research on procedures to decrease behavior. *American Journal on Mental Retardation, 96,* 121–133.

Mount, B. (1992). *Personal futures planning: A sourcebook of values, ideas, and methods to encourage person-centered development.* New York: Graphic Futures.

Mount, B. (1994). Benefits and limitations of personal futures planning. In V.J. Bradley, J.W. Ashbaugh, & B.C. Blaney (Eds.), *Creating individual supports for people with developmental disabilities: A mandate for change at many levels* (pp. 97–108). Baltimore: Paul H. Brookes Publishing Co.

O'Brien, J. (1987). A guide to life-style planning: Using The Activities Catalog to integrate services and natural support systems. In B. Wilcox & G.T. Bellamy, *A comprehensive guide to The Activities Catalog: An alternative curriculum for youth and adults with severe disabilities* (pp. 175–189). Baltimore: Paul H. Brookes Publishing Co.

Osborne, J.G. (1999). Renaissance or killer mutation? A response to Holburn. *The Behavior Analyst, 22,* 47–52.

Reid, D.H., Everson, J.M., & Green, C.W. (1999). A systematic evaluation of preferences identified through person-centered planning for people with profound multiple disabilities. *Journal of Applied Behavior Analysis, 32,* 467–476.

Risley, T. (1996). Get a life! Positive behavioral intervention for challenging behavior through life arrangement and life coaching. In L.K. Koegel, R.L. Koegel, & G. Dunlap (Eds.), *Positive behavioral support: Including people with difficult behavior in the community* (pp. 425–437). Baltimore: Paul H. Brookes Publishing Co.

Risley, T.R. (1999). Foreword. In E.G. Carr, R.H. Horner, A.P. Turnbull, J.G. Marquis, D.Magito-McLaughlin, M.L. McAtee, C.E. Smith, K.A. Ryan, M.B. Ruef, & A. Doolabh, *Positive behavior support for people with developmental disabilities: A research synthesis* (pp. xi–xiii). Washington, DC: American Association on Mental Retardation.

Rowe, D., & Rudkin, A. (1999). A systematic review of the qualitative evidence for the use of lifestyle planning in people with learning disabilities. *Journal of Learning Disabilities for Nursing, Health and Social Care, 3,* 148–158.

Rudkin, A., & Rowe, D. (1999). A systematic review of the evidence base for lifestyle planning in adults with learning disabilities: Implications for other disabled populations. *Clinical Rehabilitation, 13,* 363–372.

Schwartz, A.A., Jacobson, J.W., & Holburn, S.C. (2000). Defining person-centeredness: Results of two consensus methods. *Education and Training in Mental Retardation and Developmental Disabilities, 35*(3), 235–249.

Schwartz, I.S., & Baer, D.M. (1991). Social validity assessments: Is current practice state of the art? *Journal of Applied Behavior Analysis, 24,* 189–204.

Scotti, J.R., Evans, I.M., Meyer, L.H., & Walker, P. (1991). A meta-analysis of intervention research with problem behavior: Treatment validity and standards of practice. *American Journal on Mental Retardation, 96,* 233–256.

Smull, M.W., & Burke Harrison, S. (1992). *Supporting people with severe reputations in the community.* Alexandria, VA: National Association of State Directors of Developmental Disabilities Services.

Vollmer, T.R., Iwata, B.A., Zarcone, J.R., Smith, R.G., & Mazeleski, J.L. (1993). The role of attention in the treatment of attention-maintained self-injurious behavior: Noncontingent reinforcement and differential reinforcement of other behavior. *Journal of Applied Behavior Analysis, 26,* 9–21.

Wagner, G.A. (Chair). (1996, May). *Mixing and marketing in person-centered contexts.* Panel presented at the annual convention of the Association for Behavior Analysis, San Francisco.

Wagner, G.A. (1999). Further comments on person-centered approaches. *The Behavior Analyst, 22,* 53–54.

Wagner, G.A., & Martin, P.L. (1995). Some relationships between behavioral and person-centered approaches. *Superintendents' Digest, 14,* 15–18.

Wolf, M.M. (1978). Social validity: The case for subjective measurement, or how applied behavior analysis is finding its heart. *Journal of Applied Behavior Analysis, 11,* 315–329.

13

A Better Life for Hal

Five Years of Person-Centered Planning and Applied Behavior Analysis

Steve Holburn and Peter M. Vietze

This chapter is about Hal, an adult with autism, and a team of people who persevered through a long and sometimes difficult process of helping him change his life. The story spans Hal's 27 years in New York City institutions to his new life in a typical community neighborhood on Long Island, New York, and it describes the process that made the transition possible. From 1994 to 1998, Hal was involved in Personal Futures Planning, a variant of person-centered planning delineated by Mount (1992a; 1992b; 1994). As an outgrowth of the Personal Futures Planning, Hal and his parents also participated in an extensive behavioral intervention program employing applied behavior analysis techniques to eliminate aggressive behavior, and, as a consequence, they were able to spend time together on a regular basis. Bolstered by their participation in both Personal Futures Planning and applied behavior analysis, Hal's parents came to play a central role, if not the most central role, in helping Hal change his life.

BACKGROUND

In 1967, when Hal was 7 years old, he was admitted to Willowbrook State School on Staten Island in New York. His family could no longer manage his dangerous running away, self-injury, and other challenging behaviors related to autism. According to his mother, Hal was a "tough

This work was supported by the New York State Office of Mental Retardation and Developmental Disabilities. The authors thank Barbara Podber for her assistance in all phases of this project. Appreciation is also extended to Al Pfadt, Bernard Carabello, Aletha Bauman, and Kathy Broderick.

cookie." Some of the aides at Willowbrook took a special interest in Hal, but they could not protect him from the restraints, hunger, and abuses that befell many Willowbrook inhabitants (see Bronston, 1973). The family surmised that Hal did not like Willowbrook because at the end of the weekly car ride with his parents and older sister, he routinely fought his return to the institution and, once in the institution, immediately took refuge under a table. Back then, family members could venture no farther than the waiting room, so they could only imagine his actual living conditions. Hal's family endured the separation. They thought it was best for Hal, and there seemed to be no alternative.

Hal also endured Willowbrook. He grew up there. At age 20, after most of the residents had moved to the community as a result of the Willowbrook Consent Decree in 1975, Hal was transferred to a smaller state-operated institution in New York City. (He was deemed unable to live in the community because he was a "runner" and he had a dangerous habit of chewing discarded cigarette butts.) This smaller institution was nearer to Hal's family house. During his tenure there, Hal's parents rejected a number of community group home possibilities for reasons of safety and concerns about the stability of the nonprofit, voluntary agencies offering the living arrangements. Similarly, voluntary agencies hesitated to offer residential services to Hal because of his reputation and their fear of becoming responsible for someone whom they could not adequately support.

In 1994, after 14 years of living in the smaller developmental center, Hal became involved in Personal Futures Planning. He was the lead-off participant in a project to facilitate community transitions for 21 Willowbrook class members who still resided in institutions. For most of these people, adequate community services and supports could not be established because of their challenging behavior. This venture, the Willowbrook Futures Project, was a collaborative planning effort that brought together people from various settings, including 1) the New York State Institute for Basic Research on Staten Island, 2) the New York State Office of Mental Retardation and Developmental Disabilities in Albany, 3) the Challenging Behavior Subcommittee of the Commissioner's Task Force in Manhattan, 4) four developmental disabilities service organizations in New York City, and 5) various voluntary agencies in the New York metropolitan area. Several months before Hal's person-centered planning began, he was evaluated at the New York State Institute for Basic Research in Developmental Disabilities, where a suspected diagnosis of autism was confirmed. This information was consoling to Hal's parents, who had been baffled by how much he differed from other residents.

PERSONAL FUTURES PLANNING

Hal was the first participant in the Willowbrook Futures Project because he was considered the most challenging candidate to move into the community. Yet, the team also knew that reintroducing Hal to the community after he had spent most of his life in institutions would take the cooperation of many people over a long period of time. Indeed, before Hal actually moved to the community, his person-centered planning team formally met 34 times between 1994 and 1998, with 56 different people in attendance at one time or another during this period. The planning process tapered considerably after Hal moved, although three additional person-centered planning meetings were held during the first year following his move. Early on in the planning, an unusually large number of people were involved (the average attendance of the first five meetings was 19), and robust participation was sustained thereafter (the average attendance of follow-along meetings was 10).

Thus, Hal's person-centered planning generated a great deal of interest, and it was a highly visible process. The meetings were held in various locations, including 21 meetings at the developmental center, 8 at his parents' house, and 5 at voluntary provider agency offices or residences. Ad hoc subcommittees, such as a find-a-home committee and a behavior plan committee, were spun-off from the main meetings and were held at these and other locations. A core group of five people were present at nearly all person-centered planning meetings: Hal's mother and father, the facilitator of the meetings (the first author), a friend-advocate who had also spent most of his life at Willowbrook, and the developmental center psychologist.

Initial Preparation

Prior to the first meeting, the facilitator spent time with Hal and met the people who knew Hal well. Most of these people, including Hal's parents, had reservations about community involvement because of the severity and, in particular, the tenacity of Hal's challenging behavior. The worst fear was that Hal would dart in front of a moving car. Years earlier, he had run out of the developmental center, across a busy street, and into a grocery store where he was found sitting on the floor gorging on potato chips.

It was clear that if people were going to take seriously the idea of Hal's community inclusion, then a demonstration of a successful (safe) community outing was needed as a first step. This opportunity arose when, after a month of visiting with Hal and staff at the developmental center, the facilitator was permitted to take Hal for a walk around the block with the help of two staff members whose quickness and agility were known to effectively counter Hal's risky behavior. The venture was a success: Hal was delighted with his 20-minute walk through the neighborhood with his tense entourage, and the group returned to an applause reception. In retrospect, the brief walk was an auspicious beginning to a much longer journey.

Potential participants in Hal's person-centered planning were contacted and sent invitation letters specifying the purpose of the meetings, as well as introductory material describing the principles and process of person-centered planning. We encouraged participants to spend some time with Hal before the first meeting and to consider the following questions for later discussion:

- What past experiences have most influenced Hal's life?
- Who are the people in Hal's life, past and present? What is the nature of their relationships?
- How does Hal spend his time? How much choice does he have in what he does?
- What does Hal like to do? What frustrates him or makes him angry?
- Where does Hal spend his time, and how does he react to these places?
- What is Hal's reputation, and on what is it based?

First Three Meetings

The first three meetings were held at Hal's parents' house. At these meetings, we established ground rules and discussed the underlying philosophy of person-centered planning, using O'Brien's (1987) five essential accomplishments of person-centered planning as a guide: community presence, community participation, choice, competence, and respect. The ground rules targeted equal and courteous meeting participation, voluntary attendance, and the use of positively framed language devoid of technical jargon (see O'Brien & Mount, 1991). Later on, we dropped the language rule because it was inhibiting involvement of people who worried that they would make a verbal mistake.

Ironically, another factor interfering with meeting participation was the presence of Hal himself. Hal did not use speech and appeared to understand very little of what was said at the meetings. Nonetheless, we tried to include him. He attended the first two meetings but was clearly not interested and continually distracted his parents, so we held meetings without him thereafter. However, Hal was actively involved in many other aspects of the process, and despite his absence at the subsequent person-centered planning and ad hoc subcommitte meetings, the process remained focused on achieving a better life for Hal.

The team used the mapping process described by Mount (1992a, 1992b). First, a personal profile was developed by mapping out important events in Hal's life, places where Hal spends time, people in his life, his daily routine, choices, preferences, nonpreferences, and challenging behavior. After the meetings, these maps were photographed, attached to the minutes, and circulated to participants. In creating the profile, we learned that Hal immediately became healthier and happier when he moved from Willowbrook to the smaller facility in 1980. Even so, the smaller facility was a monolithic structure that housed 135 people at the time that person-centered planning began for Hal. It was surrounded by a high fence with a sign that read, "PROPERTY OF NEW YORK STATE: NO TRESPASSING." Hal was confined mainly to one wing of the fourth floor, where 25 direct support staff provided coverage to residents with significant behavior problems. The following excerpt from a quality of life assessment (described in detail later in this chapter) reveals the climate of the residence when person-centered planning began:

> Interior physical qualities: Most people would not consider the inside to be attractive or homey. Hal's living area is loud, open, austere. There are some bright colors. Long hallways with bedrooms off hallway. Offices and classrooms on same floor as bedroom. Yelling and running is common. Sometimes appears chaotic with staff looking exhausted, exasperated. Occasional offensive odors. Residents seen pacing, sitting. Windows do not open. Dorm-like bedroom shared with two other people. One hits Hal frequently. No obvious personal possessions demarcate bedroom as Hal's. Water fountain outside bedroom does not work.

The personal profile maps showed that throughout his life, Hal developed numerous special relationships with staff that ended abruptly when the employee moved on to another job. At the beginning of person-centered planning, Hal showed a preference for only one staff member. During family visits, he responded positively to his father, who visited frequently, but Hal vigorously hit his mother, who consequently curtailed her visits. Generally, Hal was guarded closely and had little control of his surroundings. Most of the decisions pertaining to Hal—such as who his roommates were, where his time was spent, and what he wore—were made by others. However, Hal was able to decide whether to participate in a given activity; he was given choices, although limited, at meals and snack time; and he was able to decide when he went to bed.

His likes and dislikes were clear. The preferences map indicated 16 things that Hal enjoyed, including manipulating things, listening to soft music, wearing new clothing, finishing what he started, eating sweets, and helping out. Seven nonpreferences were generated, including being around a lot of people; being in noisy situations; and encountering changes in his environment, routine, or caretakers. A map of his daily routine showed an orderly but unimaginative schedule with activity changes approximately every half hour. A respect map showed 15 characteristics that people admired about Hal, such as his physical strength, agility, persistence, alertness, and ready smile. It also listed nine characteristics that were not admired, including Hal's being impatient, ripping off his shirt, hitting his mother, and running away from staff. Hal was believed to be very healthy, if not indefatigable, and was given three milligrams (mg) of Haldol (a neuroleptic antipsychotic medication) per day to help manage his behavior.

During the first three meetings at Hal's parents' house, Hal's maps were used to envision a more desirable future for him. A new home would be near his parents and in a quiet neighborhood with minimal traffic. He would live with a few roommates with whom he could get along, and perhaps they would all share in the rent or ownership of the home. He would have a private room with a combination bathtub-shower, a stereo, a combination TV-VCR, and maybe even a pet. The group also envisioned ways in which Hal might become more involved in the community, develop more relationships, and engage in more productive work.

Roller Coaster Ride

Throughout the rest of the planning process, the team worked toward achieving the vision that we had developed. At each meeting, we reviewed our progress and adjusted our strategy, but neither the process nor the progress was smooth. We seemed either to lurch ahead or to be stymied by a setback. As Hal's father put it, "I feel like I'm on a roller coaster." As we continued to meet and as Hal's community experiences accumulated, parts of the vision were modified by a shifting consensus about what would be best for Hal, and other parts were scaled back by limitations in feasibility. Despite occasional droughts of inaction, we were buoyed by people behind the scenes who were helping us achieve the vision for Hal by pushing our ideas through different levels of the bureaucracy.

During the first 6 months, success came easily. Hal's parents had invited as participants staff from a voluntary agency specializing in autism, and the staff quickly assumed the role of providing residential and day services. The find-a-home subcommittee identified two possible houses in Bayside, Queens, as well as two prospective roommates. An employee of the voluntary agency, Bill, befriended Hal. After visiting Hal on a regular basis, he began taking Hal to various places in the local community with help from the developmental center staff. To extend these activities, a unique transitional funding grant was arranged for the agency, and Hal was soon spending 1 day per week with Bill, half of which was spent in the community and half of which was spent at the agency day program. Hal even made a few visits to his parents' house. Figure 13.1 shows how many hours per month Hal spent in the community from 1994 to 1998. The figure indicates that the hours increased during the transitional funding period but that the rate was irregular. Data for Figure 13.1 were abstracted from activity log entries and data forms that were filled out by assistants who accompanied Hal, as well as data that were recorded by his parents. For verification, log entries and data forms were compared with 1) mandatory sign-in-and-out sheets at the developmental center entrance and 2) pay vouchers indicating that the assistants were working at the dates and times of the recorded activities.

Substantial changes also occurred at the developmental center during the first 6 months. Hal was transferred to a more peaceful floor and given a private bedroom with a bathroom. The bedroom had windows that opened, a television, drapes, and a radio. He was also assigned a preferred staff member to assist him, one-to-one, throughout the evening. According to Hal's mother, "He loves it—he's a different person now!" Hal was doing more things that he enjoyed, and all who knew him unanimously agreed that he was more relaxed, better behaved, and more responsible.

Things began to get bogged down during the second 6 months. The two possible houses in Bayside fell through. One was in a "saturated area," a neighborhood that had reached the maximum level of group homes by a preestablished standard; the other required renovations that proved to be too expensive. Also, the prospective roommates were contested because they were not on a priority list for community placement (other people, most of whom lived in institutions, had been waiting longer to move and were on a "mandated placement list").

Another problem was a growing divergence between the vision developed by the person-centered planning team and the planning that was underway for Hal's day and residential services by the voluntary agency. Although Hal was learning some new skills and responsibilities at the agency day program, he did not like the cramped quarters, and he sometimes had to be coaxed out from under a table. He frequently hit himself and bit his hand during repetitive compliance activities, which were not consistent with the vocational interests and preferences identified by the planning team. Ironically, while the institutional system was adapting more to Hal's interests, the voluntary

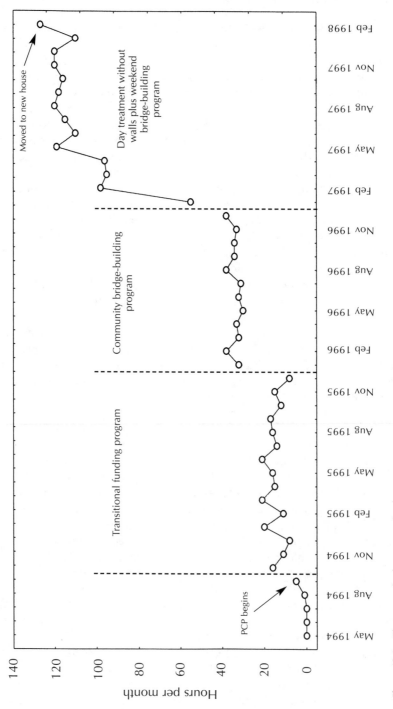

Figure 13.1. Time spent in the community. (*Key:* PCP = person-centered planning.)

agency was eager to take control of the process and demonstrate that Hal could adapt to a highly structured autism program. This disconnect remained, despite meeting reviews of the vision for Hal and the principles of autonomy and inclusion.

Community Bridge-Building Program

Planning meetings continued approximately once per month, and progress picked up again, more than a year after person-centered planning began. The planning team eventually divested the voluntary agency, and Bill gradually faded from the picture after the transitional funding was exhausted. A different voluntary agency was selected. The new agency was interested in shifting its service philosophy to a more person-centered approach. Two employees from that agency had been attending Hal's meetings from the beginning, and they enthusiastically stepped up to the challenge.

We needed to continue community experiences in a way that was more accountable to the person-centered process. To assist, the New York State Office of Mental Retardation and Developmental Disabilities established funding for a community bridge-building program. The program permitted hourly payment to an individual who accompanied a person from an institution during community outings. Hal's parents hired the bridge builder: an acquaintance named Don, who had worked with Hal in the past as an employee. Don signed an agreement that specified his responsibilities in providing truly individualized community experiences, and he was periodically paid using a voucher signed by either parent. Don submitted the voucher to the previously noted state office, which disbursed payment from the fund that was created for the bridge-building program. Twice per week, Don and two assistants supplied by the developmental center accompanied Hal to different places in the community, usually by vehicle, for a 4-hour period. Later, at person-centered planning meetings, Don shared Hal's reactions to these community experiences, and then the group planned a new, monthly bridge-building schedule of events and activities.

Figure 13.1 shows that time in the community approximately doubled after the introduction of the bridge-building program. More specifically, Figure 13.2 gives a snapshot of the types and frequency of community activities that took place during this phase of person-centered planning. The range of experiences was fairly broad, although 40% of the activities involved food consumption. Of the total 176 activities, 63 were new experiences, which suggests that about two thirds of the activities were repeats.

During the bridge-building phase, progress continued on other fronts as well. Hal's father found him a house in Long Island, which,

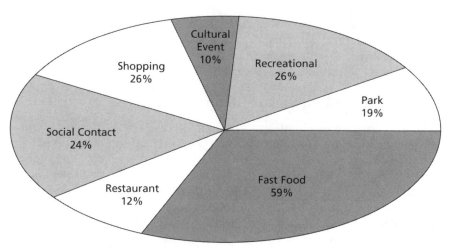

Figure 13.2. Number of community activities by category during the bridge-building program.

with renovations, appeared perfect for Hal. After 2 years, Hal eventually moved to this house. The long delay was due to a complicated process of achieving local community board approval, purchasing the house, renovating it, certifying it, negotiating a budget for agency services, and hiring the right staff. In the meantime, the person-centered planning team continued to meet. A new schedule of activities was established for Hal at the developmental center that was commensurate with his burgeoning skills and interests. A broader range of activities was made available. Hal also assumed the job of messenger, which entailed supervised delivery of items throughout the developmental center, including mail, packages, and other goods. In addition, with supervision, he learned to do his laundry, arrange his clothing, and clean his room. By the fall of 1996, Hal was visiting at his parents' house once per week.

Day Treatment Without Walls

To bridge the gap while the house was being readied, the voluntary agency proposed a community-based, Medicaid-funded day treatment program. In this atypical arrangement, which was approved in January 1997, two agency staff assisted Hal on weekdays in exploring various job possibilities and community activities in the Long Island neighborhood to which he would be moving. In addition, the bridge-building program continued in abbreviated form on weekends. These new assistants learned about Hal by their participation on the person-centered planning team and by accompanying the bridge builder in local community activities. This program continued until Hal moved, and, as Figure 13.1 shows, Hal consistently spent a large amount of time in the community for more than a year during this period.

Hal received modest compensation for various jobs, including working in a greenhouse and placing fliers on car windshields; however, he preferred a job that consisted of his picking up soda cans from agency residences on a different route each day of the week and dropping them off at a grocery store, where he fed them into a recycling machine. The increased responsibility and community exposure seemed to have a positive effect on Hal, as indicated by the following log excerpt about the voluntary agency staff's experience upon returning Hal to the developmental center after a full day in the community:

> As we prepared to leave the building, staff members who work with Hal, as well as custodial staff, commented on how much more pleasant he was upon his return from a day in the community than on days in which he does not have the opportunity to spend time in the outside world. It was music to our ears.

REUNITING THE FAMILY

Soon after person-centered planning began, the developmental center psychologist and the meeting facilitator observed Hal and his parents during visits at the developmental center. They observed that Hal frequently and forcefully hit his mother, a septuagenarian, who wore a flack jacket to protect herself. Four interaction patterns appeared problematic. First, it seemed that Hal's mother, Rita, unintentionally reinforced hitting. After a hit, she scolded him, then tried to teach an alternative response by saying, "This is how you show love to Mommy," at which point she would kiss him and occasionally offer a piece of candy. Despite Hal's barrages, Rita was reluctant to retreat. In her eyes, enduring the blows was testament of her love for him. A second complication during visits was a method that Hal's parents used for testing his memory and ingenuity. Hal loved candy, and before visits, Hal's father often hid candy in his own clothing and at strategic places on the floor where Hal lived, such as in the elevator or in the fire extinguisher case, which permitted a demonstration of Hal's memory. A find-the-candy game ensued in which Hal thoroughly searched his father's jacket, shirt, pants, and socks, until he could find no more candy. Hal sometimes became agitated at that point; however, his father always had one more hidden piece that he eventually gave up, often to pacify Hal. On the way out, when the visit was over, the candy that had been placed at various locations earlier served as a diversion for a smooth getaway.

The third problem was Hal's annoyance with changes in his routine or features of his environment during visits. His parents tried to keep visit arrangements consistent, but given the unpredictable nature of institutional conditions, consistency was rare, and Hal invariably became upset when things were not just right. Fourth, Hal's parents brought snacks for Hal to enjoy during the visits. Hal would eat ravenously; food would fly, and his drink often ended up on the floor. When finished, he would take his parents by the hand and tug them vigorously toward his bedroom, leaving a mess behind.

Behavioral Intervention

The facilitator and the psychologist proposed an extensive plan to improve the interaction between Hal and his parents during visits. The plan entailed 1) helping the parents identify key antecedents and consequences of Hal's (and their) behavior and 2) assisting them in arranging contingencies to support more appropriate behavior. New ways of interacting with Hal were to be learned through structured, regular training sessions (eventually dubbed "Mommy Visits") with the stipulation that private visits would resume only after new behavior patterns were established. It was anticipated that one consequence of hitting would be Rita's leaving the room, at least momentarily. The proposals to restrict visits and to exit contingently were initially unpopular with some members of the behavior plan subcommittee that was formed to explore a solution to the hitting: Restricting private visits was thought to be draconian, and contingent exiting would "give the wrong message." Eventually, however, the parents and the subcommittee agreed to the plan, and it was implemented several months after being proposed. By the time the plan began, Rita had not seen Hal for 6 weeks due to increased severity of hitting, and she was eager to begin visiting again.

The behavior plan was dynamic in the sense that many intervention procedures would be shaped by Hal's reactions, so the facilitator and the psychologist were unable to precisely specify all methods in advance. The plan was complex in that it included provisions to alter family interaction patterns, develop a tolerance for variation in conditions, and establish a more functional routine during visits. The facilitator and the psychologist, who served as instructors, coordinated sessions and were present during visits, and the parents had latitude to modify certain features of the plan. In fact, if Hal's parents had a strong hunch about a certain antecedent or consequence, they were guided in implementing and observing the effects, but only if the instructors believed that it would not contribute to any of the four previously discussed problems. The instructors discussed these problems extensively with Hal's parents and described elementary behavior analysis principles such as reinforcement, punishment, and stimulus control. These principles were used to explain hypotheses about why the problem behaviors were occurring and how they might be resolved.

Prior to each Mommy Visit, Hal's parents, the facilitator, and the psychologist reviewed the prior session and clarified the strategy for the imminent visit. During the sessions, the parents were often coached by reiterating the rationale for certain interventions and pointing out pertinent learning principles that were operating at the moment. After each visit, debriefing sessions were held, at which time the instructors and Hal's parents discussed the strong and weak points of the visit and formulated the strategy for the next one. Session information was recorded by the psychologist on a data sheet during the visit, and 13 sessions were videotaped and reviewed in debriefing sessions. The first 24 visits were held twice weekly, then visits were gradually interspersed to a schedule of once per month.

To address Hal's presumed need for consistency, the facilitator and the psychologist speculated that he could adapt to varied conditions, so they deliberately but gradually altered conditions throughout the visits. Accordingly, each session was systematically different from the preceding session in at least two of the following ways: session time, seating arrangements, direct-support staff, type of food, leisure items, and door of exit. Beginning with Session 10, Hal's father was occasionally excluded, and by Session 11, sessions were held in different rooms at the developmental center. During the Mommy Visits, Hal was taught to eat snacks more slowly and, when finished, to pick up food from the floor, clean the table, dispose of the trash, and wash his hands. Candy was not allowed until later in the Mommy Visits. Four months after Session 11, five visits also included car rides in which Rita would leave the car contingent on a hit, but the activity was discontinued because of the impracticality of this consequence.

Evaluation Visits There were 94 Mommy Visits from April 1995 to February 1998, the month that Hal moved to his new home in the community. The main thrust of the initial Mommy Visits was to evaluate the various antecedents and consequences of hitting while presenting Hal with various leisure activities. Rita's kisses sometimes evoked hitting, and kissing was limited. Hand mitts did not deter hitting. Various consequences of hitting were piloted: saying "No!", briefly removing food, having either Rita or both parents leave the room from 20 seconds to 5 minutes, and using combinations thereof.

During the first 11 visits, there were problems in 1) identifying a hit (Rita would not leave the room if a hit did not hurt) and 2) responding rapidly to a hit (Hal's parents sometimes vacillated and interacted with him as they left the room). To resolve these problems, the instructors and Hal's parents observed videotapes of the visits in debriefing sessions until they agreed on what constituted a hit. In addition, videotape examples of delays in exiting were noted. Figure 13.3 depicts the results of the 94 Mommy Visits by showing the frequency of hits on the left y axis and duration of session on the right y axis. The first 11 sessions were terminated arbitrarily, and as Figure 13.3 shows, decreased hitting was associated with longer visits during this period.

One Hit Ends Visit   By session 12, the instructors and Hal's parents agreed to terminate visits entirely after one hit. From that point, the duration of visits gradually increased to a peak of about 1.5 hours and eventually decreased to a relatively stable average of approximately 14 minutes per visit. Although these visits ended after one hit, some sessions showed more than one hit because Hal occasionally hit Rita with two to four rapid, successive hits—a pattern that was more pronounced beginning with session 34, when Rita began sitting next to Hal. On the day that Session 30 took place, Haldol was discontinued and then reinstated at a low dosage on the day of Session 40. This interruption roughly corresponded to the increase in both hitting and duration of visits during that time period and appeared to at least partially explain those behavior changes. (Prior to Session 30, Haldol had been tapered from 3 mg per day and remained at .5 mg per day after it was reinstated.)

Reinforcement for No Hitting   A problem with the consequence of one hit ending a visit was that it also unfortunately constituted a contingency such that if Hal wanted the visit to end, he was required to hit Rita. As an alternative, the psychologist and the facilitator taught Hal to end the visit by taking his parents by the hand and walking them to an exit door. When Hal reached the door, however, he promptly hit Rita. Although this was unnerving to Rita, the instructors had fortuitously discovered a reliable antecedent and a juncture at which they could intercede. Beginning with Session 45, they physically interrupted the anticipated last-minute hit and presented a small piece of candy if a hit did not occur at the exit. Following this procedure, many sessions ended without a hit, and as Figure 13.3 shows, from January 1997 (Session 70) to February 1998 (the month that Hal moved to his new house), only one hit occurred during the Mommy Visits. Thus, Hal was able to end visits at his discretion, without hitting Rita.

Generalization Visits   In November of 1995, 6 months after the Mommy Visits began, both of Hal's parents began visiting Hal together privately at the developmental center. (Hal's father had been visiting him alone during evenings as the Mommy Visits were taking

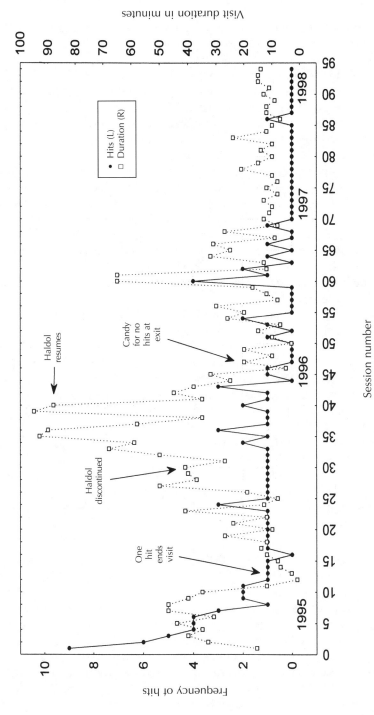

Figure 13.3. Frequency of hitting and duration of Mommy Visits.

305

place.) In relation to the Mommy Visit data, these generalization visits began between Sessions 38 and 39 in Figure 13.3. Hal's parents were asked to record the occurrence of hitting and to maintain the same procedures used in Mommy Visits. These private visits continued at a rate of approximately three times per month until Hal moved. During this 27-month period, his parents recorded 74 visits, 42 of which occurred with no hitting. As the visits accumulated, the ratio of visits without hits compared to visits with hits became more favorable.

Early on in the Mommy Visits, the facilitator and the psychologist showed Hal's parents how they could engage Hal in various activities during visits, but they preferred to just visit, which seemed to be Hal's preference as well. However, his parents enthusiastically and consistently required Hal to eat his snacks more slowly, clean up afterward, and wash his hands. This teaching appeared to generalize to other situations during visits. For example, Hal's parents began to require that he wash his hands and tuck in his shirt after using the bathroom, as well as pick up paper that he dropped on his bedroom floor and dispose of it in the wastebasket.

Summary   The facilitator and the psychologist did not expect Hal to adapt so easily to the changing conditions of the visits; fortunately, this loosened up a formerly rigid routine and made visiting more enjoyable. Before the community activities and behavioral intervention, Hal had resisted participation in activities that were new or frustrating. Hal and his caregivers had reached a behavioral gridlock in which staff and family members ensured that Hal's routine did not change because change upset Hal. Little by little, the facilitator and the psychologist observed that Hal was willing to try new things and was able to tolerate formerly frustrating circumstances. Hal's parents were proud of his expanding interests and repertoire and did not seem to miss the find-the-candy game that disrupted their former visits. In short, the Mommy Visits permitted the family to spend time together privately and peacefully.

CHANGES IN QUALITY OF LIFE

Periodically throughout the person-centered planning process, the planning team assessed Hal's overall quality of life. To quantify the degree of change that might be taking place, we assessed nine dimensions of quality of life using the Person-Centered Planning Quality of Life Indicators–Consensus Version (Holburn & Pfadt, 1995). The dimensions were derived from an evaluation component of the Positive Futures Project (Mount & Patterson, 1986). Each dimension consists of three to eight subcomponents, or aspects, the origins of which are described in Holburn, Jacobson, Vietze, Schwartz, and Sersen (2000). To complete this assessment, two or more informed respondents discuss each of 48 total aspects and, by consensus, arrive at a change score ranging from −3 (very negative change) to +3 (very positive change) for each aspect. This approach was based in part on the rationale that group discussion toward consensus is warranted because sufficient disagreement occurs among team members in evaluating the global functioning of people with developmental disabilities (Bailey, Buysse, Simeonsson, Smith, & Keys, 1995).

Each aspect of the Person-Centered Planning Quality of Life Indicators–Consensus Version is defined in the form of questions to guide respondents. For example, the quality of life dimension Home has six aspects, one of which is Neighborhood:

> *Neighborhood* (the physical qualities and ambience of the neighborhood). Is it primarily residential? Does it seem safe, attractive? Is it an industrial area? Is it a wealthy neighborhood? Sidewalks? Streetlights? Bus route nearby? Is it near community resources? Busy? Quiet? Near undesirable features like a dump, airport runway, etc.? (p. 1)

To evaluate whether change occurred in the person's neighborhood, respondents consider the noted questions in reaching agreement on the overall degree of change that might have taken place in the neighborhood within a given time period. For Hal, the assessment was completed at intervals of 9, 10, 10, 9, and 15 months, which spanned a 5-year period. In the first administration (June 1995), respondents were asked to compare the present conditions with those that existed when person-centered planning began (September 1994), thus constituting the first 9-month interval. In subsequent administrations, the prior assessment date was the comparison reference point. The final administration was conducted in February 1999, a year after Hal moved to the community. During each administration, the facilitator summarized in writing the current status for each aspect, which became a useful "look back" for subsequent administrations. The assessment required 1½–2 hours to complete, and consensus was obtained from the same four people at each administration: the facilitator, the developmental psychologist, and Hal's parents.

Figure 13.4 shows longitudinal quality of life assessment results in terms of cumulative improvement. Each part of the figure depicts profiles of one dimension, as well as the component aspects comprising the dimension, which are arranged roughly by degree of improvement. As a result, one can examine the cumulative perceived changes in each aspect across the 5-year period in addition to the moving profile of that dimension.

To stay with the example of Neighborhood, Figure 13.4e shows that no changes were recorded in this aspect until the last interval, when it was rated +3 (the highest score possible), corresponding with Hal's move to the community. Likewise, Home exterior (Figure 13.4a) had identical change scores across the five intervals, but Home interior (Figure 13.4a) was perceived to improve somewhat consistently throughout the study. The latter is consistent with the tangible improvements that occurred in Hal's living environment before he moved, which contrasted starkly to the institutional climate described previously in the "First Three Meetings" section.

Generally, the nine profiles show consistent improvement across time. Although the change scores are graphed to the same scale unit, it is difficult to make comparisons between dimensions because of the wide variation in degree and acceleration of perceived improvement of aspects within dimensions. Nonetheless, at least two dimensions showed distinctly different patterns across time. Consistently high gains were seen in aspects of Preferences (Figure 13.4i), which had the highest possible ratings at most time intervals, whereas relatively modest improvements occurred in aspects of Health (Figure 13.4c). More specifically, high positive ratings were uniformly given for the degree to which Hal liked activities, avoided annoyances, and experienced new opportunities (aspects of Preferences, Figure 13.4i). Conversely, Figure 13.4c shows that no improvement was noted at any interval in the general Health aspect, and other aspects of Health showed minimal improvement for the most part. Little or no change in health aspects was consistent with Hal's good health from the start. It is interesting to note that the only other aspects that showed no improvement were participation in Associations (an aspect of Relationships, Figure 13.4d) and choice of engagement in minor vices (e.g., alcohol, caffeine, nicotine, explicit magazines; aspect of Choices, Figure 13.4f).

The February 1997 profiles correspond in time to the day treatment without walls phase of Figure 13.1. Commensurate with this phase, distinctive gains are seen in the 1997 profiles for Day Activity (Figure 13.4b), Relationships (Figure 13.4d), and Respect (Figure 13.4g). Overall, however, it is difficult to identify the effects of any one factor on Hal's quality of life ratings because 1) the ratings themselves were subjective and 2) many things happened at the same time during the person-centered planning, some of which occurred as part of the process and some of which occurred outside of the process. For example, psychotropic medications were prescribed independently of the person-centered planning process: Trials of BuSpar, Risperdal, and Depakote were administered, usually in combination with the Haldol that resumed in December of 1995 (see Figure 13.3, Session 40).

The Person-Centered Planning Quality of Life Indicators–Consensus Version was developed to make intra-individual, criterion-referenced comparisons. Although we have quantified changes in quality of life, using this instrument to make comparisons between individuals or to sum across dimensions for a total quality of life score for one person must be done with caution. There is no way to establish true linear equivalence among aspects comprising a given dimension nor between the dimensions themselves. Thus, because the differences observed between profiles and dimensions are not absolute and because those differences do not hold the same relative importance for all individuals, the change scores must be interpreted carefully.

HAL'S MOVE TO THE COMMUNITY

On February 28, 1998, Hal officially moved to his new home after a gradual transition process of visits and overnight stays. Aside from a few nights of poor sleep, it was an easy transition. The home was on a cul-de-sac in a quiet residential neighborhood, and Hal had a private bedroom and a completely individualized home routine. His day program continued as before. Hal's parents remained very involved in his life, and the person-centered planning team continued to meet on a less frequent basis after his move. Parent-recorded data indicated that for the first 5 months, Hal's parents visited him at his new home approximately once per week, and Hal visited his parents at their home approximately 3 times per month. The last quality of life assessment was administered 1 year after Hal moved, and as the February 1999 profiles in Figure 13.1 suggest, improvement continued, if not accelerated. By that time, Haldol had been discontinued, and Hal was taking no other psychoactive medication. Many aspects of the planning team's vision of a more desirable future had been met, such as Hal's having more autonomy, better relationships, and productive community involvement; others, such as owning his own home and living close to his parents, did not happen.

Fortunately, the agency that was providing residential and day services had been involved with Hal's person-centered planning team since its inception. This involvement was consistent with the agency's effort to shift to a more person-centered model of services and supports—a model that was based on the same five essential accomplishments that guided Hal's person-centered team. Thus, when Hal moved, he was moving into a program that was transforming its principles, staffing patterns, administrative oversight, and even transportation arrangements in a way that fostered person-centered outcomes.

a. Home

b. Day Activity

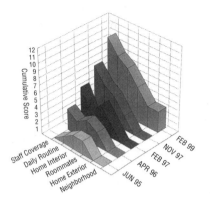
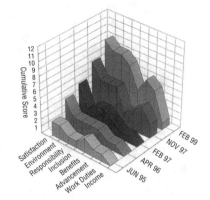

c. Health

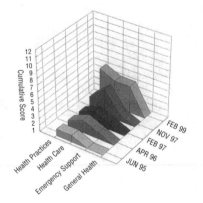

d. Relationships

e. Community Places

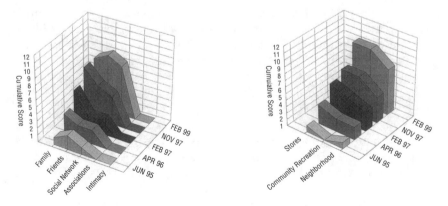

Figure 13.4. Longitudinal quality of life assessment results in terms of cumulative improvement.

f. Choices

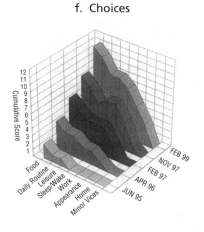

g. Respect

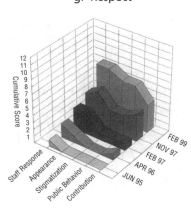

h. Capabilities

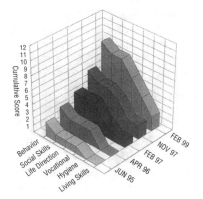

i. Preferences

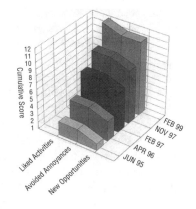

CONCLUSION

This chapter has discussed how Personal Futures Planning was implemented to facilitate community transition for a person who had spent nearly his entire life in an institution. The person-centered planning team accomplished that mission and more, but we did not expect the process to be so long, nor did we expect to encounter all of the obstacles that had to be overcome. Looking back, it is clear that the team members became adept at problem solving. As Hal's father was fond of saying, "Person-centered planning is the Liquid-Plumr of DD [developmental disabilities]!" Heavy parent involvement in both the planning process and the behavioral intervention was undoubtedly a major factor in changing Hal's life for the better. Procedurally, we believe that the blending of person-centered planning and applied behavior analysis was essential for changing the patterns of interaction that permitted reuniting the family.

Two factors that greatly facilitated Hal's planning process were the group feedback methods and the level of organizational commitment of both the state and voluntary agencies. The results of the planning group's efforts were continually fed back to the group members in various forms. After each meeting, members received copies of the minutes, which reflected discussion, strategy, and responsible parties. Reviewing the prior meeting minutes at the start of each meeting aided planning continuity and often prompted follow-up action. In addition, old maps were retained and used extensively throughout the planning. They were hung up and reviewed at strategic points in the process, such as when a new phase of planning was at hand or when new members joined the team. Contrasting former maps with updated maps served to reinforce the team's progress, especially when examining new relationships, preferences, and community activities.

Often, when the team seemed to be drifting in the wrong direction, we assessed Hal's progress in light of the five essential accomplishments of person-centered planning (O'Brien, 1987). This exercise also proved useful if a significant controversy emerged. In such situations, the essential accomplishments served as reference points in facilitating resolution. Two other forms of information that helped guide the group were the quality of life assessment results and the videotapes of Hal interacting during Mommy Visits, practicing new routines at the developmental center, and enjoying the community. These two types of feedback confirmed the team's progress, but they also generated discussion about how we could do certain things better.

Probably the most significant factor in contributing to the outcomes that were achieved was the extent to which the developmental center and its parent office facilitated the process. The team anticipated bureaucratic resistance but instead received flexible funding to accommodate its ideas, as well as additional staff and transportation when necessary. The three initiatives in Figure 13.1 that made community inclusion possible—transitional funding, the community bridge-building program, and day treatment without walls—were unique arrangements that required significant fiscal and procedural negotiation behind the scenes.

An example of modification in organizational protocol is illustrated by the selection of a residential agency for Hal after the trial run with the initial agency failed. Typically, finding a residential agency for a person moving out of a developmental center is a matter of negotiation between the developmental center and the potential agency. In Hal's case, however, the core planning team, which included his parents, became the selection committee, with guidance from administrative staff who better understood technical procedures. The team interviewed representatives from five agencies, and one of the interview questions was "How would you feel about members of the person-centered planning team hiring and firing staff in the home?" Some agencies actually responded positively to this suggestion, but it was soon obvious that this was an unfeasible idea. Nonetheless, it illustrates the degree to which the larger system was willing to break protocol to accommodate the process and how far the team had come as a result.

Some of our colleagues have registered concern about the amount of time it took to find a community living arrangement for Hal. We too were concerned about this delay. Surely, other available methods would have been more efficient in terms of time and resources. However, we tried to remain faithful to the person-centered process and the vision that it generated. The pace of working toward the goals was sometimes frustrating, and we could have accelerated the transition by short-cutting parts of the process, but doing so probably would have resulted in less constructive changes in Hal's lifestyle and family relationships. It also should be noted that Hal was not the only beneficiary of this endeavor. As the planning proceeded, we observed positive changes in organizational responsiveness, team effectiveness, and staff attitudes in both the state and voluntary agencies, although data were not systematically collected in these areas. An especially gratifying observation was that as Hal's behavior improved and his capabilities grew, the people around him raised their expectations, and the process seemed to cycle upward. In short, it was a productive 5 years. Against the background of 31 years of institutionalization, that does not seem so long.

REFERENCES

Bailey, D.B., Buysse, V., Simeonsson, R.J., Smith, T., & Keys, L. (1995). Individual and team consensus ratings of child functioning. *Developmental Medicine and Child Neurology, 37*, 246–259.

Bronston, B. (1973). Willowbrook. (Testimony to the New York State Joint Legislative Committee for Mental and Physical Handicaps, February 17, 1972.) In B. Blatt (Ed.), *Souls in extremis: An anthology of victims and victimizers* (pp. 351–356). Needham Heights, MA: Allyn & Bacon.

Holburn, C.S., Jacobson, J.W., Vietze, P.M., Schwartz, A., & Sersen, E. (2000). Quantifying the process and outcomes of person-centered planning. *American Journal on Mental Retardation, 105*, 402–416.

Holburn, C.S., & Pfadt, A. (1995). *Person Centered Planning Quality of Life Indicators–Consensus Version*. Staten Island: New York State Institute for Basic Research in Developmental Disabilities.

Mount, B. (1992a). *Mapping transitions: A workbook for helping people move*. New York: Graphic Futures.

Mount, B. (1992b). *Personal futures planning: A sourcebook of values, ideals, and methods to encourage person-centered development*. New York: Graphic Futures.

Mount, B. (1994). Benefits and limitations of personal futures planning. In V.J. Bradley, J.W. Ashbaugh, & B.C. Blaney (Eds.), *Creating individual supports for people with developmental disabilities: A mandate for change at many levels* (pp. 97–108). Baltimore: Paul H. Brookes Publishing Co.

Mount, B., & Patterson, J. (1986). *Update of the positive futures project: Initial outcomes and implications*. Hartford: Connecticut Department of Mental Retardation.

O'Brien, J. (1987). A guide to life-style planning: Using The Activities Catalog to integrate services and natural support systems. In B. Wilcox & G.T. Bellamy, *A comprehensive guide to The Activities Catalog: An alternative curriculum for youth and adults with severe disabilities* (pp. 175–189). Baltimore: Paul H. Brookes Publishing Co.

O'Brien, J., & Mount, B. (1991). Telling new stories: The search for capacity among people with severe handicaps. In L.H. Meyer, C.A. Peck, & L. Brown (Eds.), *Critical issues in the lives of people with severe disabilities* (pp. 89–92). Baltimore: Paul H. Brookes Publishing Co.

14

Evaluating Preferred Activities and Challenging Behavior Through Person-Centered Planning

Kevin P. Klatt, Diane Bannerman Juracek, K. Renee Norman, David B. McAdam, James A. Sherman, and Jan Bowen Sheldon

The strategies, interventions, programs, and theoretical orientations that are important in serving people with developmental disabilities have continually changed and evolved since the 1960s (Favell, 1999; Horner, 2000). Person-centered planning is one of the strategies exemplifying this evolution. Though descriptions vary, researchers and implementers of person-centered planning agree the essence of the process is supporting a person in building a lifestyle defined by his or her preferences and ongoing choices (Mount, 1997).

Person-centered planning is conducted for several purposes, as reviewed throughout this book. One of the primary purposes is to provide opportunities for individuals to identify preferences and make choices in everyday life (Anderson, Bahl, & Kincaid, 1999). Providing preferred activities to people with developmental disabilities is critical for several reasons, including the obvious ethical and moral obligations. Another important reason is that providing preferred activities may have corollary effects on challenging behaviors. That is, providing opportunities to engage in preferred activities, in lieu of formal interventions targeting behavior reduction, may result in a reduction of challenging behaviors (Holburn, 1997). (See Harchik, Sherman, Sheldon, & Bannerman, 1993, and Lancioni, O'Reilly, & Emerson, 1996, for comprehensive reviews of the research on preference and choice.)

Therefore, person-centered planning is a process in which individual preferences are initially identified and continually updated. Several questions, however, remain to be investigated pertaining to person-centered planning, preferred activities, and the effects on challenging behavior. For instance, how often do preferred activities, once identified through person-centered planning, occur for a person with a developmental disability? Do challenging behaviors occur more or less often during preferred activities compared with all other activities? Does providing a greater number of preferred activities result in less challenging behavior—that is, is more better? Finally, is it necessary or sufficient to provide preferred activities to reduce or eliminate challenging behaviors?

This chapter describes how we conducted person-centered planning, embedded preferred activities within a daily activity schedule, and tracked the relationship between preferred activities and challenging behavior at a community-based agency that serves people with severe developmental disabilities. The entire process is illustrated for three individuals with developmental disabilities.

THE QUALITY OF LIFE PLANNING PROCESS

The Quality of Life Planning process is a person-centered approach that includes a person with developmental disabilities and a support team to develop and implement a plan for a lifestyle that is consistent with a person's preferences and needs. The Quality of Life Planning process was developed at Community Living Opportunities (CLO), a nonprofit program in northeast Kansas providing community services to people with severe developmental disabilities in conjunction with faculty and graduate students at The University of Kansas.

The Quality of Life Planning process was developed specifically for people with severe developmental disabilities who have difficulty communicating their preferences and making choices by traditional modes of communication (e.g., verbal communication). The values on which the process is based are represented by the following desired outcomes:

- Opportunities for choice and self-determination
- Effective learning opportunities
- Effective communication
- Active participation in the community
- Positive relationships with others
- Pleasant social and living environment
- High level of participation in daily experiences
- Healthy lifestyle
- Understanding and exercising legal and personal rights

The Quality of Life Planning process includes five components: 1) building the Quality of Life Planning team, 2) assessment, 3) the

Quality of Life Planning meeting, 4) implementation of the Quality of Life Plan (QLP), and 5) regular review of the QLP implementation and outcomes. These components are detailed in the following subsections.

Building the Quality of Life Planning Team

People who are central to the focus person and committed to the development and implementation of Quality of Life Planning (e.g., family members, friends) are organized into a team. The team should also include people from other organizations who can provide supports that are not available within the agency. For example, an employee from the focus person's favorite store might be involved as a link to the community.

Assessment

The critical initial step in the Quality of Life Planning process is conducting assessments to identify a person's needs and preferences. Depending on the individual, the assessment process might include a medical evaluation that identifies physical causes of challenging behavior or a communication skills evaluation. One of the most important assessments in Quality of Life Planning, however, is called "And Here's What I Want."

The And Here's What I Want assessment process includes interviewing team members and observing the focus person to obtain the following information:

- Identification of strengths and areas of need
- The individual's satisfaction with current lifestyle and services (e.g., living arrangement, employment, leisure activities)
- Identification of both broad and specific daily living preferences (e.g., where to live and with whom, what to do during the day)
- Identification of hopes and dreams for the future

During the interview process, all team members and others who know and care about the person are individually interviewed. The interviews are based on a protocol consisting of questions that range from broad and open ended to specific. Interviewees are urged to respond about preferences and needs from the focus person's point of view (e.g., "Put yourself in Smitty's shoes").

The second phase entails interviewing and/or observing the focus person to identify individual needs and preferences. This can be challenging if the person has difficulty communicating verbally. In these cases, various procedures are used (see Reid, Everson, & Green, 1999). For example, the observer provides opportunities for the person to participate in activities and then measures the extent to which the individual participates in the activities, the type and degree of challenging behavior that occurs during and after the activities, and the extent to which the individual moves toward the activity when the activity materials are moved a short distance away. The observer also assesses the person's preferences in a number of new situations. For example, the person might be observed participating in new community activities, visiting another type of living arrangement, engaging in different leisure activities, working at a new job, or eating new foods. Data from the interviews and observations are integrated to create a *proposed* list of preferences, needs, hopes, dreams, and so forth. These lists are used throughout the next part of the Quality of Life Planning process—the Quality of Life Planning meeting.

Quality of Life Planning Meeting

The Quality of Life Planning meeting is attended by team members and friends and led by a trained facilitator. It is an annual celebration of the person's accomplishments and a time to generate goals and build on the person's vision for the future. The meeting is typically held at a favorite restaurant or other community environment. Posters are displayed that review the person's accomplishments and strengths, as well as positive comments that people have made about the person. During this celebration of accomplishments, the group reviews the And Here's What I Want evaluations. Finally, team members discuss, prioritize, and reach a consensus on recommendations for the coming year. These include preferences that are both broad (e.g., "I want to get a job") and very specific (e.g., "I want to be able to eat Moon Pies, drink soda, and use my rocking chair").

Implementation of Quality of Life Planning

Keeping the promises of the QLP requires day-to-day vigilance. It is one thing to generate a life plan and another to implement it. One purpose of the QLP is the promise of daily access to preferred activities, items, choices, friends, and routines. To illustrate, quality of life for our friend Jack translates into getting hot cocoa in the morning, taking a long bath, getting groceries for older women at the assisted living apartments, not having to climb too many stairs, spending time with his favorite teacher, and going to the farmers' market with his parents on Saturday. We have often noticed that if these preferences are not available for any reason, then Jack is not happy and may express his discontent by displaying aggressive behavior. Yet, when Jack's preferences are respected, he is likely to be a happy participant in his daily activities and can handle everyday frustrations much better.

An effective strategy for keeping the QLP promises is a written individualized daily activity schedule. For people with severe disabilities who cannot communicate well, a schedule becomes critical because it informs those who support them of important routines, preferences, commitments, and activities (Anderson, Sherman, Sheldon, & McAdam, 1997). It is a road map to a successful, satisfying day.

The schedules that we use are individualized written lists of chronologically ordered daily routines and activities. Schedules indicate 1) the activity, 2) the approximate time that the activity should occur, 3) who will accompany the person, 4) the means of transportation, and 5) any other details that are required for the schedule to match the person's needs and wants. Schedules are developed to contextually fit the individual's QLP. Because most people have roommates or live with family members who may have conflicting commitments or preferences, it is impossible to have everything that they want in their schedules. Rather, preferences, responsibilities, and conflicts are weighed to generate a schedule that is as satisfying and realistic as possible. The following factors are taken into consideration for schedule development:

- Preferred activities, people, and places
- Responsibilities (e.g., employment, self-care, chores)
- Opportunities for learning (as recommended in the QLP for the focus person)
- Opportunities to make choices within the schedule
- Health concerns (e.g., likelihood of seizures)
- Community accessibility
- Competing schedules, preferences, and needs of family members or roommates
- Order of activities (e.g., whether preferred activities should follow less preferred activities)
- Functions of challenging behaviors

Schedules are computer generated so that they can be modified as needed. These written schedules are used by family and support staff, but they are not useful to people with severe disabilities who cannot read. In such cases, we create parallel schedules to facilitate understanding and self-initiation. For instance, a parallel schedule might consist of photographs or line drawings of activities or perhaps an audio or video schedule. For instance, Jack has a small notebook schedule that contains photographs of him engaged in his schedule's various activities.

Regular Review of Quality of Life Planning Implementation and Outcomes

An important aspect of the Quality of Life Planning process includes data-based evaluation and review. Data are collected to analyze progress and to troubleshoot areas in need of revision. The most important data to collect are summarized next.

Collecting Individualized Outcome Data   Part of the day-to-day vigilance required to implement the QLP includes the measurement and review of outcomes. Staff and families use a daily data card to collect individualized data on the people whom they directly support. These data include

- Incidences of challenging behavior
- Degree of engagement in activities
- Delivery of preferences described in the QLP
- Implementation of all scheduled activities
- Degree to which critical issues for a particular person (e.g., medical symptoms, satisfaction ratings) are addressed

These data are summarized and reviewed quarterly to assess whether the QLP priorities are being implemented and whether the QLP has had any effect on behaviors.

Quality-at-a-Glance Evaluations   Another direct assessment of the implementation of the QLP should come from people who know and care about the person but do not live with the person (e.g., family members, advocates). We use at-a-glance checklist evaluations (available from the authors upon request) to assess the implementation of the daily schedule, the appearance and safety of the home, the quality of teaching, and the quality of the program. The results of these easy-to-use rating checklists allow ongoing outside evaluations of a person's quality of life.

Team Review of the Quality of Life Plan   The support team that developed the QLP should convene as frequently as necessary (at least quarterly) to update and assess the outcomes and implementation of the plan. Because preferences change, each person's QLP may need to be revised. For example, Jack's lifestyle preferences, including activities and priorities, changed significantly when he acquired a girlfriend. If his QLP had remained as it was, then he likely would have been unhappy.

APPLIED ANALYSES

Using the QLP, we conducted three analyses pertaining to preferred activities and challenging behaviors for three men with severe developmental disabilities. The analyses were conducted to answer the following three questions:

1. How often do people with developmental disabilities engage in preferred activities?

2. Do challenging behaviors occur less often during preferred activities than during all other activities combined?

3. Does access to more preferred activities per day result in fewer challenging behaviors?

Participants

Carl was 34 years old with a primary diagnosis of profound mental retardation. He generally spoke in two- or three-word phrases and had good receptive language. Carl loved to play practical jokes on his roommates and direct care providers. He liked to spend time riding his bicycle, listening to his radio, using the vacuum cleaner, and going to convenience stores to buy soda. His challenging behaviors included hitting others, engaging in property destruction, and slapping his face.

Smitty was 41 years old with a primary diagnosis of profound mental retardation. He had poor receptive and no expressive language. Smitty enjoyed eating Moon Pies and doughnuts, going to the library to listen to music, and eating at local restaurants. His challenging behaviors were biting his hand, rubbing his foot firmly against his shoe, and property destruction.

John was 43 years old and had a primary diagnosis of severe mental retardation. He used limited words and phrases and had good receptive language. John enjoyed going to a nearby airport to watch planes, visiting the staff at a local hotel, and going to look at flowers in city parks and at florist shops. His challenging behaviors consisted of biting his arm, exhibiting aggression toward others, insisting that others repeat him, and invading others' privacy.

All three men had previously lived in various state institutions before moving to their residences at the time of the study, which were eight-person group homes located in residential neighborhoods of a mid-size city. Smitty and Carl lived in the same home and worked at various jobs within a supported work environment. John lived in a group home with seven other individuals and his schedule consisted of work and leisure activities within his home and community.

Person-Centered Planning

The previously described Quality of Life of Planning process was implemented for the three men. Several preferred activities and items were selected from each individual's QLP. The activities and items selected did not include an exhaustive list from the QLP. Activities and items were selected only if they could be presented or not presented daily (e.g., living in a preferred apartment could not be changed on a daily basis). In addition, challenging behaviors were identified for each individual.

Data Collection

Data were collected on both challenging behaviors and the type of activity for each participant. Data were recorded by direct support staff working within each participant's group home. On each individual's personalized data card, direct support staff recorded the frequency of challenging behaviors and the ongoing activity in 15-minute blocks throughout each day. During the investigation, all of the preferred activities were listed on the front or back of the data cards to prompt direct support staff to make the activities available and to record when they occurred.

At 3:00 P.M., the participants were finished with their work responsibilities and a different group of direct support staff started their shift. Therefore, only challenging behaviors and activities occurring between 3:00 P.M. and 8:00 P.M. (for Carl and Smitty) or between 3:00 P.M. and 11:00 P.M. (for John) were analyzed.

Procedures

At approximately 3:00 P.M. each day, the participants used their parallel schedules to plan their afternoon and evening activities with assistance from direct support staff. The direct support staff helped the participants decide which activities were possible each day. The direct support staff were instructed to help the participants participate in as many preferred activities as possible. After arranging the activities to be completed, the direct support staff supervised the participants in implementing their schedules by assisting in the completion of as many activities as possible. Preferred activities could also be obtained at unscheduled times if the participants made a request and the direct support staff could provide them (e.g., a trip to get a soda). The number of preferred activities completed within a daily schedule were affected by several factors, including the availability of transportation, weather conditions, the amount of money required, and store hours.

Data Analyses

Several within-person comparisons were made to analyze challenging behaviors in relation to preferred versus all other activities. The analyses were conducted by reviewing the data cards used each day by the direct support staff who were responsible for each specific participant. Only data recorded during the 15-minute blocks on the data cards were used in each analysis. Intervals that a participant's direct support staff left blank were not used in the analyses. The analyses were conducted after collecting data for 103, 111, and 83 days for Carl, Smitty, and John, respectively.

The first analysis compared the percent of intervals containing preferred activities to intervals with all other activities (i.e., no preferred activities). The second analysis analyzed the proportion of challenging behaviors occurring during preferred versus all other activities. In the third analysis, the average rate per day of challenging behaviors was assessed according to the number of different preferred activities provided. That is, challenging behaviors were averaged across all days on which a participant engaged in one, two, three, four, or five *different* preferred activities.

Interobserver Agreement

We evaluated interobserver agreement for challenging behaviors and the type of activity (preferred or other) by observing the direct support staff and participants on several occasions for 30–90 minutes. During these times, challenging behaviors and the type of activities were recorded during 15-minute intervals. These data were then compared with the direct support staff data. Observations were conducted during 3% of the total intervals for Carl, during 2% of the total intervals for Smitty, and during none of the intervals for John (no observer was available). Interobserver agreement for challenging behaviors and the type of activities was calculated by dividing the number of agreements by the number of agreements and disagreements combined and then multiplying by 100%.

Interobserver agreement on the type of activities (preferred or other) averaged 97% for Carl and 100% for Smitty. Agreement on the occurrence of challenging behavior averaged 87% for Carl. For Smitty, agreement on the nonoccurrence of challenging behavior was 100%. Only nonoccurrence agreement was obtained for Smitty because no challenging behaviors occurred when the observers were present, although agreement on occurrence of challenging behavior during other time periods unrelated to this study was usually close to 100%. For John, interobserver agreement was not obtained during the study, although agreement on challenging behaviors outside the study was usually at or near 100%. (Data were routinely collected as part of the intervention; reliability was usually high during these observations.)

Results

The first analysis, depicted in Figure 14.1, was a comparison of the percent of intervals for which each participant engaged in a preferred activity versus all other activities combined. For Carl, preferred activities occurred in an average of 44% of 15-minute intervals, ranging daily from 0% to 90%. The number of intervals included in Carl's analysis was 1,791 (across 103 days). Preferred activities for Smitty occurred in an average of 33% of the 15-minute intervals, ranging daily from 0% to 83%, with 1,988 intervals (across 111 days) included in the analysis. John's data showed that preferred activities occurred in an average of 26% of the intervals, ranging daily from 0% to 88%, with 2,213 intervals (across 83 days) included in the analysis.

The second analysis, shown in Figure 14.2, depicts the average percent of challenging behaviors across all intervals and the proportion of challenging behaviors that occurred during preferred activities versus other activities combined. The third bar in Figure 14.2 is the proportion of preferred activities versus other activities (also depicted in Figure 14.1). For Carl, challenging behaviors occurred in 14% of all intervals. The proportion of challenging behaviors during preferred activities versus other activities combined was 39% and 61%, respectively. For Smitty, challenging behaviors occurred in 6% of all intervals. The proportion of challenging behaviors during preferred activities versus other activities was 4% and 96%, respectively. For John, challenging behaviors occurred in 50% of all intervals. The proportion of challenging behaviors during preferred activities versus other activities was 15% and 85%, respectively.

The third analysis, shown in Figure 14.3, assessed the number of challenging behaviors in relation to the number of different preferred activities per day. For Carl, the average number of challenging behaviors was 2.5, 1.4, 3.0, and 5.1 on days with 1, 2, 3, or 4 preferred activities, respectively. For Smitty, an average of 1.1, .9, .8, 1.6, and 2.0 challenging behaviors occurred on days with 1, 2, 3, 4, or 5 preferred activities, respectively. For John, an average of 18, 18, 9.8, 8.2, and 3.3 challenging behaviors occurred on days with 1, 2, 3, 4, or 5 preferred activities, respectively.

To summarize, it appears that for the three participants, less time was spent doing preferred activities than other activities, the proportion of challenging behaviors was lower during preferred activities for Smitty and John, and the association between the number of preferred

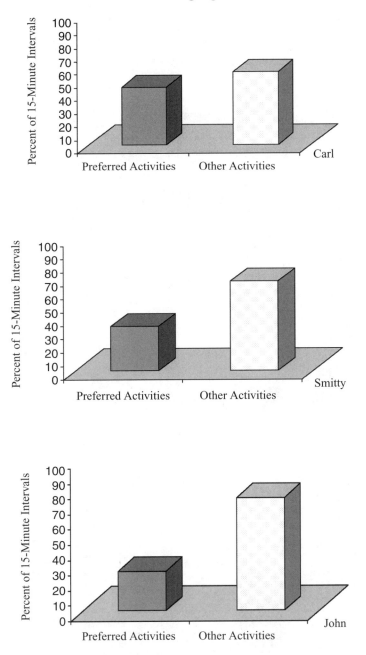

Figure 14.1. The average proportion of preferred activities versus all other activities combined.

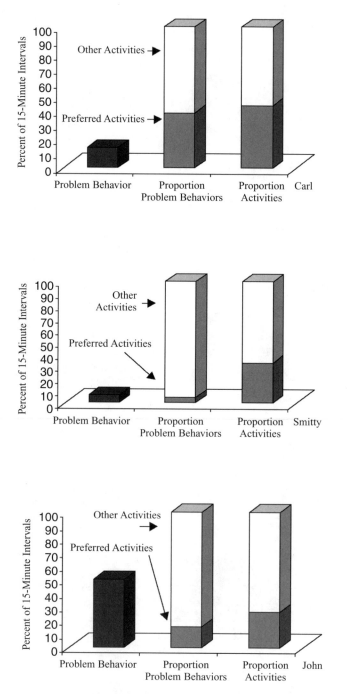

Figure 14.2. The average percentage of challenging behavior overall, the proportion of challenging behavior during preferred activities versus other activities, and the average proportion of preferred activities versus all other activities combined.

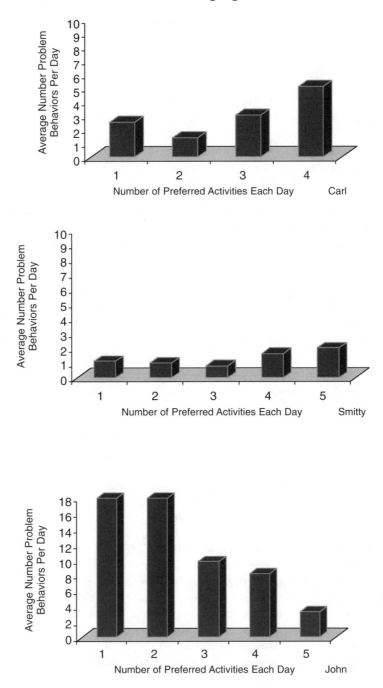

Figure 14.3. The average number of challenging behaviors per day across the number of different preferred activities provided per day.

activities per day and challenging behaviors differed across the three participants.

DISCUSSION

We conducted three analyses to investigate the effects of preferred activities on challenging behaviors for three people with severe developmental disabilities in their community-based group home. In the first analysis, the amount of time engaged in preferred activities (as identified by Quality of Life Planning, a person-centered planning approach) ranged across participants from 26% to 44% of assessed intervals. Engagement in preferred activities within days, however, varied greatly for all three participants. In fact, on some days the participants did not engage in any preferred activities. Although refusal to engage in preferred activities was not recorded, the participants were anecdotally observed to rarely refuse participation in a preferred activity. Hence, the variability of engagement in preferred activities was most likely due to other factors such as illness, challenging behaviors, and/or inconsistencies in the participants' programming (e.g., schedules, staff turnover). Much variability exists in the extent to which these data are representative of engagement in preferred activities for people with developmental disabilities in general. This variability may be problematic if engagement in preferred activities is desired or appears to positively affect challenging behaviors. Identifying the factors that affect the variability of engagement in preferred activities (e.g., money, transportation) requires additional research.

The second analysis measured the proportion of challenging behaviors that occurred between preferred activities and other activities. If challenging behaviors were distributed randomly, then the proportion of challenging behaviors between preferred activities versus all other activities would have been equal to the proportion of time engaged in preferred activities versus all other activities (i.e., in Figure 14.2, the middle and far-right bars would be equal). This proved to be the case only for Carl. For Carl, then, challenging behaviors did not appear to be related to whether the activity was preferred. For Smitty and John, the proportion of challenging behaviors was lower during preferred activities than the proportion of time that each spent engaged in preferred activities. Thus, for Smitty and John, fewer challenging behaviors occurred during preferred activities. Data from this analysis corroborate previous research showing that engaging in preferred activities affects challenging behaviors for some individuals with developmental disabilities (Clarke et al., 1995). Although these data

suggest that engagement in preferred activities results in fewer challenging behaviors for some individuals, the specific variables affecting
challenging behaviors were not identified. Without identifying such
variables, a strong argument cannot be made that the preferred activities alone reduced a participant's challenging behaviors. It is possible,
for example, that during preferred activities, the stimuli that set the
occasion for challenging behaviors were not present (e.g., instructions
to complete a task). In this case, it would not have been the preferred
activity affecting challenging behaviors but, rather, the absence of the
stimuli that set the occasion for the challenging behavior. This is an
important distinction to make when addressing challenging behaviors
because recommendations to provide more preferred activities might
not result in fewer challenging behaviors if the variables affecting a
person's challenging behaviors are not addressed.

The third analysis was conducted to determine whether providing
several different preferred activities per day would differentially affect
challenging behaviors. For Carl, a greater variety of preferred activities
per day were associated with more challenging behavior; for John, the
relationship was reversed; and for Smitty, there was no difference. One
possible hypothesis that may explain these results is that the challenging
behaviors were affected by variables other than merely preferred activities. Challenging behaviors typically have a purpose: They either serve a
socially mediating function (e.g., obtain or avoid something) or occur in
the absence of social contingencies (e.g., provide self-stimulation or
automatic reinforcement) (Carr, 1977; Iwata, Dorsey, Slifer, Bauman, &
Richman, 1982/1994). Accordingly, a person whose challenging behaviors function to avoid a particular stimulus (e.g., an instruction) would
most likely have fewer stimuli to avoid during preferred activities. In
this case, fewer challenging behaviors would occur because of the
absence of stimuli that set the occasion for the challenging behaviors
rather than anything inherent in the preferred activity.

To illustrate, Carl's proportion of challenging behaviors was
approximately the same between preferred activities and other activities, suggesting that preferred activities had little to no effect on his
challenging behaviors. When Carl engaged in a greater variety of preferred activities per day, however, his challenging behaviors actually
increased. An ongoing functional assessment suggested that his challenging behaviors functioned to gain access to a preferred activity or to
protest when an activity that he enjoyed was terminated. For instance,
one of his most preferred activities was vacuuming. Yet, Carl often
engaged in challenging behaviors when he had difficulty running the
vacuum cleaner (e.g., if it came unplugged when he went further than
the cord reached) or when a direct support staff terminated a preferred

activity to prompt him to engage in another activity in his schedule. Consequently, the more opportunities that Carl had to engage in preferred activities, the more opportunities that he had to engage in challenging behaviors when he had difficulty performing an activity or when the activity was terminated. In his case, then, challenging behaviors may have been maintained when he protested and was able to participate in the preferred activity for a longer duration of time (e.g., direct support staff plugged in the vacuum cleaner).

The conclusions reached from our data should be interpreted with caution due to several experimental shortcomings. In this study, person-centered planning was conducted to identify preferred activities. Although all the team members for each participant had developed close relationships with the participants, had known the participants for many years, and had agreed that the selected activities were preferred by the individual, a data-based preference assessment would have been necessary to confirm whether the chosen activities were high preferences. Another potential weakness in this study is the extent of the personal preferences that were measured. Preferred items that could be presented or absent each day were included in the study, whereas other preferences—such as place to live, type of job, and choice of roommates—were not included. These other preferences likely affect challenging behavior but are not amenable to direct experimental manipulation. Other types of research methods will need to be incorporated in future studies to analyze the effects of these preferences. A final caution is that interobserver agreement on challenging behaviors and preferred activities was collected for only two participants and for relatively few intervals. This lack of interobserver agreement prevents strong conclusions concerning the reliability of the data. For each of the participants, however, interobserver agreement scores for challenging behaviors apart from the study were typically high.

CONCLUSION

Despite the limitations of the study described in this chapter, analyses from the study suggest that conducting person-centered planning to identify and provide preferred activities might result in fewer challenging behaviors for some but not all people with severe developmental disabilities. Although developing preferences and making choices are important behaviors in their own right for people with developmental disabilities regardless of the effects on challenging behavior (Bannerman, Sheldon, Sherman, & Harchik, 1990), these analyses have shown that simply providing high-preference activities is not always sufficient to reduce challenging behaviors. Therefore, developing a preferred lifestyle by using strategies such as person-centered planning is perhaps necessary but may not be sufficient to reduce the challenging behaviors of all people with severe developmental disabilities.

The results reported in this study add to the growing literature pertaining to person-centered planning, preferences, and challenging behaviors. As people with developmental disabilities continue to move to less restrictive environments and an emphasis is placed on improving quality of life, efforts to reduce challenging behaviors should consist of several steps. First, person-centered planning should be conducted to identify and provide opportunities to develop preferences by experiencing various living conditions, community activities, and other aspects of daily life. Second, preferences need to be continually assessed. Third, activity schedules that are tailored to individualized preferences must be implemented. Finally, if challenging behaviors continue to impede progress, then a functional assessment and/or analysis should be conducted to identify the functions of the behavior so that appropriate strategies can be implemented.

REFERENCES

Anderson, C.M., Bahl, A.B., & Kincaid, D.W. (1999). A person-centered approach to providing support to an adolescent with a history of parental abuse. In J.R. Scotti & L.H. Meyer (Eds.), *Behavioral intervention: Principles, models, and practices* (pp. 385–396). Baltimore: Paul H. Brookes Publishing Co.

Anderson, M.D., Sherman, J.A., Sheldon, J.B., & McAdam, D. (1997). Picture activity schedules and engagement of adults with mental retardation in a group home. *Research in Developmental Disabilities, 18,* 231–250.

Bannerman, D.J., Sheldon, J.B., Sherman, J.A., & Harchik, A.E. (1990). Balancing the right to habilitation with the right to personal liberties: The rights of people with developmental disabilities to eat too many doughnuts and take a nap. *Journal of Applied Behavior Analysis, 23,* 79–89.

Carr, E.G. (1977). The motivation of self-injurious behavior: A review of some hypotheses. *Psychological Bulletin, 84,* 800–816.

Clarke, S., Dunlap, G., Foster-Johnson, L., Childs, K.E., Wilson, D., White, R., & Vera, A. (1995). Improving the conduct of students with behavioral disorders by incorporating student interests into curricular activities. *Behavioral Disorders, 20,* 221–237.

Favell, J.E. (1999). Foreword. In J.R. Scotti & L.H. Meyer (Eds.), *Behavioral intervention: Principles, models, and practices* (pp. xiii–xvi). Baltimore: Paul H. Brookes Publishing Co.

Harchik, A.E., Sherman, J.A., Sheldon, J.B., & Bannerman, D.J. (1993). Choice and control: New opportunities for people with developmental disabilities. *Annals of Clinical Psychiatry, 5*(3), 151–161.

Holburn, S. (1997). A renaissance in residential behavior analysis? A historical perspective and a better way to help people with challenging behavior. *Behavior Analyst, 20,* 61–85.

Horner, R.H. (2000). Positive behavior supports. In M. Wehmeyer & J. Patton (Eds.), *Mental retardation in the 21st century* (pp. 181–196). Austin, TX: PRO-ED.

Iwata, B.A., Dorsey, M.F., Slifer, K.J., Bauman, K.E., & Richman, G.S. (1994). Toward a functional analysis of self-injury. *Journal of Applied Behavior Analysis, 27,* 197–209. (Reprinted from *Analysis and Intervention in Developmental Disabilities, 2,* 3–20, 1982)

Lancioni, G.E., O'Reilly, M.F., & Emerson, E. (1996). A review of choice research with people with severe and profound developmental disabilities. *Research in Developmental Disabilities, 17*(5), 391–411.

Mount, B. (1997). *Person-centered planning: Finding directions for change using personal futures planning.* New York: Graphic Futures.

Reid, D.H., Everson, J.M., & Green, C.W. (1999). A systematic evaluation of preferences identified through person-centered planning for people with profound multiple disabilities. *Journal of Applied Behavior Analysis, 32,* 467–477.

V

Training and Policy

15

Implementing Person-Centered Planning on a Statewide Basis

Leadership, Training, and Satisfaction Issues

Stan Butkus, David A. Rotholz,
Kathi Kelly Lacy, Brian Abery, and Sarah Elkin

Person-centered planning was introduced in 1998 on a statewide basis in South Carolina's Department of Disabilities and Special Needs (DDSN). Implementing this change in the planning and provision of supports and services for people with developmental and other disabilities required changes in guiding policies, practices, and expectations. It also required the development of new resources and processes (i.e., trained person-centered planning facilitators and the person-centered meeting process) to translate the philosophy into practice. This chapter contains three sections that describe 1) systems change issues from the perspective of those who direct the statewide system of supports and services, 2) the process and content for training person-centered planning facilitators and their role in the delivery of supports and services, and 3) assessment of participants' initial satisfaction with person-centered planning. The work on which this chapter is based also highlights an effective collaboration among a state agency and two University Centers for Excellence in Developmental Disabilities Education, Research and Service (i.e., the Center for Disability Resources at the University of South Carolina and the Institute on Community Integration at the University of Minnesota. This multidimensional information provides a unique overview of one state's effort to implement person-centered planning on a statewide basis.

Preparation of this chapter was supported by multiple cooperative agreements, including agreements between 1) the South Carolina Department of Disabilities and Special Needs (DDSN) and the Center for Disability Resources (CDR) at the University of South Carolina and 2) the National Institute on Disability and Rehabilitation Research (NIDRR), the U.S. Department of Education (Grant No. H133B980047), the South Carolina DDSN, and the Research and Training Center on Community Living (RRTC) at the University of Minnesota's Institute on Community Integration.

SYSTEMS CHANGE ISSUES

Services to people with mental retardation in the United States have evolved dramatically since the 1970s. Key elements of this evolution have been the enhancement of service and support quality and the methods through which this has occurred (Bradley, 1994). Traditionally, the development and implementation of supports and services for people with mental retardation and related disabilities have been the territory of "experts." However, descriptive studies indicate that such planning processes foster little participation on the part of people with disabilities, their family, or their friends and are often viewed in a negative manner (e.g., Gallivan-Fenlon, 1994; Lichtenstein & Michaelides, 1993; Stancliffe, Hayden, & Lakin, 1999). In addition, it appears that traditional approaches to service planning are unsuccessful in stimulating changes in outcomes that are associated with service plan goals and objectives (Stancliffe et al., 1999).

In the 1990s, increasing self-determination, choice, and control for people with disabilities became a rallying point to examine public policy and the essential elements of how public resources are used to assist people with disabilities (O'Brien & Lyle O'Brien, 1998). Increasing self-determination is a major goal of person-centered planning. It provides a vehicle through which people can articulate their vision for the future. This vision may include equal opportunity in employment, social inclusion, personal control, and a chance to live as independently as possible within the community (Stancliffe, Abery, & Smith, 2000). The person's hopes and dreams—as well as his or her gifts, talents, and abilities—are articulated, and the individual and his or her family and friends voice their preferences in how services and supports can be most appropriately incorporated into the person's life.

One problem in increasing self-determination is the difference between knowledge about self-determination and the actual implementation of practices that support it. A number of experts have focused on enhancing the control that consumers exercise over the support planning process. This includes people determining the types of service that they receive, where these supports are delivered, and from whom they are obtained. Current approaches to service planning, however, seldom take these factors into account and typically focus on placing individuals into programs. Rarely are the people for whom the system was developed asked what they desire, and even less frequently are those desires taken into account when programs are designed. This occurs despite research showing that professionals make poor predictions about the preferences of the people whom they support (Green, Reid, Canipe, & Gardner, 1991; Parsons & Reid, 1990).

Achieving self-determination through person-centered services has many challenges. Person-centered planning is a concept that is at once easy to embrace and complex to initiate. A number of articles on person-centered planning point to some of these problems. Lyle O'Brien, O'Brien, and Mount (1997), who have been instrumental in the development of person-centered planning, expressed concern that it might become a fad. They emphasized that mindlessly implementing person-centered planning will dilute its efficacy. At the practice level, Holburn and Vietze identified a number of potential obstacles to implementation that are related to employee behavior and "role clarity, language, regulation compliance, and funding" (1999, p. 122). Thus, there appears to be a dilemma: Systemwide implementation seems antithetical to the roots of person-centered planning, yet person-centered planning targets the need for change in practice, which almost by definition involves systems and the policies that guide those systems.

This dilemma was exemplified through a series of self-determination pilot projects, which were funded by the Robert Wood Johnson Foundation, to stimulate system change efforts. The projects were grant funded, small in scope, and limited to a few individuals. Running 2–3 years in length, they sought to demonstrate innovative approaches to increasing self-determination. However, they all faced a challenge that is common to pilot projects—that of translating local success to statewide policy and practice (Schorr, 1997). Schorr noted that pilots or demonstrations often experience success because the normal rules of operation and practice are suspended while enthusiastic practitioners apply new concepts and practices.

South Carolina's self-determination initiative is going forward in a way that anticipates concerns raised by Lyle O'Brien and colleagues (1997) and others but also takes into account limitations that are inherent in moving successful pilot projects to a statewide level. More specifically, for change to take root on a broad scale, new policies, practices, and expectations are required. What follows is a description of South Carolina's changes in policy, practice, and expectations to increase self-determination for consumers with lifelong disabilities.

In South Carolina, services to people with disabilities are led by the South Carolina Commission on Disabilities and Special Needs (called "the Commission" hereafter), which sets policy and oversees DDSN. In early 1997, the Commission determined that DDSN should change service policy and increase self-determination through person-centered practices and should do so in a gradual and planful way. It was decided that phased-in, statewide implementation should begin by July 1, 1998.

To properly plan for increased self-determination, a series of meetings were held to discuss key elements of change with major stakeholders in the process. These participants included consumers, family members, advocates, Disability and Special Needs (DSN) Board staff (i.e., staff at the local disability service agencies), and DDSN staff. From these meetings, a Concept and Preliminary Implementation Plan was developed. It identified forces driving the change, described South Carolina's person-centered philosophy, and outlined three primary changes. First, person-centered planning was separated from and made independent of a service coordinator's customary role of developing individual service plans. Second, an agreement was forged to simplify and equalize the service funding process by shifting to a model that is tied to an individual's level of need. Third, a decision was made to shift from a process-oriented standards approach to an outcome-based performance measurement system. Although these three changes were essential steps, the change in expectations was just as significant. This was not a pilot project of self-determination practices; it was the beginning of statewide policy implementation. The phased-in approach over a 3-year period was designed to give local service providers the opportunity and flexibility to make the necessary changes in their procedures and practices to meet the new expectations.

Background and System Framework

DDSN is designated as South Carolina's authority on services for people with mental retardation, autism, and brain and spinal cord injuries. DDSN is an independent agency in the state government and serves 23,000 people with disabilities through local disabilities boards (approximately 94%) and regional centers (i.e., institutions; approximately 6%). DDSN has contracts with 37 local disability service agencies covering all 46 counties in the state. These agencies, the DSN Boards, are the administrative, planning, coordinating, and service delivery bodies for services funded by DDSN. The DSN Boards provide most services directly, including residential, day and employment services, individual and family support, early intervention, and service coordination. Service coordinators work directly for the DSN Boards. Until July 1, 1998, they were responsible for developing service plans for consumers who were eligible for DDSN services. After July 1998, a gradually increasing number of consumers in the DDSN system had their service plans developed by a person-centered planning team led by a facilitator who was trained in person-centered planning techniques.

Critics across the United States have argued that service plans tend to match what the agency provides (e.g., program-centered services) and that there has been little opportunity for consumers to express interest in a different way of being served (e.g., person-centered services). Regional offices of the Centers for Medicare & Medicaid Services (formerly the Health Care Financing Administration) have referred to this problem, cautioning providers to avoid "the cookie-cutter approach" to service plans (Morris & Kelley, 1999, p. 5). In some states, such issues prompted calls for service coordination to be independent of agencies providing direct service.

In South Carolina, DDSN believed that developing service plans was the key to initiating person-centered planning, supports, and services. Therefore, policy and resources were shifted to create the capacity to develop plans independent of agencies providing direct services. The policy intent was for services to be responsive to the needs and interests of the individual by giving consumers and their families increased choice and control. A request for proposals was issued in the Spring of 1998 to train in person-centered plan facilitation a cadre of people who were independent of DDSN, the DSN Boards, and the DSN Boards' service providers. These facilitators would assume the planning role previously held by service coordinators. The contract was awarded to the University of Minnesota's Institute on Community Integration via its Research and Training Center on Community Living (RRTC). A description of the training process is outlined in the "Training for Facilitators" section of this chapter.

The shift to independent facilitators created a situation in which the facilitator took the lead role in guiding the planning process, although the service coordinator was still involved in coordinating and assisting with plan implementation. This initially caused many concerns. Most prominent among these was the decision to shift the planning responsibility away from service coordination and the DSN Boards. Service providers worried that consumers would ask for things that they did not need. There were fears that consumers would make poor decisions. There were questions regarding the independence of the plan developer in that he or she would not know the focus person and, therefore, would develop poor-quality plans.

In July 1999, a year after shifting policy to develop plans independent of agencies providing services (i.e., shifting to person-centered planning), DDSN and the Center for Disability Resources at the University of South Carolina conducted an initial evaluation of satisfaction with the person-centered planning process. This process included a telephone survey in which participants in planning meetings were asked how they felt about the planning process and the independent facilitator who led the meeting(s). This process and its results are reported in the "Assessment of Participants' Initial Satisfaction with Person-Centered Planning" section of this chapter.

TRAINING FACILITATORS

We created a network of independent, highly trained, and well-supported person-centered planning facilitators. Working under contract in South Carolina, RRTC staff trained 41 facilitators. The facilitators were recruited through a fixed-price competitive bid process that was administered by the South Carolina Budget and Control Board (the state office which publishes such notices). Additional recruitment was conducted through parent and professional newsletters, conferences, and word of mouth. At some time, 14 of the 41 facilitators had previously worked for DDSN or for a county DSN Board. The facilitators had various vocational backgrounds, including special education teacher, minister, parent of a child with a disability, legislator, physician, attorney, music therapist, service coordinator, home health care professional, and secretary. During the first year, four facilitators gave up this role for a variety of reasons, leaving 37 trained facilitators.

On the one hand, person-centered planning facilitation is as much (if not more) of an art than a science. Consequently, some people with even minimal training and little supervision can become excellent facilitators. On the other hand, if individuals do not possess the personality, motivation, or willingness to take risks needed to succeed— or if they find it difficult to fully embrace the core values underlying person-centered planning—then no amount of training will result in their serving effectively in this role. Most individuals with an interest in person-centered planning facilitation, however, fall into neither of these groups. Instead, they embrace the idea of person-centered planning and are looking for the appropriate tools to improve the lives of people with developmental disabilities.

Person-Centered Principles and the Facilitator Role

Person-centered approaches to service planning have been developed to empower individuals with disabilities to take greater control over the supports that they receive and to enhance their quality of life. These processes are based on the assumption that individualization, flexibility, collaboration, and the involvement of family and friends are necessary for creating a desirable future. All of these processes begin with the recruitment of family members, friends, and others who are significant in the individual's life. The members of this group, or circle of support, work together to share their knowledge, better understand the focus person, and envision a desirable future. Action plans, which are designed to make the individual's personal vision a reality, are then developed and implemented.

The process of person-centered planning is flexible by nature. The planning group may vary in size and membership according to the goals at a given point in time. New people are invited in as they express an interest in participation. The goals and needs of the focus person may change over time. The group may dissolve after a period and form again at a later date. The circle, however, is united in its commitment to assisting individuals in achieving their desired lifestyle. The members' commitment to and knowledge of the focus person make it possible for person-centered planning to be successful for people with even the most severe disabilities (Pearpoint & Forest, 1998; Sanderson, Kennedy, Ritchie, & Goodwin, 1997).

The role of person-centered planning facilitators is complex. As a starting point, they must understand and embrace the values underlying person-centered planning. Facilitators must also possess skills and knowledge in several essential areas. They need well-developed social and communication skills and the ability to apply these skills in understanding other people and in making themselves understood. Facilitators must have knowledge of the community and its supports that may be relevant to the focus person. In addition, facilitators need 1) skills to effectively mediate differences and facilitate consensus in a group, 2) creativity and the capacity to stimulate it in others, 3) the ability to remain focused on the role of facilitator (i.e., assisting people in building quality lives), and 4) the capacity to monitor and evaluate outcomes. Finally, the facilitator must employ strategies to involve all participants with a particular focus on self-determination.

If person-centered planning is to be an effective alternative to traditional approaches to support services development, then sufficient numbers of individuals will need to be trained to facilitate the process. Far too often, efforts to train individuals to serve in this capacity have provided only short-term instruction with little technical assistance or follow-up. For person-centered planning to become an option for *all* people with disabilities, an integrated, comprehensive, and competency-based approach to training and technical assistance needs to be employed.

Training and Technical Assistance Components

The University of Minnesota's RRTC has developed an instructional and technical assistance program for training facilitators in Essential Lifestyle Planning (ELP; Smull, 1989; Smull & Burke Harrison, 1992). The advanced training component integrates additional person-centered approaches (e.g., PATH, Pearpoint, O'Brien, & Forest, 1993; Personal Futures Planning, Mount, 1994). The program combines two levels of classroom training with supervision and mentoring, as well as continuing education and technical assistance. It is designed to build the capacity of human service systems in supporting people with disabilities to exercise greater control over their lives and to achieve their personal visions for the future. Upon completion of training, facilitators have the tools necessary to individualize planning for service provision based on the unique characteristics of focus people and their environments.

Research and Training Center on Community Living's Facilitator Training Program   RRTC's facilitator training consisted of two levels of classroom training, followed by an extended period during which participants received technical assistance and supervision from trainers. Participants were introduced to the basic assumptions, values, and concepts underlying person-centered planning in 3 days of Level 1 training. During this time, trainees became aware of the process to which they were committing themselves by exploring the benefits and challenges of person-centered planning. The remainder of Level 1 training provided a comprehensive understanding of the philosophy, background, and process of ELP.

Conducted during a 4-day period, Level 2 training expanded the strategies available to facilitators for individualizing the person-centered planning process; supporting focus people and their circles; and facilitating the development, implementation, and monitoring of supports that are designed to help make each individual's vision a reality. Among the topics covered were

- Determining effective strategies for facilitation
- Building circles of support
- Individualizing the planning process
- Using graphics effectively
- Articulating a vision for the future
- Reaching a consensus and gaining support for the vision
- Developing, implementing, and monitoring plan outcomes
- Evaluating program integrity
- Reenergizing circles of support
- Ensuring that person-centered planning enhances self-determination
- Dealing with roadblocks

Level 2 training was initiated approximately 3 weeks following the completion of Level 1 instruction. The time between trainings provided trainees with an opportunity to more fully absorb information from Level 1 training and to read additional materials provided at the conclusion of that training. It also permitted time for the trainee to locate a consumer for whom they would facilitate a plan during Level 2 training.

The first 2 days of Level 2 instruction built on Level 1 training, providing trainees with additional tools that would allow them to effectively individualize their planning approach to meet the unique needs of consumers. During the second 2 days, trainees worked in teams to conduct initial person-centered planning meetings with selected consumers and their circles of support. Trainees were closely supervised and supported in these sessions by trainers from RRTC. Following this 4-day instructional period, facilitators worked in teams to initiate a second supervised person-centered plan with focus people of their choice. During this period, ongoing support and technical assistance were also provided.

Within 3 months of the completion of classroom instruction, trainers supervised an additional person-centered plan for each trainee. Instructors then provided ongoing follow-up, technical assistance, and supervision to facilitator trainees for a 24-month period to ensure the effective implementation of, monitoring of, and amendments to action plans, goals, and visions. Following their training, facilitator trainees were required to submit a minimum of three additional person-centered plans per year to RRTC instructors for evaluation, comment, and feedback.

Continuing Education and Technical Assistance   In the mid-1990s, the provision of technical assistance and support to individuals dispersed throughout an entire state would have been impossible. Given improvements in technology, however, long-distance technical assistance is not only possible but is also, in some situations, the most accessible and cost-effective strategy. Throughout the first 2½ years of this project, the RRTC Facilitator Training Program provided technical assistance to trainees. This included individual technical assistance/mentoring, group-based continuing education and technical assistance, and facilitator support networks, all of which are described in the following sections.

At the beginning of the third year of the person-centered facilitator training effort and as part of the process to build an infrastructure for person-centered planning in South Carolina, facilitator trainers and providers of technical assistance were trained and mentored at the University of South Carolina's Center for Disability Resources (CDR). This process involved shifting RRTC's role to CDR, resulting in a well-established technical assistance and continuing education system in place at CDR in collaboration with DDSN.

Individual Technical Assistance   Immediately after the completion of Level 2 training, individual technical assistance was provided to facilitator trainees on an as-needed basis. Assistance was available through on-site support, regularly scheduled telephone conferences between instructors and facilitators, and e-mail correspondence. The vast majority of this technical assistance focused on instructors working with trainees to review initial facilitated plans and to support problem solving related to specific focus persons.

Instructors who conducted the initial training provided on-site support to facilitator trainees on multiple occasions during the course of the first year following initial training. This assistance was tailored to fit the needs of facilitators and sometimes included the direct observation of trainees facilitating plans, evaluating and suggesting improvements to facilitation strategies that had been implemented, and providing detailed feedback on particularly challenging plans. Trainers were also available for telephone consultation and technical assistance on an ongoing basis. A third technical assistance option was a person-centered planning technical assistance web site (http://www.cdd.sc.edu/pcp/). Through this web site, trainees were able to confidentially submit questions to instructors, who provided written responses within 3 days.

Group-Based Continuing Education and Technical Assistance   Group-format continuing education and technical assistance ensured that trainees kept up-to-date with new developments and maintained ongoing access to experts in the field. Several avenues were used to provide continuing education and support to facilitator trainees, including interactive television (ITV) and the technical assistance web site.

ITV provided a cost-effective strategy to reach large numbers of individuals who resided and worked within different locations. The ITV sessions occurred bimonthly and consisted of continuing education and technical assistance seminars that efficiently supplied new facilitators with up-to-date information on changes and developments in the field, as well an opportunity to meet as a group and discuss issues pertinent to their work. The sessions were simultaneously telecast to multiple sites, with all participants linked with live video and sound. This not only allowed instructors to interact with trainees at multiple locations, but also permitted trainees to interact with each other. Each 2-hour session was composed of two components. The first focused on trainers presenting new developments within the field and providing trainees with additional strategies to enhance their ability to serve as facilitators. The specific strategy areas were selected on the basis of feedback from trainees. The second portion of each session was a discussion about common areas of concern, which were determined by questions that trainees submitted via the web site.

Another critical component of the continuing education and technical assistance offered to facilitator trainees consisted of the person-centered planning technical assistance web site. In addition to its use in individual technical assistance, the site provided the following:

- Question-and-answer page
- Exemplary practices page
- Resources page
- Facilitator chat room
- Family information page
- Support provider information page
- Links page
- Training and activities calendar page
- An online user survey

One of the most widely used features of the web site was the facilitator chat room. On three to four regularly scheduled dates each month, facilitator trainees logged-in to the chat room and took part in interactive, real-time discussions of various issues critical to the facilitation of person-centered planning. Each chat room was scheduled with a specific topic for discussion and was facilitated by one or more instructors working with the RRTC. Although not all trainees had ongoing access to the Internet at home or at work, most of them still had access through community sources (e.g., public libraries).

Facilitator Support Networks Research on adult learning indicates that professionals retain significantly more of what they are taught when teaching strategies include group discussion, practice through experience, and teaching others (Sparks & Loucks-Horsley, 1990). Person-Centered Planning Support Groups were created to ensure that such experiences were available to facilitator trainees. These groups met on a quarterly basis and were initially facilitated by instructional staff. Over the course of the project, trainees gradually assumed responsibility for running these groups. Prior to each meeting, group members decided on a topic for discussion, and one or more trainees developed an informal presentation on that topic. Instructors provided support and resources to individuals serving in this role on an as-needed basis. A portion of each meeting was devoted to the presentation and discussion of this information. During the remainder of the session, facilitators discussed challenging plans that they had developed or were in the process of developing, brainstormed creative solutions to barriers, and solicited feedback from their peers.

ASSESSMENT OF PARTICIPANTS'
INITIAL SATISFACTION
WITH PERSON-CENTERED PLANNING

We assumed that participant satisfaction would significantly affect the implementation of a statewide effort to introduce person-centered planning in the DDSN system. To assess the satisfaction with the planning meetings, DDSN arranged to have CDR take responsibility for this effort. Building on the relationship between CDR and RRTC, a collaborative project to evaluate satisfaction was initiated. This involved all three organizations, with CDR taking responsibility for implementation of the project and integration of activities and information across the three groups.

The purpose of the satisfaction survey was to learn about the views of the people who were actually involved in the planning process. (It was necessary to differentiate survey respondents from others in the service system who had opinions that were not based on actual experience in planning for a consumer's supports/services.) The survey was viewed as a means to assess one aspect of person-centered planning's effectiveness and the degree to which participants felt that the process differed from previous experiences in support/service planning for the focus person.

A telephone survey (The Person-Centered Planning Process Satisfaction Survey [PCP-SS], Abery, McBride, & Rotholz, 1999) was developed by RRTC and CDR to assess the initial levels of satisfaction with person-centered planning among a representative sample of people directly involved in the process (see the appendix at the end of this chapter). It was 1) developed with feedback and input from developmental disabilities professionals and family members, 2) pilot tested, and 3) revised based on additional feedback. The survey assessed quantitative and qualitative information from family members, friends, and support staff who participated in the meetings. Interviews with consumers are planned for a later phase of satisfaction evaluation.

The PCP-SS consists of 36 Likert-type, closed-ended questions and two open-ended ones. All respondents were asked 31 of the closed-ended questions. The remaining questions were used with family and friends (i.e., Questions 34–36) or with family only (i.e., Questions 37–38). Respondents indicated the extent to which each statement accurately described their experience in a person-centered planning process.

Prior to analysis of survey results, the 36 closed-ended items that compose the PCP-SS (Abery et al., 1999) were independently grouped on a conceptual basis into 11 subscales by three people who were intimately familiar with person-centered planning. Table 15.1 lists each subscale and its representative items.

An attempt was made to survey individuals who had taken part in all person-centered planning meetings in the DDSN system conducted over a 30-day period of time in Spring of 1999. To help ensure that the responses of survey participants accurately reflected their experiences in person-centered planning, all surveys were conducted within 14 days of initial planning meetings.

Administration of the survey took approximately 10 minutes to complete by telephone. Nine staff from DDSN and CDR were selected to become interviewers based on their communication and interpersonal skills, and they were trained to conduct the survey. The interviewer provided instructions and also explained up front that participation was voluntary, responses would be kept confidential, and only summarized information would be disseminated. An overwhelming majority (96%) of those contacted agreed to participate.

Table 15.1. Satisfaction subscale and overall satisfaction of item, mean, and standard deviation

Subscale	PCP-SS item	Mean	Standard deviation
Premeeting preparation	1, 2, 3, 9, 28	3.13	.44
Meeting process	4, 7, 8, 10	3.49	.36
Facilitator skill	5, 6, 10, 11, 14, 17, 20, 30	3.58	.35
Coverage of important issues	15, 22	3.54	.50
Teamwork and participation	12, 14, 17, 20	3.49	.41
Participation of the focus person	13, 19	2.88	.85
Informative about the focus person's needs and wants	13, 16, 18, 21	3.21	.52
Uniqueness of the process	31	3.03	.83
Adequacy of resources	27	2.86	.77
Support from service coordinator	28, 34, 35, 36	3.21	.72
Overall plan quality	21, 23, 24, 25, 26, 29	3.42	.44
Overall satisfaction	All except 27 and 31	3.37	.33

Note: PCP-SS items 37 and 38 were included in the premeeting preparation and adequacy of resources subscales for computation of overall satisfaction. They were omitted from group comparisons because they were asked only to family members.

(*Key:* PCP-SS = The Person-Centered Planning Process Satisfaction Survey.)

Results

Interviewers spoke with 242 circle of support members representing 141 consumers. Participants included 68 family members or friends and 174 staff. Approximately one half ($N = 91$) of the staff interviewed were service coordinators. The remainder were direct service or support staff.

Quantitative Analyses   Descriptive analyses were conducted on all Likert-type questions for all stakeholder groups combined, resulting in a separate set of satisfaction ratings for each subscale and an overall satisfaction rating (see Table 15.1). Satisfaction scores for each consumer were derived by averaging the responses of a given consumer's circle of support (respondents per circle of support ranged from 1 to 3). Examination of Table 15.1 shows that overall levels of satisfaction ($x = 3.37$, standard deviation = .33 on a 1- to 4-point Likert-type scale), as well as satisfaction ratings for the majority of subscales, were uniformly high for all stakeholder groups. Subscale mean scores ranged from $x = 2.86$ (adequacy of resources) to $x = 3.58$ (facilitator skill).

To further examine the results, satisfaction ratings were calculated for family/friends and staff (i.e., direct support and service coordinators). Thus, in addition to the above ratings at the focus person level, scores were also summed by type of participant. They represent the average ratings of all family/friends and staff interviewed. An independent t-test (the commonly used method to evaluate the differences in means between two groups) comparing the overall satisfaction ratings of family/friends versus staff revealed a significant difference ($t (239) = -2.33$, $p < .05$) indicating that staff perceived greater levels of satisfaction overall. It is important to note, however, that both stakeholder groups reported moderate to high levels of overall satisfaction in all categories. Specifically, subscale means were above 3.0 (quite a bit satisfied) on 9 of 11 subscales for family/friends and on 8 of 9 subscales for staff. (Only 9 subscales for staff are reported because "support from service coordinator" and "adequacy of resources" were comprised either completely or substantially of questions not asked of staff respondents.) Therefore, although family and friends were less satisfied with the process, respondents in general were quite a bit to completely satisfied with the person-centered planning in which they had taken part.

To examine for possible differences in type of satisfaction within each of the two groups, ANOVAs (analyses of variance) were conducted. They indicated that satisfaction ratings were significantly higher in some areas than others for both family/friends ($F (9,659) = 11.81$, $p \leq .001$) and staff ($F (8, 1515) = 26.38$, $p \geq .001$). The Tukey

Honestly Significant Different Test (Tukey HSD) provides a powerful and conservative (i.e., low chance of error) test of statistical significance between a dependent variable and two groups. Tukey HSD multiple comparison tests were conducted to determine which areas of satisfaction varied in each of the two groups. Family/friends reported significantly lower levels of satisfaction with premeeting preparation, participation of the focus person, and the extent to which the person-centered planning meeting was informative about the focus person's needs and wants.

For staff, the Tukey HSD tests showed similarly that satisfaction was lower in areas of premeeting preparation, participation of the focus person, and uniqueness of the process than in other areas. Family/friends and staff expressed lower levels of satisfaction with premeeting preparation and with participation of the focus person, which suggests that facilitators and trainers should pay particular attention to these areas to enhance the quality of person-centered planning facilitation.

A single-factor ANOVA was conducted to determine the extent to which overall levels of satisfaction with person-centered planning varied across the various regions of the state taking part in this evaluation. This analysis did not reveal significant differences across the four regions of the state in which person-centered planning had been implemented.

Qualitative Analyses   Qualitative procedures were used to analyze two open-ended questions of the PCP-SS. Question 32, "What did you like most about the planning process in which you recently took part?" and Question 33, "What did you like least about the planning process in which you recently took part?" were analyzed via an inductive procedure referred to as *constant comparative analysis* (CCA; Miles & Huberman, 1994). CCA consists of closely examining qualitative data to identify common themes and the linkages between them.

Responses, which included more than one per respondent, were first transcribed, and a rough "sort" was undertaken by grouping together answers with similar content. Two raters independently assigned each answer to a response category. Response discrepancies were resolved through discussion and consensus among raters. A detailed description of responses to the open-ended questions is presented in Figure 15.1.

Responses to what was liked most were grouped into 21 categories. Respondents generally showed a high level of enthusiasm about the person-centered planning in which they had participated. For example, one sibling commented,

> I learned a lot about my brother that I never knew before—it was wonderful. I thought I really knew him, but now I really know what he likes

and prefers. It was innovative, a breath of fresh air—this type of planning should have occurred a long time ago.

As Figure 15.1 shows, respondents most frequently commented on the facilitator's skill in leading the meeting and on the meeting's focus on the individual rather than programs or services provided. Facilitator comments ranged from general enthusiasm about the facilitator (e.g., "I was very impressed with the facilitation and the process," "The facilitator was very knowledgeable and very impressive") to more specific statements about the facilitator's performance (e.g., "The way the facilitator gave LaTisha choices and discussed her likes and dislikes was great. The facilitator was very patient and everyone was included."). Respondents' comments pertaining to an appreciation for the focus on the individual's dreams, goals, and needs included, "The real difference is that we are now getting the focus person's input versus basing plans on a set of predetermined ideas," "The whole meeting was focused on Robert," and "We learned new information about Angela's dreams. Her dreams are achievable!"

A third prevalent observation was that the person-centered planning process allowed the focus person to express him- or herself during the meeting. One respondent noted that the meeting "allowed Barbara the opportunity to express her views on what she wants—information that has never come out before." Similarly, people liked the fact that focus persons were involved and included in the process rather than simply observing it. One participant liked the meeting because it gave the focus person more involvement in his plan. Some participants appreciated the fact that all topics, including concerns, could be discussed freely. A number of them noted that planning meetings were open and gave everyone a chance to have input and express concerns. People also liked the fact that the meetings were positive and focused on capacities and strengths rather than on deficits. Others simply favored the process itself or how the meeting was run (e.g., "I liked the planning process, which included drawing pictures and writing on pads"). Figure 15.1 reveals other less common categories of what people liked about their person-centered planning experiences. Only 3 out of the 242 respondents responded that they did not like the person-centered planning process.

Responses to the question "What did you like least about the planning process in which you recently took part?" were grouped into 17 content categories. When asked this question, almost one quarter of staff and half of the family and friends responded to this question by saying that they liked everything about the process. The two most common criticisms were that the logistics of the meeting (e.g., time,

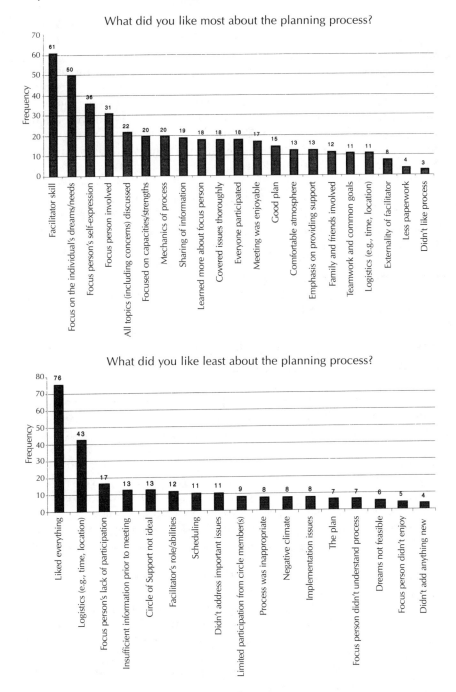

Figure 15.1. Summary of responses to open-ended survey questions.

location) were not ideal and that the focus person did not participate as much as possible. Comments about meeting logistics often centered on the length of the meetings, which tended to last longer than traditional planning meetings. One person noted, "It was rather long because there were a lot of people there and they all participated." Remarks concerning a lack of participation on the part of the focus person often referred to the individual's skill level (e.g., "James is nonverbal and could not express his wants at the meeting") and other times referred to the fact that it was difficult for meeting participants to draw answers from the focus person (e.g., "Pamela is young and a lot of the questions were above her head").

Other negative comments about the planning meetings presented the following views: the circle of support was not the ideal group, insufficient information was available prior to the meeting, the facilitator's role and/or abilities were not satisfactory, scheduling was difficult, and the meeting did not address important issues or it addressed inappropriate issues. Although the negative comments varied, examination of Figure 15.1 and Table 15.1 indicates a relatively small degree of dissatisfaction with the process.

DISCUSSION AND SUGGESTED AREAS FOR FUTURE STUDY

In the late 1990s, person-centered planning was implemented on a statewide basis in the system of supports and services provided by the South Carolina DDSN. Many people may wonder about the dilemma of systemwide implementation apparently being antithetical to the fundamental principles of person-centered planning. Yet, at the heart of person-centered planning is the need for change in practice, which is bound to the systems and the policies by which they are guided. This chapter has been based on the development of thousands of person-centered plans by people independent of DDSN and its provider network, as well as the very positive initial feedback from circle of support members.

South Carolina DDSN has implemented person-centered planning by changing policies, practices, and expectations. This has involved the collaboration of DDSN with the University of Minnesota's RRTC and the University of South Carolina's CDR. This collaboration included the development and implementation of training for facilitators, the development of an infrastructure to provide continuing support for facilitators, and the initial evaluation of participant satisfaction with the person-centered planning process.

The survey on initial satisfaction with person-centered planning in South Carolina's DDSN system clearly demonstrated a high level of satisfaction with person-centered planning regardless of one's role (i.e., family member/friends or staff), although staff registered significantly higher levels of satisfaction with the planning process. No differences were observed between the four regions of the state in which the planning was undertaken.

The work reflected in this chapter has addressed many areas essential to implementing person-centered planning on a statewide basis. In any ongoing process, however, there are always issues that remain on the horizon. Three of these issues, some of which are being addressed, include assessment of consumer satisfaction with person-centered planning, evaluation of person-centered plan quality, and measurement of the degree to which personal outcomes are achieved through person-centered plan implementation.

Furthermore, several questions remain to be answered about statewide implementation of person-centered planning. They may serve as suggestions for future research by those with the interest and opportunity to answer them. These questions, in addition to the previously stated need for satisfaction information directly from consumers, include the comparative levels of satisfaction for person-centered and program-centered styles of planning and the comparative quality of service plans under person-centered and other models of planning. It would also be useful to collect satisfaction data from consumers and their circles of support at multiple points in time.

CONCLUSION

No model for large-scale systems change is perfect, but the information provided in this chapter may help others who are interested in introducing person-centered planning on a statewide level. This chapter has focused on issues that involve the individual consumer, facilitator training and support, evaluation of satisfaction, and the systems necessary to encourage and support the effort. Having a plan of support that is authentic to the individual is a necessary starting point. Implementation requires resources and a method for defining, assessing, and ensuring person-specific outcomes. The current system in South Carolina allocates resources on an individual basis and has shifted from process evaluation to results assessment based on the goals that consumers have identified in their plans. Although the process described in this chapter involves significant work at many levels, it is essential to keep the primary focus on the one issue that counts most: the individual who is the focus of any given person-centered planning meeting. As noted by Smull (1998), having a terrific plan means little unless there is the will and capacity to implement it with a high level of integrity.

REFERENCES

Abery, B.H., McBride, M.J., & Rotholz, D.A. (1999). *The Person-Centered Planning Process Satisfaction Survey (PCP-SS)*. Minneapolis: University of Minnesota, Institute on Community Integration.

Bradley, V.J. (1994). Evolution of a new service paradigm. In V.J. Bradley, J.W. Ashbaugh, & B.C. Blaney (Eds.), *Creating individual supports for people with developmental disabilities: A mandate for change at many levels* (pp. 11–32). Baltimore: Paul H. Brookes Publishing Co.

Gallivan-Fenlon, A. (1994). Their senior year: Family and service provider perspectives on the transition from school to adult life for young adults with disabilities. *Journal of The Association for Persons with Severe Handicaps, 19*, 11–23.

Green, C.W., Reid, D.H., Canipe, V.S., & Gardner, S.M. (1991). A comprehensive evaluation of reinforcer identification processes for persons with profound mental handicaps. *Journal of Applied Behavior Analysis, 24*, 537–552.

Holburn, S., & Vietze, P. (1999). Acknowledging barriers in adopting person-centered planning. *Mental Retardation, 37*(2), 117–124.

Lichtenstein, S., & Michaelides, N. (1993). Transition from school to young adulthood: Four case studies of young adults labeled mentally retarded. *Career Development for Exceptional Individuals, 16*(2), 183–195.

Lyle O'Brien, C., O'Brien, J., & Mount, B. (1997). Person-centered planning has arrived . . . or has it? *Mental Retardation, 35*, 480–484.

Miles, M.B., & Huberman, A.M. (1994). *Qualitative data analysis*. Thousand Oaks, CA: Sage Publications.

Morris, T., & Kelley, R. (1999). *South Carolina home and community based waiver for persons with mental retardation and related conditions: Compliance review*. Atlanta, GA: Department of Health and Human Services, Region IV Health Care Financing Administration, Medicaid Operations Branch.

Mount, B. (1994). Benefits and limitations of personal futures planning. In V.J. Bradley, J.W. Ashbaugh, & B.C. Blaney (Eds.), *Creating individual supports for people with developmental disabilities: A mandate for change at many levels* (pp. 97–108). Baltimore: Paul H. Brookes Publishing Co.

O'Brien, J., & Lyle O'Brien, C. (1998). *A little book about person-centered planning*. Toronto: Inclusion Press.

Parsons, M.B., & Reid, D.H. (1990). Assessing food preferences among persons with profound mental retardation: Providing opportunities to make choices. *Journal of Applied Behavior Analysis, 23*, 183–195.

Pearpoint, J., & Forest, M. (1998). Person-centered planning: MAPS and PATH. *Impact, 11*(2), 4–5.

Pearpoint, J., O'Brien, J., & Forest, M. (1993). *PATH (Planning Alternative Tomorrows with Hope): A workbook for planning positive futures*. Toronto: Inclusion Press.

Sanderson, H., Kennedy J., Ritchie P., & Goodwin, G. (1997). *People, plans and possibilities: Exploring person centered planning*. Edinburgh, United Kingdom: SHS Ltd.

Schorr, L. (1997). *Common purpose.* New York: Anchor Books.

Smull, M. (1989). *A blueprint for Essential Lifestyle Planning.* Napa, CA: Allen, Shea & Associates.

Smull, M. (1998). A plan is not an outcome. *Impact, 11*(2), 17, 27.

Smull, M., & Burke Harrison, S. (1992). *Supporting people with severe reputations in the community.* Alexandria, VA: National Association of State Mental Retardation Program Directors.

Sparks, D., & Loucks-Horsley, S. (1990). Models of staff development. In W.R. Houston, M. Haberman, & J. Sikula (Eds.), *Handbook of research on teacher education* (pp. 234–250). New York: Macmillan.

Stancliffe, R.J., Abery, B.H., & Smith, J. (2000). Personal control and the ecology of community living settings: Beyond living-unit size and type. *American Journal on Mental Retardation, 105*(6), 431–454.

Stancliffe, R.J., Hayden, M.F., & Lakin, K.C. (1999). Effectiveness and quality of individual planning in residential settings: An analysis of outcomes. *Mental Retardation, 37*(2), 104–116.

Appendix: The Person-Centered Planning Process Satisfaction Survey

	Not at all	A little bit	Quite a bit	Completely
1. How well prepared was the facilitator to conduct the meeting?	1	2	3	4
2. How well did (name of focus person) appear to be prepared for his/her planning meeting?	1	2	3	4
3. How well did the facilitator appear to know and have an understanding of (name of focus person)?	1	2	3	4
4. How much was the pace of the meeting appropriate for people there?	1	2	3	4
5. How well did the facilitator make clear the roles and responsibilities of people at the meeting for developing the plan?	1	2	3	4
6. How well did the facilitator keep the meeting focused on the positive?	1	2	3	4
7. How well did the planning process "flow" at a pace comfortable for (name of focus person)?	1	2	3	4
8. To what extent was enough time spent in the planning session for (name of focus person) and his/her team to develop a good plan?	1	2	3	4
9. How flexible was the facilitator in scheduling a meeting that was convenient for you?	1	2	3	4
10. How satisfied were you with the way the facilitator ran the meeting?	1	2	3	4
11. How well did the facilitator make sure that (name of focus person)'s choices and points of view were listened to and considered by others?	1	2	3	4

From Abery, B.H., McBride, M.J., & Rotholz, D.A. (1999). *The Person-Centered Planning Process Satisfaction Survey (PCP-SS)*. Minneapolis: University of Minnesota, Institute on Community Integration; adapted by permission.

	Not at all	A little bit	Quite a bit	Completely
12. How much were the points of view of other people at the meeting listened to and considered?	1	2	3	4
13. How well did (name of focus person) share his/her ideas, preferences, and dreams about the future?	1	2	3	4
14. How well was the facilitator able to get everyone working together to help make sure the planning process worked well?	1	2	3	4
15. How well did the planning session cover all of the important information about (name of focus person)?	1	2	3	4
16. How well did the meeting give you an idea about what (name of focus person) would like his/her future to be like?	1	2	3	4
17. How well did the facilitator make sure that all of the people at the planning meeting other than (name of focus person) took part in developing the plan?	1	2	3	4
18. How well did the meeting identify what is most important to (name of focus person)?	1	2	3	4
19. How active was (name of focus person) in developing his/her own plan?	1	2	3	4
20. How well did the facilitator encourage the group to be creative and think about nontraditional ways of supporting (name of focus person)?	1	2	3	4
21. Based on what (name of focus person) said during the meeting, how well does the plan developed reflect what he/she wants?	1	2	3	4

	Not at all	A little bit	Quite a bit	Completely
22. How well did the facilitator address issues of health and safety during the meeting?	1	2	3	4
23. How well do you think the plan developed will help (name of focus person) make progress toward reaching his/her personal dreams and goals?	1	2	3	4
24. How clear are you about what you need to do to put the plan into action?	1	2	3	4
25. How easy is the plan to understand?	1	2	3	4
26. How satisfied are you with the plan that was developed?	1	2	3	4
27. How much did money, finances, or a lack of these things play a role in the plan that was developed?	1	2	3	4
28. How much was the financial information needed to make decisions about supports available at the planning meeting?	1	2	3	4
29. How hopeful and excited for (name of focus person) were you when you left the meeting?	1	2	3	4
30. How willing would you be to recommend this facilitator to other people with disabilities and their families?	1	2	3	4
31. How different was the process used in this meeting from planning meetings you have attended for (name of focus person) in the past?	1	2	3	4

32. What did you like most about the planning process in which you recently took part?

33. What did you like least about the planning process in which you recently took part?

	Not at all	A little bit	Quite a bit	Completely
34. How helpful was (name of focus person)'s Service Coordinator in providing information during the planning meeting?	1	2	3	4
35. How flexible was the Service Coordinator about scheduling the meeting at a time that was convenient for you?	1	2	3	4
36. How well did the Service Coordinator answer questions you had about the process or its outcomes before and after the meeting?	1	2	3	4

37. Were the people you wanted to be members of (person's name) circle there at the meeting?   Yes   No

Why do you think this happened?

38. Were you given a list of facilitators to choose from?   Yes   No

16

Realizing Individual, Organizational, and Systems Change

Lessons Learned in 15 Years of Training About Person-Centered Planning and Principles

Angela Novak Amado and Marijo W. McBride

As formal methods of person-centered planning developed in the early 1980s, some people in Minnesota made a commitment to introducing and providing training on the use of these new planning methods. From these beginning steps, efforts continued to expand. This chapter describes the lessons learned in five major Minnesota projects that spanned 15 years. Several different types of person-centered planning methods were used in these projects, and different types of project design supported different degrees of organizational and systems change. Significant lessons have been learned about factors that appear to result in more effective realization of the concepts of person-centered principles, as reflected in the quality of lives of individuals who receive services, the values of staff, and the degree and process of change in agencies and systems moving toward more person-centered support.

Experiences in these five projects indicate that training in person-centered planning and principles can result in substantial changes for individuals with disabilities, staff, agencies, organizations, and communities. However, some of the most powerful lessons are how training and projects can be designed to more effectively realize change. These experiences with a number of agencies, projects, and facilitators in one state provide valuable information and lessons about the process of development from agency-centered and system-centered processes to more person-centered methods, values, and thinking.

BRIEF DESCRIPTION OF THE FIVE PROJECTS

The five projects described in this chapter span the time period of 1985–2000. Prior to this period, in the early 1980s, a number of 5-day PASS-3 (Program Analysis of Service Systems, Third Edition; Wolfensberger & Glenn, 1975) trainings about the principle of normalization had been conducted in Minnesota; those workshop ideas laid a foundation for many emerging new ways of understanding the lives of people with disabilities and new ways of thinking about service design.

Project 1: Training Personal Futures Planning Facilitators, 1985–1991

In the early 1980s, when Mount and O'Brien formally developed Personal Futures Planning (1997; see also Chapter 1), the Minnesota Governor's Planning Council on Developmental Disabilities funded three distinct projects to train facilitators in this new planning method. In the first project in 1985, Mount conducted formal facilitator training with 17 people from 17 different agencies, including staff from the University of Minnesota, the Metropolitan Council, and residential and day program service agencies in the Minneapolis-St. Paul area. In 1989–1990 and 1990–1991, another 105 people were trained in two additional projects that were targeted to reach other geographical regions in the smaller cities and more rural areas of Minnesota.

The training components in all three projects were 2 days of initial training with practice groups of consumers and their support circles. Then, each facilitator was expected to facilitate another circle on his or her own, with a follow-up training day approximately 3 months later.

Project 2: Person-Centered Agency Design, 1991–1994

While Project 1 was underway, another Council-funded, 1-year project called Friends was being conducted to examine how staff and agencies could help people with developmental disabilities have more community friends. From this project, it was learned that an agency could not work on the issues of friendship and community inclusion in isolation from larger organizational design issues and that these processes took longer than a year. Partly due to these lessons and to the previous experiences in PASS workshops of conducting intensive 5-day evaluations with no follow-up, a longer-term project of broader scope was designed.

Consequently, the Person-Centered Agency Design project (Amado, 1994) was conducted from 1991 to 1994 with eight agencies, including residential services and day program/employment providers in larger, intermediate, and more rural areas of the state. Whereas Project 1 was designed only to train people in facilitating Personal Futures Planning, Project 2 was meant to identify a person-centered agency design and to work with organizations over a longer, 3-year time period to determine processes of implementing person-centered principles throughout each agency.

To determine the degree of person-centered agency design at that time and to train participants in person-centered planning methods, this project used Framework for Accomplishment, which was designed by O'Brien and Lyle O'Brien (1989). Framework for Accomplishment is a 5-day workshop that can be used to evaluate the degree to which an agency is person-centered, and it includes processes to identify constructive actions for more person-centered directions. The workshop's definition of *person-centered* rests on a framework for genuine accomplishment within services, which is based on the realization of three specific purposes for all human services for people who require long-term support:

1. To help people discover and move toward a more desirable future

2. To protect and promote five valued experiences now: sharing ordinary community places and activities, contribution, expanding relationships, being treated with respect and having a valued social role, and choice

3. To offer needed help in ways that support and strengthen community competence

The personal planning method used in Framework for Accomplishment is a Personal Profile, and it uses a booklet to gather information in topic areas similar to the Personal Profile in Personal Futures Planning. During Framework for Accomplishment, however, a small number of "focal individuals" are selected from the agency being evaluated. Workshop participants each spend a "day in the life" with one of these focal individuals. The workshop participant observes daily life for that person receiving support and interviews people who are significant to the person by using the questions in the Personal Profile booklet. (Sample questions include "What have the person's life experiences been like?" "What losses and separations has the person experienced?" "What does the person enjoy doing?") The following day, the participant draws two posters regarding the person's life: one regarding who the person is and what his or her life is like, the second about a desirable future for that person. In the remaining days of the workshop, an agency's strengths and weaknesses are analyzed according to the themes identified in the lives of the focal people as compared with the three purposes of human services, and constructive action plans for the future are made. Each of these eight agencies also developed a Backward Plan, using a process adapted from Russell Ackoff (1986) to develop a long-range vision for a person-centered agency design and to make specific time commitments toward that vision, such as 10-, 5-, 2-, and 1-year goals.

The Person-Centered Agency Design project was structured as a 3-year project for agencies to evaluate themselves by using Framework for Accomplishment and then to work with agencies to actually develop the ideas discovered during this evaluation process. Organizational change issues were directly addressed at monthly meetings, and additional training was held with staff who did not participate in Framework for Accomplishment and on related topics, such as supporting relationships with community members. One advantage of this project was that because eight agencies participated, it was possible to identify some of the agency factors that seemed to lead to success and to inhibit success.

Project 3: Person-Centered System Design, 1994–1996

One of the eight agencies that participated in the Person-Centered Agency Design project (Project 2) was clear that it could only go so far in truly implementing person-centered principles without more involvement and significant change by other agencies in its system. The agency staff requested that Framework for Accomplishment be conducted with all of the agencies in their region. In 1994, a 2-year project began with all 12 agencies providing service to people with developmental disabilities in a two-county area in south-central Minnesota. The participants included

- Staff from five residential services providers
- Two providers of day habilitation/sheltered work/supported employment
- Staff from a county office of the state Department of Rehabilitation Services
- Staff from each county's Department of Social Services
- Members of The Arc of the United States and People First (advocacy organizations)
- Representatives of the school district's special education program

Framework for Accomplishment was conducted with 47 participants from these 12 organizations, and plans were made to implement the ideas originating from the process. In addition, representatives from all of the agencies jointly developed a region-wide Backward Plan with a long-range vision. After the initial Framework for Accomplishment training, other staff attended 2-day facilitator training on Personal Futures Planning and on additional topics such as community inclusion. This was the only project in which all system agencies participated together in the same training.

Project 4: Performance-Based Contracting Demonstration, 1995–1998

As knowledge about person-centered planning spread, it began to be recognized that the implementation of person-centered principles required a different focus for state quality assurance and quality monitoring. In 1995, Minnesota received a waiver from the federal Centers for Medicare & Medicaid Services (formerly the Health Care Financing Administration) for residential services agencies that provided support in intermediate care facilities for people with mental retardation (ICFs/MR) to pilot alternative quality assurance methods. In place of the traditional ICF/MR guidelines, which mainly emphasized "paper compliance" through the completion of forms and documents, this waiver allowed participating agencies to be reviewed and licensed based on the achievement of personal outcomes by the individuals who received services. The state selected the personal outcome system developed by the Council on Quality and Leadership (Accreditation Council, 1995) as its alternative quality assurance method. The Accreditation Council had found that an agency's success in the fulfillment of personal outcomes depended on the quality of the person-centered planning processes utilized; hence, plans for training about person-centered planning were part of the design of this Performance-Based Contracting Demonstration project.

Over the course of 2 years, project participants attended various trainings on three different specific person-centered planning methods, including Personal Futures Planning (Mount, 1997), Essential Lifestyle Planning (Smull & Burke Harrison, 1992), and PATH (Planning Alternative Tomorrows with Hope; Pearpoint, O'Brien, & Forest, 1993). An independent evaluation of the entire project (Hewitt et al., 1998) found that the person-centered planning training was critical to the success of the overall project.

Project 5: State-Operated Community Services Training Projects, 1998–2000

Training about person-centered principles was also conducted with staff of five state regional agencies that supported individuals who had been previously institutionalized. In the late 1980s, when Minnesota's state institutions housed approximately 2,200 individuals with developmental disabilities, the state made a commitment to substantially downsize these facilities. This initiative resulted in the eventual closure of all six large state facilities, with the last one closing in June 2000.

Although many of these residents moved into privately run group and foster homes and other living situations, the downsizing and closure processes included opening some state-operated community services. Approximately 375 individuals moved into the state-operated community services system, which operates both residential and day programs through five state regional agencies that are staffed primarily by former state institution employees.

Managers of these state-operated residential and day program services knew about the Person-Centered Agency Design Project (Project 2) and requested Framework for Accomplishment training for the staff of these state-operated programs. In 1998, two agencies participated in the Framework for Accomplishment training and found it to be so useful that they requested similar training for the remaining three agencies. These agencies also developed a Backward Plan (described previously in the section on Project 2) to generate a long-range vision for a person-centered design and to make specific time commitments and goals to reach that vision. Again, sample time frames included 10-, 5-, 2-, and 1-year goals.

LESSONS LEARNED

Full organizational implementation of person-centered principles can be challenging. The experiences and results from these projects provide lessons for other organizations seeking greater success in implementing these ideas and in overcoming barriers. Lessons from these projects are grouped into two categories: 1) lessons about the planning process itself and 2) lessons about organizational, systems, and community change.

Lessons About the Planning Process Itself

Numerous lessons were learned about this planning process, including preferences for this type of process compared with traditional ones. Other lessons concerned the benefits and challenges of the process, as well as the importance of the quality and scope of facilitator training.

Lesson 1: Person-Centered Planning Processes Are Preferred to Traditional Ones   Many project participants noted that person-centered planning meetings resulted in increased happiness for the consumer and that consumers and their families were better able to participate in and had more voice in these processes than in traditional ones. The individuals' sense of self, personal satisfaction, and self-determination improved.

Other group members were more responsive to and pleased with person-centered planning processes than with traditional methods. Meetings became more upbeat and positive, and new, more positive relationships developed between team members. Teams became more actively focused on the individual's preferences, choices, and goals, and people who were not service providers increasingly took active roles. Planning meetings became more social and less formal (Hewitt et al., 1998). They took place in nontraditional places, such as restaurants and coffee shops, and usually included some form of refreshments. The focus individuals invited whomever they wished to attend support network meetings, including girlfriends, boyfriends, siblings, and other friends. Some assisted in the process of sending out invitations, and some facilitated their own meetings. Agency staff spent time with each person before the actual planning meeting to find out what was most important to that person. Participants reported that meetings focused on "identifying important values and quality of life issues for the individual rather than the findings of assessments or meeting other regulatory requirements" (Hewitt et al., 1998, p. 5). Agencies that had used Framework for Accomplishment's Personal Profiles adapted their planning processes to emphasize desirable personal futures and the five valued experiences.

Participants' responses in different projects included the following:

- "Everyone looks forward to meetings more. It used to be said after meetings, you'd hear, 'That wasn't so bad, was it?' Now meetings are more darn fun. They're a heck of a lot more meaningful."

- "People are happy to go to meetings—we don't see behaviors 2 weeks ahead of time like we used to."

- "A lot of consumers have talked to me about their annual meetings—they never talked about it before; they were summoned."

Lesson 2: These Processes Can Foster Dramatic Changes in People's Lives Results reported at the project conclusions and in post-project follow-up surveys indicated the positive impact of these processes on people with disabilities, facilitators, organizations, and systems. Person-centered planning led to improved quality of life, significant life changes, desired lifestyle outcomes, and increased motivation for individuals to work toward their stated preferences (Hewitt et al., 1998, pp. 8–9).

As of 2002, more people in Minnesota are living in their own places and with people whom they chose. Individuals purchased their own homes and moved into truly accessible apartments. More people are employed in community jobs and are making more money. Individuals went on dates for the first time, and some got married. Many joined community organizations (e.g., the Knights of Columbus, a tractor club, an arthritis support group, an informal line-dancing group, a church group) and started volunteering (e.g., the opera house, the public library, a preschool, a volunteer fire department, the Big Sister/Little Sister program). Many either started self-advocacy organizations or joined existing ones. Staff summarized the situation with comments such as, "People's lives are more real" and "We hear more [of] what their wants really are; they're asking about what's available . . . that never used to come out at all."

In the projects using Framework for Accomplishment, the 5 workshop days occurred during the time frame of a month or so. As noted previously, many of the Framework for Accomplishment questions were about an individual's life history. During these month-long training periods, some staff worked vigorously to find parents, siblings, or cousins who had not seen their relatives in 20, 30, or even 60 years. For several individuals who had lived in state institutions most of their lives, there were numerous dramatic instances of reconnecting with siblings and cousins and expanding relationships with parents. One person's family got together for the first time in 20 years. In another case, a person's twin brother without disabilities was accidentally discovered, and the siblings reconnected—the staff did not know that the man with disabilities had a twin, and the twin thought that his brother had died years ago. These dramatic results often came about during the initial training itself, without any additional organizational changes. One outcome of these results during the initial training was an increased alignment of participants and other stakeholders with the value of using person-centered planning ideas and methods.

Many changes in staff attitudes, which staff themselves reported, contributed to these changes. Staff saw people with disabilities in a new light, began to see services from a new perspective, and became more open and sensitive to the needs and the individual rights of the people they supported. Staff reported that they got out of a rut, started thinking more in terms of things that people can do, and stopped getting bogged down in the day-to-day life of documentation. Other outcomes are shown by the following staff comments:

- "We used to make people work at things they were not good at and did not want to do. We now assist people to do things they want to do."

- "People are seen as people more—not as their diagnosis or as 'special.'"
- "Our thinking has kind of turned."
- "We've gone further, never looked at it that way before."

One discovery was that agencies could tremendously increase the five valued experiences from Framework for Accomplishment: relationships, contribution, valued roles, community presence, and choice. The agencies could increase people's experiences in all of these areas without increased funding, additional staff, and changes in rules and regulations.

Lesson 3: There Will Be Difficulties Implementing the Process as Intended A common misconception was that person-centered planning meant asking the person, "What do you want?" Many planning teams implemented it that way, which gave people with disabilities more opportunities to express themselves but missed the larger picture of deeper thinking about the possibilities of people's lives. In many cases, planning groups did not generate desirable futures for individuals with disabilities that stretched beyond current service system options to lives as full community citizens. Many changes were at "level one"—increased choices and better life experiences within the same models of service delivery.

Some participants reported that it was difficult to empower consumers who had no history of being able to make their own choices. In addition, they reported that it was difficult to learn not to lead the person in answering, to provide enough information so that the person had a real concept of what was available, and to encourage the person to answer honestly. In many cases, members of the planning team still tended to be the members of a traditional planning team—people came to the planning meetings because of their traditional roles (e.g., county case managers, guardians, other family members), regardless of the consumer's wish for them to attend. For some people, person-centered planning methods became a new and different way to have interdisciplinary team meetings or annual meetings.

Lesson 4: Planning Facilitators Need to Do More Than Attend One Training Session The first projects about person-centered planning in Minnesota began with training facilitators in these planning methods. As implementation of the methods evolved from this starting point, it became obvious from both these early projects and the later ones that effective implementation involved more than simply training facilitators in "doing a method." Facilitators were more successful when they were grounded in the philosophy of person-centered thinking. Rather than merely attending a single training, facilitators were more successful when they practiced methods, received ongoing technical assistance to expand skills and understanding of person-centered principles, stayed connected with others who facilitate the process, and continued to learn new techniques. One project had ongoing meetings and get-togethers for the facilitators, and the facilitators reported that this was the most helpful element of the training (Hewitt et al., 1998).

Lessons About Organizational, Systems, and Community Changes

A common weakness was the perception that person-centered planning is a different kind of planning process that can be undertaken in a vacuum without significant organizational change. Mount noted, "Almost every personal futures plan that is true to the person challenges the existing organizational process and structure in some way" (1994, p. 100). Effective person-centered planning is not limited to the planning process itself; it also demands organizational, systems, and community changes.

Lesson 5: Effective Implementation Affects, Challenges, and Requires the Need to Change Internal Agency Infrastructures When comparing the progress of agencies within the same project, more positive results with individual plans and for people's lives were experienced by agencies that developed consistent internal structures for plan follow-through. Common reported barriers to implementation of person-centered plans were described as follows: "No follow-through by the interdisciplinary team" and "We're given the opportunities and freedom to be flexible but not given the support." In follow-up surveys to projects that focused only on facilitator training, all of the parents who responded complained that the initial meetings were great but that nothing had happened afterward; there had been no follow-up.

Serious implementation of these ideas also requires follow-up and redesign of many organizational structures (Amado, 1994). For the more successful agencies, changes in internal organizational design included the following:

- Closing 6-, 8-, and 12-bed group homes
- Closing segregated day center programs
- Changing agency mission statements, job descriptions, and staff orientation training to reflect a more person-centered approach
- Assisting in the development of new self-advocacy groups or assisting people to join existing ones

- Changing staff meetings to emphasize individual desirable futures and ways for staff to assist people in making community connections

- Requesting variances from licensing boards to allow individuals more control over their lives

- Establishing internal committees to generate, implement, and review action steps toward the short-term and long-term visions

Lesson 6: The Degree of Long-Term Organizational Commitment and Longer-Term Project Design Affects the Degree of Change Although there were some specific examples of immediate, dramatic results for some consumers, these projects indicated the need for long-term commitment. Comparison of all five projects demonstrates that the degree of organizational commitment and project design for long-term implementation greatly affected the degree of change in people's lives. When a project design included specific structures to support long-term change, there was more organizational change. If a staff member attended facilitator training without the entire agency and lead management being committed to the change process, then the degree of change was limited.

Three of the five projects used Framework for Accomplishment for their initial training. Two of these three projects were designed with 3-year and 2-year time frames respectively, with distinct goals for project-end and monthly implementation meetings. One project was begun without this type of specific long-term project time frame, and after the initial training, the five sites that participated varied in their degree of implementation and follow-through. Of these five sites, the agency that has experienced the most progress as of 2002 is the one that has established the most internal structures committed to implementation of project goals. These structures include a cross-facility team which meets monthly, additional training for all direct support staff, and the integration of project goals into job descriptions and internal planning mechanisms. It is obvious that training in person-centered principles and facilitation cannot stand alone to create large-scale organizational or systems change.

Lesson 7: Various Factors Affect Successful Organizational Implementation At the same time, a longer-term project design is not in itself sufficient to guarantee change, nor is simply stating a commitment to move to person-centered design. In the longer-term projects that involved multiple agencies, results could be compared among the agencies that were more and less successful. In some cases, members of a support circle could implement changes in certain aspects of daily life—such as simple choices and more opportunities for community participation—but major life changes needed more significant organizational effort and commitment. For instance, whereas one agency only implemented changes within its group home (e.g., choices over meals), another agency in the same project closed a group home of the same size and moved people to more individualized support situations, with the people choosing their own homes and roommates.

In early stages of projects, it was often surprising how easy it was to implement internal and simple changes. Then, the agencies typically reached the limit, or "the ceiling," of their existing service model and had to confront far more difficult issues. This ceiling was easy to see in some planning meetings for focus individuals who lived in group homes. When these individuals were asked about their desires for the future, they often responded with ideas for more fun activities. Because members of the planning teams ostensibly wanted to honor the individuals' preferences, they thought that they were fulfilling the intention of the planning if they helped the person engage in those fun activities. Yet, the team members often did not think beyond that point. All of the agencies were challenged by how seriously and extensively they would go in implementing these principles.

Elements that were similar among the agencies that experienced the most change and were lacking (in various degrees) among the agencies that experienced the least change included

- The understanding and commitment of the executive director
- The degree of commitment at the program director/coordinator level
- An agency's self-perceived capacity to change, atmosphere of creativity, and willingness to take risks
- Cohesive teams for which all members were involved, understood the process, worked together, and were enthusiastic about making changes
- Involvement with or start-up of self-advocacy groups
- Whether staff members became significantly involved in connecting consumers to community members
- Support by governing boards, other county agencies, families, and the community
- Systematic internal organizational changes in mission statements, job descriptions, and so forth

Lesson 8: Common Attitudinal, Organizational, and Systems Barriers Need to Be Addressed   The degree of change was limited in each project by attitudinal, organizational, and structural factors.

Participants perceived time and attitude as the main internal barriers to implementation of these principles. Time concerns included 1) the lengthier process required to engage in person-centered planning rather than in traditional planning, 2) the high level of "paper pushing" or busy work that some staff experienced in their jobs, and 3) the perception that the system did not view this type of planning as necessary.

Three categories of attitudinal barriers included 1) the view that "we're already doing it," 2) a lack of alignment among all participants, and 3) resistance to change. As person-centered planning has become so familiar recently, many people responded, "We're already doing it" without understanding the fundamental shifts in values and support structures that true person-centered planning demands. Some people thought the planning process ended as soon as the meeting was over, did not really buy into or believe in the concepts, or just "went along" without really changing. Some resisted change in terms of not getting out of their "ruts," finding the change process overwhelming, or thinking that change was unnecessary because "everyone was already person-centered." A particular problem was noted as "staff talking the talk but not walking the walk."

Truly implementing person-centered plans in all of the projects also demanded more serious system change efforts. Some of the identified system barriers were funding and specific rules, as well as the need for more housing options and increased overall creativity. Financing that increased flexibility and the person's control was necessary. Rules that were identified as barriers compartmentalized individuals, promoted turf battles between agencies, promoted overprotectiveness, and limited risk. It was necessary to develop rules that separated housing from the provision of support. There was a need for licensing that increased flexibility and recognized the balance between risk and opportunity. In terms of the need for more creativity, participants felt that person-centered planning identifies what needs to be done but not how to do it. Thus, providers had to develop new strategies for providing support based on different expectations.

Lesson 9: Agencies Need Outside Input These projects provided some evidence that when an agency evaluates its own progress, it sees and reports a degree of improvement from system-centered to person-centered principles that others outside the agency do not see. For instance, although residential providers in one project reported that consumers were happier, had more control over their lives, and experienced more freedom and growth, day habilitation providers who served the same individuals reported that in some cases, the residential providers were not even meeting basic care needs.

One project evaluation (Hewitt et al., 1998) noted many agency "blind spots"—common and everyday examples of lingering agency-centered or system-centered practices to which agencies seemed blind but could easily change. Examples included time clocks, clipboards, certificates of occupancy, licenses and house rules posted prominently in living areas; commercial paper towel and soap dispensers in home bathrooms; staff talking about focus individuals in front of them; staff drinking soda and eating food in front of consumers on restricted diets or who did not have access to the same soda and food; home telephone answering machines that identified program names; and staff entering homes without knocking. Another example of agency blind spots in the implementation of person-centered principles included the closures of eight-bed or six-bed group homes, then opening four-bed homes.

Facilitator trainees who were not from provider agencies, such as staff of self-advocacy organizations and self-determination projects, perceived that agencies were still very traditional and system-centered and provided less control to the people with disabilities than they thought. These blind spots indicate that if an agency wants an honest appraisal of its implementation of person-centered principles and values, then it should include outside evaluation and not limit itself to internal assessments.

Lesson 10: Include All of the Major Players in the System

When more stakeholders in the system participated in a project, greater system impact resulted. In addition, an agency could only go so far in its implementation of a person-centered design without participation from other agencies in the larger system.

Two of the five projects involved many more system "players" and elicited commitment from multiple agencies. Only one of these projects simultaneously trained staff from all of the groups that supported individuals with developmental disabilities in the same geographical area (i.e., residential agencies, day habilitation/employment programs, schools, county social services). Two different cross-agency committees were set up to continue implementation. At the end of this 2-year project, the participants reported more impact on interagency cooperation, agreed-on goals, and systemwide changes than reported in any other project. These participants felt that the system was becoming more consumer friendly, that the agencies had better working relationships, and that staff were talking with each other as people rather than as agencies. The bonding between the agencies meant an increased focus on the individual with disabilities rather than against each other. One such participant reported, "Case managers and the county are more open to trying things. Money used to be a stop; now it's, 'Let's try to find the money somewhere.'" Participants felt that boundaries were being pushed and that brand new things were occurring.

The importance of involving all system players was also reflected in the other project that included numerous system players; however, this project did not include all of the relevant agencies. In the final evaluation, 98% of those responding said that it would be important in future projects to have all parts of the service delivery system change together (Hewitt et al., 1998). In contrast to some of the other projects that were more local, this project had many formal commitments from the state and federal government, the University of Minnesota, and both local and statewide chapters of The Arc of the United States. More elements of the larger system were influenced by this project, such as the state licensing and funding rules for all provider agencies, as well as initiatives such as a managed care demonstration project and the Robert Wood Johnson Self-Determination project (Hewitt et al., 1998).

Lesson 11: True Implementation Means Conscious Involvement of Community Members The goals of person-centered planning include life as a full community citizen, greater community member involvement in a person's life, and "changing common patterns of community life" (O'Brien & Lovett, 1992, p. 3). When people with disabilities were asked what they wanted for their lives, however, they typically did not mention community friends. Most planning groups did not invite or were not successful in recruiting community members, nor did they spontaneously pursue community friendships for the focus individuals. Most circles of support did not include anyone beyond family members and staff.

In and of itself, the person-centered planning training did not usually assist staff in reaching out to community members. Yet, several of the projects included specific efforts and a great deal of additional training about building community and promoting friendship (Amado, 1993). As a result of this focus, many community members befriended individuals who received services. Some staff found it easier to understand and grasp the larger person-centered vision through this more specific and concrete training about community belonging and friendship.

There were other examples of how pursuing the individuals' desired futures had an impact on community members. Realtors and developers provided increased rental and purchase options for consumer-controlled housing, including adaptations to rental property, contracts for deeds, and so forth. Employers hired more individuals with disabilities and featured them in their company newsletters. Local newspapers also carried stories about individuals with disabilities. Community education programs and community associations included individuals with disabilities in their general classes and meetings, and some community associations even changed their meeting locations to be more accessible for their new members with physical disabilities. Some of the most successful efforts in different projects came about through Community Member Forums (Amado & Victorian-Blaney, 2000), which gathered community members together to share with them the vision of a fully inclusive community and to enlist them in seeing and taking action on their role in realizing that vision.

CONCLUSION

Since Minnesota's first training session about person-centered planning in 1985, many other initiatives have contributed to the changing face of the services system, including the closure of the state institutions, large ICFs/MR, and large residential and day training facilities; a stipulation that new residential facilities be limited to four beds or less; the creation of major projects to expand supported employment; and the implementation of the Robert Wood Johnson Self-Determination Initiative, Partners in Policy-Making, and major advances in school inclusion. As of 2002, person-centered planning is part of the state's rules governing the interdisciplinary planning process.

Yet, despite much progress in the implementation of person-centered ideas, service provision is still very traditional in many cases, and many people with disabilities still find the system to be very facility- and system-centered. We have learned that no matter how much person-centered planning training occurs, it often seems as if the system-based way of thinking and doing things is like a vacuum cleaner, sucking everything up into itself. New models may come along, but they get vacuumed into system thinking and system-defined ways of doing things. Although support has definitely improved and is more individualized, a great deal of agency control and a lack of community continue to exist in many cases. People may even live in their own homes and have community jobs but still belong to the system rather than to the community. Like many others in the field, we have learned that it takes an enormous amount of effort to stand in the face of the vacuum cleaner's draw and resist the pull. Finally, we have learned that a professional's or program's claiming to be "person-centered" is a danger sign. Being "person-centered" is not a place at which one ever arrives, like an end point; it means always evolving, growing, developing, and stretching. It means always asking, "What else is possible?"—not just for this individual, but also for our communities. What is possible today is far beyond our thinking of even a few years ago. We have learned that support can never be completely person-centered, but it can only continue to become more and more so.

REFERENCES

Accreditation Council on Services for People with Disabilities. (1995). *Outcome-based performance measures: A procedures manual.* Towson, MD: Author.

Ackoff, R. (1986). *Management in small doses.* New York: John Wiley & Sons.

Amado, A.N. (Ed.). (1993). *Friendships and community connections between people with and without developmental disabilities.* Baltimore: Paul H. Brookes Publishing Co.

Amado, A.N. (1994). *Person-centered agency design: A three year project 1991–1994.* St. Paul, MN: Human Services Research and Development Center.

Amado, A.N., & Victorian-Blaney, J. (2000). Requesting inclusion from the community: The necessity of asking. *TASH Newsletter, 26*(5), 15–17.

Hewitt, A., O'Nell, S., Smith, J., Bast, J., Larson, S., & Lakin, K.C. (1998). *An evaluation of alternative methods to assure and enhance the quality of long-term care services for persons with developmental disabilities through performance-based contracts (PBC Project).* Minneapolis: University of Minnesota, Institute on Community Integration.

Mount, B. (1994). Benefits and limitations of personal futures planning. In V.J. Bradley, J.W. Ashbaugh, & B.C. Blaney (Eds.), *Creating individual supports for people with developmental disabilities: A mandate for change at many levels* (pp. 97–108). Baltimore: Paul H. Brookes Publishing Co.

Mount, B. (1997). *Person-centered planning: Finding directions for change using personal futures planning.* New York: Graphic Futures.

O'Brien, J., & Lovett, H. (1992). *Finding a way toward everyday lives.* Harrisburg: Pennsylvania Office of Mental Retardation.

O'Brien, J., & Lyle O'Brien, C. (1989). *Framework for accomplishment.* Decatur, GA: Responsive Systems Associates.

Pearpoint, J., O'Brien, J., & Forest, M. (1993). *PATH (Planning Alternative Tomorrows with Hope).* Toronto: Inclusion Press.

Smull, M., & Burke Harrison, S. (1992). *Supporting people with severe reputations in the community.* Alexandria, VA: National Association of State Directors of Developmental Disabilities Services.

Wolfensberger, W., & Glenn, L. (1975). *Program Analysis of Service Systems (PASS)* (3rd ed.). Toronto: National Institute on Mental Retardation.

17

Public Policy and Person-Centered Planning

Michael Smull and K. Charlie Lakin

Person-centered planning has moved from the fringes of service systems to the center. It has gone from being a way to help people move to a desired future with minimal public service involvement to being a way to organize and direct publicly funded services. When person-centered planning occurred in a small number of agencies with relatively few people, it was not an issue that concerned those who make public policy. At that time, the role of policy makers was largely limited to allowing (and on occasion financing) while staying out of the way of the efforts. Through these initiatives, a perception was established that the development and implementation of person-centered plans contributed to an enhanced quality of life. These pilot efforts also demonstrated that person-centered planning could be accommodated within existing structures of regulation and reimbursement. As person-centered planning becomes expected and even required practice, however, it is necessary to examine the roles of public policy and public policy makers in providing person-centered planning services.

PUBLIC POLICY DEFINED

Public policy reflects decisions that are typically made by elected officials or by people who have been appointed by publicly elected officials. The primary purpose of most of these decisions is to promote the public welfare of a segment of society (e.g., people who are older than 65 years, people with disabilities, people in school). Most public policy has a direct or indirect impact on the use of resources. For example, the policies of the federal Medicaid program derive their power from the fact that states gain (and can then use) resources by agreeing to follow the policy requirements. In an ideal system, all public policy decisions would be rooted in knowing the effects of the decisions on the people who are the focus of the decisions. If public policies were based on such an ideal, then the policy makers would have answers to important questions before making decisions: What is the decision intended to do, and does it actually do it? Who are the judges and what are the measures of success? Is individual welfare substantially improved for sufficient numbers of people as a result of the decision? If so, in what ways?

It turns out that this decision-making process is rarely possible and rarely done. Public policy is created to promote a particular vision of public welfare; then, as it is implemented, the effects emerge. As the vision of what constitutes public welfare shifts, the public policies follow. The consequences, intended and unintended, emerge with the application of the policies. Although how well a policy will work cannot be fully anticipated, thinking through its implications in the light of current knowledge is likely to increase the probability of success. Increasing the probability of success, then, requires the following:

- Careful review of the prior effects of public policy within the area under consideration
- An understanding of current circumstances and their implications in achieving the outcome
- A clear vision of the desired outcome
- Clarity regarding the skills, structures, and organizational culture that would make achieving the desired outcome more likely
- An understanding of the role, potential, and limitations of public policy in creating favorable circumstances and achieving the outcome

HISTORY OF SERVICE PLANNING

In the 1960s, a century of medical and institutional dominance of services for people with developmental disabilities began to erode. Alarm and discouragement about the squalor of institutions and medicine's limited capacity to respond effectively to the primary needs of people with developmental disabilities resulted in heightened attention to the possibilities of psychology. There were at the time two emerging schools of psychology: humanistic and behavioral. McCandless and Evans's textbook, a standard in 1973, noted that humanistic psychology focused on "man's potential, his uniqueness and dignity" and operated from a perspective that "individuals are basically self-determining, rational and active in shaping their own growth" (pp. 46–57), whereas behavioral psychology focused on people as learners and viewed "[man] as a product of his learning" and "changing as a result of experiences within the environment" (pp. 54–55).

There was not much competition between these two schools regarding the treatment of developmental disabilities. Humanistic psychologists seldom saw applications of their self-determining, self-actualizing approaches to human development. Yet, behavioral psychologists had enormous confidence in the power of their science and argued that with appropriate analysis of a task's components, appropriate discriminative stimuli around those tasks, and appropriate reinforcement of desired performance or approximations of it, people with severe cognitive limitations could learn sophisticated tasks. As a result, cognitive disabilities became commonly addressed through a learning regimen based on the principles of behavioral psychology. Basic aspects of task and behavior analysis became foundational expectations for those who provided services. Such expectations were integrated into regulations that governed service delivery. For example, in the federal government's first effort to support residential care of people with intellectual disabilities through the intermediate care facility for people with mental retardation program, regulations issued in 1974 (42 CFR 405.1009) specified "active treatment" which

> Requires the following:
>   (a) The individual's regular participation, in accordance with an individual plan of care, in professionally developed and supervised activities, experiences, or therapies.
>   (b) An individual written plan of care that sets forth measurable goals or objectives stated in terms of desirable behavior and that prescribes an integrated program of activities, experiences or therapies necessary for the individual to reach those goals and objectives.

Sturmey noted, "There have been few studies of the application of goal planning within the context of routine services" (1992, p. 99). Although Sturmey went on to conclude that available research indicated that studies showed that approximately 50% of short-term objectives were acquired, these were "short-term objectives" that were merely steps in a task analysis rather than complete functional skills (p. 94). Other research is both equivocal and incredibly scanty given the massive amounts of resources allocated to developing and implementing the more traditional individual program plans (IPPs). Fleming and Stenfert-Kroese (1990) reported that people with IPPs had better skill acquisition than comparison group members without IPPs. Yet, Felce, deKock, Mansell, and Jenkins (1984) found minimal evidence of skill acquisition and no evidence of goal acquisition associated with whether people had IPPs. Of course, it might be hypothesized that equivocal results may come from varying quality in the IPPs themselves.

The adoption of individual program planning around behavioral principles prompted a number of efforts to specify the characteristics of plans and the component goals and objectives that reflect best practice in developing IPPs. Many criteria have been proposed as features of good program plans and component goals (DePaepe, Reichle, Doss, Shriner, & Cameron, 1994; Fleming & Stenfert-Kroese, 1990; Legal Advocacy for Persons with Developmental Disabilities, 1989). Typical of these efforts were the 23 criteria in five domains specified and defined by Legal Advocacy for Persons with Developmental Disabilities in its 1989 guidebook *Individual Habilitation Plan Review*. These domains included

1. Functionality: contains functional (useful) objectives, is age appropriate, addresses a variety of natural environments

2. Community focus: promotes community participation and inclusion

3. Technical adequacy: has sequential steps to annual goals and objectives that are observable and measurable; specifies conditions in which behavior should occur; specifies the level of performance to achieve objectives; sets deadlines for achievement; specifies initiation and review dates; delineates criteria for continuing or modifying objectives; names people responsible for writing, implementing, and monitoring objectives

4. Teaching methods: performs task analysis, specifies the steps of task analysis to be taught, provides learning opportunities that are adequate in terms of frequency and length, uses clear and detailed teaching methods, contains teaching that provides for motivation and reinforcement, specifies prompts and fading

5. Data collection: selects objective baseline data, delineates a method of collecting progress data, collects progress data as specified, evaluates data at least monthly

Given such standards and their detailed specifications, researchers at the University of Minnesota investigated the correspondence between relatively well-written and implemented IPPs and actual outcomes for people with cognitive disabilities. The raters agreed on more than 90% of the criteria to use for IPP quality. Then, they reviewed the IPPs of 126 individuals living in institutions and in the community to determine the presence of an IPP goal or objective and the quality of that goal or objective. Quality was determined in each of five areas: 1) communication, 2) self-care, 3) household chores, 4) leisure and recreation activities, and 5) community participation. This research found that having goals or objectives in one of five areas was unrelated to improved outcomes in those areas, the rated quality in any domain was unrelated to outcomes in that domain, and the only domains of IPP quality showing any signs of validity were the weak and inconsistent relationships between the IPP technical adequacy and data collection and individual outcomes (Stancliffe, Hayden, & Lakin, 1999a, 2000).

Existing research provides little support for the basic processes and preferred practices in IPP development. IPPs have been implemented as a component of a favored psychological and/or philosophical orientation. They have persisted as a standard expectation and even as a regulatory requirement of service delivery. IPPs are popular because they specify what will be done, where it will be done, who will do it, how it will be demonstrated, and so forth. IPPs have meshed well with demands of policy in that accountability is achieved even if individual outcomes are not.

Despite the absence of research supporting its efficacy, when the IPP process began, it provided a structure and a focus that benefited people who had been receiving custodial care. Once the shift from custodial care was completed, it could be argued that the utility of IPPs for those who receive services dropped radically. This meant that "defensive" planning became the order of the day. Plans began to be written to the rule—not to help the person achieve a desired lifestyle. Goals were written vaguely by interdisciplinary teams to pass inspection in quality assurance reviews and to avoid modification when changes in a person's life required new learning. It became important for plans to meet criteria, not for them to be useful.

There seemed to be universal requirements for goals to be measurable and for data to document progress. As a result, many people who created the plans learned how to write goals that were measurable but not meaningful. Vague goals such as "one community outing weekly of his choosing" were met by activities like going through the drive-through window at a fast-food restaurant. Requirements to record more and more data have resulted in data sheets that were filled in based on memory at the end of shifts; sometimes they were even completed before the shift started. Some direct support staff learned from each other how to create "reliable" data rather than to record data as it happened. Plans increasingly became something that was done for the sake of compliance, and they were not often seen as being relevant to the person's life. This gradual loss of faith in the value of planning resulted in an organizational culture that saw the plans as outcomes, not as vehicles for helping people achieve desired lifestyles. The limits of this approach became evident at the end of the 20th century. As policy and practice continue to move from dictating traditional IPPs to person-centered planning, policy makers and service providers need to remember the context in which this change is occurring.

SHIFT IN VISION

The spread of person-centered planning represents a fundamental shift in the definition of *welfare* for people with disabilities, as well as a shift in the roles of those who fund and inspect planning. The prior vision for service planning required only that people with disabilities were kept healthy and safe, were taught skills to promote independence, and received services in the least restrictive environment. In the early 1990s, however, this vision began to evolve. As of 2002, the vision is to support people with disabilities in moving toward their desired lifestyles and in becoming valued community members while 1) addressing health and safety issues in the context of desired lifestyles, 2) offering opportunities for learning to help people better achieve their goals, and 3) making the best use of all available resources to accomplish these goals.

Thus, the vision has shifted from describing how to provide services to supporting people in achieving desired lifestyles. Issues of health and safety continue to be addressed, but it has been recognized that these issues always have a context: what is important to the person. Learning is still expected, but instead of professionals deciding what someone will learn, they are looking for ways to help the person acquire skills that he or she believes are important. The final and most important vision shift is that professionals are moving from determining the least restrictive environment and then placing the person in that environment to supporting a person in exploring how he or she wants to live within the community and then helping the individual move toward that life.

This "new" vision is both more complex and less resolved than it was just presented. The vision is being stated in a number of ways, and although the new vision statement includes person-centered planning, the adoption of person-centered practices lags behind. An example of this complexity is found in the view of control. In the old vision, control was vested in professionals who were assumed to know what was best for people. In the new vision, the direction—the vision of the future—is determined by the person (or the people who are closest to the person), whereas control over implementation is shared. Consciously sharing control is inherently more complex and challenging than asserting control.

As this shift continues to take place, those who are developing public policy need to keep in mind that a plan is not an outcome. An excessive emphasis on planning can result in overlooking the desired outcome of changes in people's lives. Plans should be seen as a way to record learning and to determine what to do with what has been learned. Thus, planning is really a set of skills, and each person-centered planning process requires a somewhat different set of skills. For all but a small minority of "naturals," acquiring those skills requires structured practice with mentoring and coaching. In addition, although the various processes share underlying values, they require sufficiently different skills; knowing one process does not take away the need for training or support in another. In fact, when the people developing plans lack the needed skills, this absence can destroy the trust required for good planning and implementation and can present unnecessary risks to health and safety.

Determining which process to use can be challenging. The planning processes have various strengths and work best in different circumstances. This area is largely unexplored in terms of research. The absence of organized learning about which processes work best in which circumstances has resulted in different "camps." That is, different groups claim that their process is better than the others. Those who are leading efforts for broad implementation of person-centered planning also need to see that the challenges in implementation will show what to foster and what to change within their organizations. These leaders must recognize the need for a system that is person centered, not simply a system that supports person-centered planning.

CURRENT POLICY CIRCUMSTANCES AND PERSON-CENTERED PLANNING

Many consequences of new public policy cannot be anticipated. However, the probability of achieving the desired results increases if the circumstances in which the policies are to be implemented are taken into account. Within the service system at the beginning of the 21st century, there are significant positive outcomes of and formidable obstacles to broad implementation of person-centered planning.

Positive Outcomes

The favorable circumstances are rooted in 15 years of development regarding best practice models. These models began with efforts to apply Personal Futures Planning (Mount, 1987) to services within small agencies and led to broader efforts to develop supported living. In a parallel development, supported employment spread across the country (Kiernan & Stark, 1986; Wehman & Moon, 1988). A later effort, self-determination, added the important component of control over resources. These efforts have had many results. First, a diverse and widely scattered set of best practice models, which provide local examples of how organizations can support people who have person-centered plans, are being implemented. Second, a smaller but still widely distributed set of examples exists regarding how rules, structures, and organizations can support people in having positive control over their lives. Third, people throughout the United States are skilled in one or more forms of person-centered planning. Fourth, broadening perceptions have led to the assumption that helping people have positive control over their lives is the right thing to do. Fifth, increasing numbers of people in positions of power and authority have experience in developing and implementing person-centered plans, including people who are employed in the public agencies that fund, regulate, and license the services provided to people with disabilities. Sixth, service provision rules are changing not only to require person-centered planning but also to support person-centered practices. All of these outcomes provide opportunities for implementing person-centered public policy.

Obstacles

In 2002, best practice continues to rapidly evolve, but typical practice is changing at a slower pace. Thus, the gap between best practice and typical practice is widening. There are still numerous examples of typical practice that reflect recommended practice from the late 1980s. In addition, many organizations that provide services have adopted person-centered language without any substantive change in practice. Public policy makers need to confront systems in which plans are created to meet compliance requirements rather than to serve as road maps for people's futures. On a similar note, policy makers commonly face a culture in which

- Good plans on paper are considered more important than good lives

- Blame rather than accountability is prevalent, so responsibility is avoided and creative ideas that fail result in punishment

- Those who spend the most time with the focus person are consulted the least, and their input is not recorded

- Organization administrators increasingly operate in a chronic state of crisis as they try to cope with the stresses of high staff turnover, difficulties in recruiting qualified applicants, and other challenges of organizational business; thus, temporary solutions are permanent and having time to think is a luxury

Another obstacle pertains to service/support coordinators who are required to develop plans and to ensure plan implementation. They typically work with large numbers of people and face frequent personnel changes. When these factors are combined with paperwork requirements, service/support coordinators simply do not have the time to develop good person-centered plans. Furthermore, their distress over time limitations and low pay results in a high turnover rate. This means that it is not possible to create the trust that arises from relationships built over time.

In fact, increasing turnover within service providing agencies has spread to all but the most senior levels of staff. At the same time, educational levels for direct support staff are falling, as is the percentage of staff who are internally motivated. Increasing numbers of immigrants are being recruited into direct support roles and are particularly challenged to help people with disabilities become part of communities to which the immigrant workers are not yet well connected themselves and which they are seeking to understand. All of management's time is spent on recruitment of staff, retention of staff, and compliance to rules. Managers say that they do not have time to do more than ensure that plans guard health and safety.

An additional obstacle to implementing person-centered policies involves those who license and inspect service providers. These individuals often seek compliance with old and new paradigms simultaneously and unintentionally reinforce the blame culture. Person-centered planning also is not typically seen as a skill or a competency. The result is plans that have person-centered labels but lack person-centered content.

Strategy for Change

The opportunities will be seized and the obstacles will be addressed only within a comprehensive strategy for change. Those who develop public policy need to recognize three things that must be dealt with simultaneously. As shown in Figure 17.1, policy makers must work not only to establish best practice but also to push incremental changes in typical practice and to create positive pressure for change. Those who are attempting to lead systems change often forget that successful examples of best practice are typically created by people who have a passion for what they are doing. Such passion allows them to overcome any and all obstacles. Those who follow are generally caring but do not have the same passion. As Fritz (1999) noted, those who come later tend to follow the "path of least resistance" in trying to change practices. Making incremental change is even more challenging because of the unfortunate tendency of those who engage in best practice to have their justifiable pride turn into elitism. In too many places,

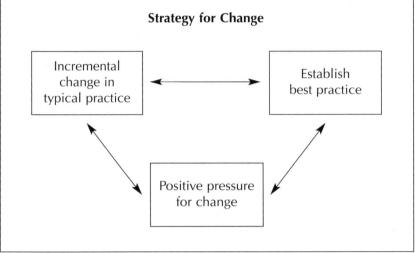

Source: Smull & Allen (2001b); Copyright 2002 Smull & Allen.

Figure 17.1. Ways for policy makers to create positive pressure for change.

people who are making incremental changes get little credit. It seems that in those places, people's work is considered either best practice or worthless.

Nonetheless, neither creating best practice models nor supporting incremental change is sufficient. The organizational change literature clearly shows that change requires pressure (Kanter, Stein, & Jick, 1992; Kotter, 1996). The pressure created by simply requiring person-centered planning changes plans; those plans affect lives but do not appear to create the level of change desired. Positive pressure for pervasive substantive change will come in part when those who inspect plans are as skilled as those who teach planning. More pressure for large-scale change will come from teaching those who use the services and their families how to develop plans and implement them. As is shown in Figure 17.2 this first requires teaching individuals and families how to develop a basic plan that describes what is important to and what is important for the focus person and the balance between them. Then, those leading the planning (i.e., the focus person and/or his or her family) must be able to explore what is conceivable (including what has happened in other places, not just locally) and decide on the best option. Finally, they need sufficient control over the available public resources and assistance in navigating the system to make it happen.

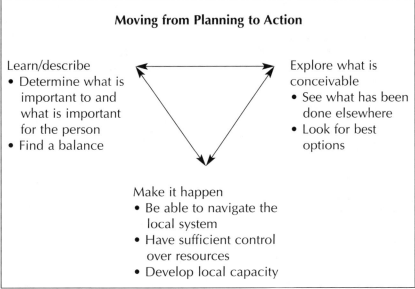

Moving from Planning to Action

Learn/describe
• Determine what is important to and what is important for the person
• Find a balance

Explore what is conceivable
• See what has been done elsewhere
• Look for best options

Make it happen
• Be able to navigate the local system
• Have sufficient control over resources
• Develop local capacity

Source: Smull & Allen (2001a); Copyright 2002 Smull & Allen.

Figure 17.2. Ways to move from planning to action.

Public Policy's Role

There are a number of ways in which public policy makers can address inadequacies in present policy to achieve better outcomes. The approaches generally reflect different levels of certainty (not necessarily justified certainty) that the decision will promote the welfare of the targeted individuals and/or society. An overarching need exists for a coherent set of policies that help create win-win situations. For example, part of creating positive pressure for change is showing those who provide services how person-centered practices will contribute to solving critical problems such as reducing turnover among direct support staff. Public policy makers also need to keep in mind that senior management of organizations providing services has finite time to devote to any effort and that a series of disconnected requirements results in fragmented compliance efforts. Those mandating the efforts must see the change as being analogous to weaving a new cloth, with each effort being a thread. Within this analogy, those directing the efforts need to give instructions on weaving or the result will be a pile of disconnected threads.

While keeping an eye on "the whole cloth," those in positions of authority need to remember what public policy can accomplish and what it should avoid. There are four ways that policy can change practice. First, it can require actions to be taken, which then make change occur. Second, it can pay for actions to happen. Third, it can promote certain actions or values. Fourth, it can reduce and/or remove barriers to change. Each factor is discussed in the following subsections.

Require Actions to Be Taken   Public policy can seek better outcomes by requiring people to perform in specified ways. The argument for requiring someone to do things in a certain way is strongest when the consequences of not doing so are substantially detrimental to the individual receiving services and/or when the evidence that doing things in a certain ways has significant benefit. Licensing standards are an example of requiring actions to be taken. Depending on the standards, service providers may have to respect certain rights, provide certain amounts and quality of living space and food, ensure certain aspects of a safe physical environment, and undertake certain professional practices if they are to be allowed to serve people with developmental disabilities. Requiring particular things to happen through policy obviously necessitates a basis of substantial conviction that those things will benefit people. The dangers of changing public policy without evidence of likely success are reduced when 1) the policy poses little risk, 2) the policy being replaced is supported by little evidence of benefit, and 3) the policy change is accompanied by an effort to gather information to substantiate its effectiveness.

With regard to such conditions, participation in person-centered planning poses few risks to people with developmental disabilities. The primary risks appear to be wasted time and unfulfilled expectations, deriving from planning sessions that define more desirable futures but accomplish little in achieving them. As for the possibility that requiring person-centered planning would replace other effective approaches to planning, the limited available research suggests relatively little cause for concern. A set of studies focused on the content of traditional IPPs and their association with people's lives and skills. These studies found no relationship between people's IPPs and relative engagement in activities at home and in the community or accomplishment of real-life habilitative outcomes (Stancliffe et al., 1999a, 1999b, 2000). As of 2002, "The vast majority of states are requiring planning that reflects the values and principles of person-centered planning in their home and community-based waivers and/or in regulation. It is the norm" (R. Cooper, personal communication, January 4, 2002). Although there is little evidence that these requirements will deprive people of otherwise effective planning programs, failing to evaluate the effects of policies that require person-centered planning is unacceptable.

Given these caveats and the possibility that person-centered planning is or will be required, what else must be addressed? The following suggestions are not rooted in research, but they are based on what we have seen and heard in our travels across the United States in conducting training and evaluations.

First, those who are paid to develop and/or review person-centered plans should have the necessary skills. Developing person-centered plans has been seen as something that anyone with good intentions can do by attending overview training, watching a video, and/or reading a few example plans. Each person-centered planning process has a set of embedded skills, and each requires training and structured practice for the practitioner to become skilled. When person-centered planning was conducted either outside or on the fringes of the system, it made sense to exclude the system from determining the necessary skills for planners. If good plans are to be created inside the system, then competencies must be met. People should learn not only what a good plan looks like but also how a good development process is more important to implementation than the format. Planners need to know that good process goes far beyond simply asking the person with whom they are planning who should be present when the plan is developed. Inspectors must be able to determine whether the plan's content and process make sense for the focus person.

Second, person-centered plans that are used to direct the paid services that people receive must have a required minimum content. An example of such requirements would be that plans address the following seven questions:

1. **What is important to the person?** What is important to the focus person only includes what the person expresses with words or behavior.

2. **What is important for the person?** What others believe is important for the focus person includes issues of health and safety. It also includes things that others who know the individual well believe will contribute to his or her being a valued community member.

3. **Is what is important for the person addressed in the context of what is important to the person?** Many problems in dealing with health and safety issues stem from treating the issues as if they have no context. When what is important to a person is largely ignored, it is more difficult to have that person's support in addressing what is important for him or her.

4. **Is there a good balance between what is important to the person and what is important for the person?** The balance between what is important to a person and what is important for that person is determined individually. What is important to each person influences how that person copes with what is important for him or her.

Conversely, changes in what is important for each person often alter part of what is important to him or her. The balance between them is shifting and interactive and only becomes a problem for a person (or for those who love the person) when there is an unresolved conflict between what is important to that person and what is important for him or her. The challenge for those who are making (or influencing) decisions on behalf of people who use disabilities services is to recognize that this is just as true for these individuals as it is for people without disabilities. In seeking this balance, those family and support team members should start by looking at what is important to the focus person.

5. **What does the person want to learn, and what else do those who are planning learn about the person?** Helping the focus person acquire new skills has the same issues of context. Rather than simply helping the person acquire the next skill in a hierarchy, planners should consider what the focus person needs to learn to help him or her achieve lifestyle goals. In addition, planners are never finished learning about a focus person's preferences and support needs. Planners should be able to say what they do not know, what they are seeking to learn, and/or what they need to learn.

6. **What needs to stay the same, to be maintained or enhanced?** Planners need to look for those things that are working, as well as those things that are not working, within the focus person's life. Planners need to do this so that while helping the focus person make a change in one area, there will not be an unintended loss in another area. They need to determine whether there are areas in which what is working can be built on and enhanced. Planners also need to ensure that those who are providing the support get credit for what is going well while they look at what needs to change.

7. **What needs to change?** Plans that help people move toward lives that they want and reflect a balance between what is important to and what is important for them should have goals and actions that address needed changes. Two ways to consider needed changes involve answering these additional questions: What does the focus person and those who support him or her need to do to maintain or enhance what is working? Given differences between how the person lives and how the person wants to live, as well as what else the person wants to learn (or planners need to learn), what should happen to create needed change?

A third action that public policy can require is paperwork reduction. There is a natural tendency to add any planning or other documentation requirements to those that already exist. Those who plan and those who document what is happening report spending disproportionate amounts of time on paperwork. As new documentation requirements are added, the time that is spent on paperwork must not increase. Note that the volume of paperwork is not the issue but, rather, the time spent completing it—especially the time that doing so takes away from time with people who use services. Every effort should be made to reduce these time requirements to a minimum.

Fourth, if plans are to be implemented, then focus individuals (or their representatives) need sufficient control over the public resources that allow changes in which services are received and who provides them. Yet, simply giving people control over resources is not sufficient. This leads to the fifth and final change that public policy should require: People must be able to describe how they want to live before they are asked where they want to live. They need to make informed choices about desired services and delivery agents. People using services and their families have to be supported as leaders in developing their own plans.

Pay for Actions to Happen One way to get people to take desired actions is to create financial incentives for doing so. Financial incentives are economic benefits that are experienced by individuals or organizations in return for defined actions or outcomes. Payments for actions are instituted because of an assumption that the action is related to desired outcomes. Because a consistent relationship between service actions and individual outcomes is lacking, many policy advocates argue that policies focused on paying for things to happen should emphasize ultimate outcomes, not the practices (e.g., person-centered planning) that are assumed to help achieve those outcomes. In such incentive systems, however, person-centered planning would be a tool to assist in achieving the paid-for outcome. Whether person-centered planning in general or in one of its varieties contributed to achieving such outcomes would dictate its continued use.

This chapter asserts that consistent funding in a few key areas could make substantial differences in outcomes. First, support the training for plan writers to achieve competence in whichever planning format they use. Second, support the training of self-advocates and family members in learning how to write plans with others. Third, reimburse plan development regardless of who (other than the focus person or a close relative) developed them. This assumes that there are criteria for acceptable plans. Part of this suggestion's intent is to ensure that self-advocates and family members are able to spend the time needed to help others in developing plans. Fourth, provide funding for the technical assistance necessary to change practices within organizations. Efforts at helping organizations change their practices and structures—from offering programs to providing support—have shown that assistance is typically needed in changing not just the policies but also the underlying structures and organizational culture (Gardner & Nudler, 1999). Fifth and finally, support the training of frontline managers so that they can be good managers. Buckingham and Coffman's research showed that "it is her relationship with her immediate manager that will determine *how long she stays* and *how productive* she is while she is there" (1999, p. 36). Paying attention to the skills of managers can reduce turnover and increase the implementation of the person-centered plans.

Promote Certain Actions or Things   Another way to get people to take desired actions is to promote those actions as being desirable and preferred—as being best practice and what good organizations routinely do. Given the limited empirical evidence that person-centered planning itself yields results that are consistently better for people with developmental disabilities, policy makers might feel justifiably reluctant to demand the use of person-centered planning approaches. They may, however, feel more justified in promoting practices such as reflecting an orientation and searching for ways to realize desired social outcomes. Promoting ways of doing things can include providing 1) forums for training; 2) infrastructures for ongoing technical assistance; and 3) sources of informational support—whether in written, video, CD-ROM, Internet, or other formats—to make the approach easily, widely, and skillfully adopted. In addition to promoting the training of person-centered planning facilitators, policy makers may establish a network for ongoing communication and information sharing among facilitators to sustain and refine the collective skills and enhance planning capacity. Person-centered planning practices can be supported by informing consumers of such practices as well as their purposes and their availability. In short, policies that promote rather than require certain approaches or related outcomes can have a substantial influence on common practice. Equally important, promotion of practices can avoid the frequent outcome of requirements that establish legally compliant but less-than-effective applications.

Remove Barriers to Change   There are substantial disincentives to using person-centered planning approaches. Policies that are instituted to make person-centered planning approaches available can reduce these disincentives. One disincentive is that person-centered planning must take place when key people in a person's life are available to come together. Unlike traditional planning, which is dominated by professionals, person-centered planning is dominated by friends, family members, and neighbors. Thus, accommodations must be met for planning that takes place in different times, ways, and places. This sometimes involves funding for food, transportation, child care, and so forth because participants have other work, community, and family commitments that must be accommodated. In turn, this factor may require the allocation of staff support to help focus individuals pick those who they want to come to their meetings and then to help the selected people attend the meeting. It may involve flexibility to pay facilitators who have special skills but may not have the formal professional degrees of people traditionally involved in interdisciplinary assessment and planning and for whom payment is easily processed. The flexible availability of people, services, and other resources is an important way to remove disincentives to person-centered planning. Regardless of the efforts to accommodate the selected people's schedules, some will not be able to attend the meetings. In these instances, support must be offered to make sure that the person's input is still represented.

Two other disincentives must be addressed. People across the United States with whom we talk commonly cite as barriers to person-centered planning the lack of time needed to do it well and the paperwork burden involved. If these disincentives are to be removed, then roles will have to redefined and practices changed. Those who have been given the task of writing plans need to see themselves as coaches and mentors first. They help the focus person (and those closest to him or her) to develop the plan. In addition, they look for time-efficient ways to do this. Planners need to 1) support others in developing plans; 2) view planning as a partnership; and 3) consider their first role quality assurance, not plan writing. Only when there are no other resources do they write the plan. Once a good first plan has been written, these people should support its ongoing development rather than create a new plan annually. Those who oversee the planners need to ruthlessly eliminate paperwork. It is too easy to add just one more form, and it is difficult to get rid of the old forms.

CONCLUSION

Public policy makers appear to have already decided that person-centered planning is required to improve the lives of people with disabilities. Their present task is to ensure that plans represent the focus person and are implemented. They need to take the steps necessary to make plans reflect what is important to the person. In addition, policy makers need to describe what others need to know or do to have a reasonable balance among competing pressures such as the focus person's happiness, safety, and health; the focus person's preferences and what others want for the person; and the focus person's preferences and available public resources.

Policy makers must also require plans that provide a framework for continuous cycles of learning, acting, and reflecting while meeting all of the requirements for continued funding. They must also realize that plans do not create outcomes and are not self-implementing. A mediocre plan that is well implemented is better than a great plan that is ignored. Furthermore, policy makers must recognize that people want lives—knowing that specific, acknowledged processes were engaged in will not satisfy them. In fact, good person-centered plans increase expectations and bring to awareness what should be reality. Failure to act on them causes disappointment, reinforces cynicism, and destroys trust in the system that is supposed to support and protect.

Consequently, the larger challenge is to provide the leadership and structures needed to emphasize helping people achieve the lives that they want within their communities rather than to emphasize producing better plans. To do this, public policy makers need to remember that although what is required matters greatly, creating positive pressure for change matters even more. Finally, they need to keep in mind much is still unknown about policy making for person-centered planning. Much of what we recommend in this chapter is based on our experiences and remains untested in large-scale application. Those who are ultimately successful in implementing public policy on person-centered planning will be those who continue to learn and act on what is learned.

REFERENCES

Buckingham, M., & Coffman, C. (1999). *First break all the rules: What the world's greatest managers do differently.* New York: Simon & Schuster.

DePaepe, P., Reichle, J., Doss, S., Shriner, C., & Cameron, J. (1994). A preliminary evaluation of written individualized habilitation objectives and their correspondence with direct implementation. *Journal of The Association for Persons with Severe Handicaps, 19*, 94–104.

Felce, D., deKock, U., Mansell, J., & Jenkins, J. (1984). Providing systematic individual teaching for severely disturbed and profoundly mentally handicapped adults in residential care. *Behavior, Research and Therapy, 22*, 229–309.

Fleming, I., & Stenfert-Kroese, B. (1990). Evaluation of a community care project for people with learning difficulties. *Journal of Mental Deficiency Research, 34*, 451–464.

Fritz, R. (1999). *The path of least resistance for managers: Designing organizations to succeed.* San Francisco: Berrett-Koehler.

Gardner, J.F., & Nudler, S. (Eds.). (1999). *Quality and performance in human services: Leadership, values, and vision.* Baltimore: Paul H. Brookes Publishing Co.

Health Care Financing Administration. (1974). Medicaid program: Conditions for intermediate care facilities for the mentally retarded: Final rule (42 CFR 405.1009).

Kanter, R., Stein, B., & Jick, T. (1992). *The challenge of organizational change: How companies experience it and leaders guide it.* New York: The Free Press.

Kiernan, W.E., & Stark, J.A. (Eds.). (1986). *Pathways to employment for adults with developmental disabilities.* Baltimore: Paul H. Brookes Publishing Co.

Kotter, J. (1996). *Leading change.* Boston: Harvard Business School Press.

Legal Advocacy for Persons with Developmental Disabilities. (1989). *Individual habilitation plan review.* Minneapolis: Minnesota Disability Law Center.

McCandless, B., & Evans, E. (1973). *Children and youth: Psychosocial development.* Fort Worth, TX: The Dryden Press.

Mount, B. (1987). *Personal futures planning: Finding directions for change* (Doctoral dissertation, University of Georgia). Ann Arbor: University of Michigan Dissertation Information Service.

Smull, M., & Allen, W. (2001a). *Families planning together: An introduction.* Workshop and slide show.

Smull, M., & Allen, W. (2001b). *Going from programs to supports: Why organizational change is so damned hard.* Workshop and slide show.

Stancliffe, R.J., Hayden, M.F., & Lakin, K.C. (1999a). Effectiveness and quality of individual planning in residential settings: An analysis of outcomes. *Mental Retardation, 37*(2), 104–116.

Stancliffe, R.J., Hayden, M.F., & Lakin, K.C. (1999b). Effectiveness of challenging behavior IHP objectives in residential settings: A longitudinal study. *Mental Retardation, 37*(6), 482–493.

Stancliffe, R.J., Hayden, M.F., & Lakin, K.C. (2000). Quality and content of individualized habilitation plan objectives in residential settings. *Education and Training in Mental Retardation, 35*(2), 191–207.

Sturmey, P. (1992). Goal planning for adults with mental handicap: Outcome research, staff training and management. *Mental Handicap Research, 5,* 92–108.

Wehman, P., & Moon, M.S. (Eds.). (1988). *Vocational rehabilitation and supported employment.* Baltimore: Paul H. Brookes Publishing Co.

18

Numbers and Faces

The Ethics of Person-Centered Planning

John O'Brien

> *The Kingdom of Number is all boundaries*
> *Which may be beautiful and must be true;*
> *To ask if it is big or small proclaims one*
> *The sort of lover who should stick to faces . . .*
> *—W.H. Auden*

Many of the chapters in this book come from what Auden called "the Kingdom of Number" in the first line of his poem "Numbers and Faces" (1991, p. 623). These chapters aspire to a scientific answer to the question, "Does person-centered planning work?" The residents of the Kingdom of Number are properly concerned to define person-centered planning within quantitatively measurable boundaries and to calculate whether treatment effects are quantitatively big enough to establish its validity. What interests me about person-centered planning proclaims me a student of faces, privileged by the editors to reflect on this book from the perspective of one who does not work in the Kingdom of Number. I have read this book to find some of the stories it tells about the ethical decisions that challenge practitioners of person-centered planning and have thought about how practitioners might respond to these challenges as well. In pursuing my inquiry, I have borrowed Auden's notion of asking whether some matter "is big or small" in human terms because I think that practitioners of person-centered

Preparation of this chapter was partially supported through a subcontract to Responsive Systems Associates from the Center on Human Policy, Syracuse University for the Research and Training Center on Community Living. The Research and Training Center on Community Living is supported through a cooperative agreement (No. H133B980047) between the National Institute on Disability and Rehabilitation Research (NIDRR) and the University of Minnesota Institute on Community Integration. Members of the Center are encouraged to express their opinions; these do not necessarily represent the official position of NIDRR.

planning face many decisions about whether some aspect of a person's life is big enough to demand action or small enough to ignore.

Person-centered planning challenges the ethics of its practitioners because it creates a context for the kind of listening that invites engagement in another person's life. Ethical challenges also arise when listening to a person with a developmental disability puts a human face on a contradiction between a service's espoused values and its actual performance. Listening reveals personal interests. Meeting such interests fits the system's stated commitment to values of individualization, self-determination, and inclusion; however, the system's attempts at action may reveal a considerable lag in its capacity to respond. Ethical challenges take the form of deciding whether a contradiction is big enough to call for action or small enough for the practitioner to pass by without active concern. The ethical challenges deepen with recognition of the power difference between the practitioner and the person to whom he or she listens. The person with a developmental disability has little chance of favorably resolving the contradiction without mobilized allies who will act with him or her. The practitioner can easily walk away from this person's situation after completing the meeting and its related paperwork.

In Chapter 13, noting that Hal liked soft music and disliked noisy situations and being around lots of people put a face on commitment to individualized supports. Are the discoveries big or small in the following description of Hal's living area?

> Loud, open, austere . . . yelling and running is [sic] common . . . appears chaotic with staff looking exhausted, exasperated . . . dorm-like bedroom shared with two other people, one hits Hal frequently; no obvious personal possessions.

Those involved in person-centered planning for Hal treated the conflict between his interests and his living arrangements as big enough to call for immediate action. Short-term changes hugely improved his institutional living conditions, and he later moved into a home with features and routines designed specifically for him.

Chapter 10 (see also Becker, Dumas, Houser, & Seay, 2000) puts listening in the context of discovering people's lifestyle preferences. Listening to Scott, a 52-year-old with minimal support needs, identify the goal of moving from his parents' house into his own apartment put a face on an agency's verbal commitment to enhance self-determination. Is it big or small that after a year, he was still waiting for his service coordinator to act and had no idea of why no progress toward his move had been made? Johnny was a 35-year-old who had lived in an institution. Listening to his pride in his apartment explained why having a vacuum cleaner to keep his place clean was highly desirable to him; this put a face on an agency's verbal commitment to assist people to live in ways that make sense to them. Is it big or small that getting a vacuum cleaner took 9 months and that the agency had difficulty supplying replacement bags? Helen, a 42-year-old with infrequent support needs, identified a love for animals and a strong preference for working in a pet store. Listening to her preferences put a face on an agency's verbal commitment to serve people in a person-centered way. Is it big or small that Helen was placed in a janitorial job at the provider agency that agreed help her get a job working with animals? These agencies chose to participate in a nationally funded demonstration of self-determination, but the service coordinators apparently decided that the identified preferences were small things. It was not worth collaborating with the people involved to find creative ways to orchestrate Scott's move from his parents' home, to ensure that Johnny had a functioning vacuum cleaner, or to assist Helen in getting a job at a pet store.

Chapter 9 describes a process to support people moving out of congregate facilities to specify preferences and to use these preferences to guide their selection of a group home. More than 60% of the people moving wanted a job with pay, which highlights the intention to empower people. Is it big or small to discover that only one of the available placements had paid community jobs open to residents and that at nearly half of the available facilities even segregated work for pay was out of the question? Helping people obtain paying jobs was apparently outside the scope of the preference assessment, as was the choice of any living option other than traditional supervised group living. These system-imposed boundaries defined some big personal preferences as small and, thus, irrelevant.

RESPONSIBILITY OF PERSON-CENTERED PLANNERS

Practitioners of person-centered planning do not cause contradictions between service values and service capacities; they encounter these contradictions in the lives and futures of the people with whom they choose to plan. They did not cause and cannot single-handedly dissolve the service realities that inhibit people from moving toward the lives they want. In services that require person-centered plans for everyone, practitioners may experience a contradiction between an attractive value (discovering and honoring people's preferences) and the pressures of their work.

It is not fair to blame practitioners of person-centered planning for contradictions between service values and service capacities. It is not fair for service managers to mindlessly assign accountability for person-centered outcomes to practitioners without accepting responsibility for necessary changes in their organization's structure and culture. Yet, what is at stake is not blame or organizational accountability but personal responsibility. Practitioners of person-centered planning who accept responsibility for living in the tension between service values and service capacity support the development of more competent services. Those who shy away from living with the tension become part of the barrier separating people with developmental disabilities from inclusion and self-determination.

Person-centered planning contributes to developing service capacity when its practitioners mobilize people to do the hard, sustained, creative work necessary for a service organization to live up to its commitments to human development, inclusion, and self-determination. People are mobilized when they take responsibility for the tension between what they want—such as actively and competently supporting Helen to work in a pet store—and their current reality—a service that places people in jobs it already has rather than develop jobs around people's interests. Those who can hold the tension between their values and current activities are more likely to find creative ways to resolve it than people who walk away from the tension by scaling down what they want to match what they can do—such as placing Helen in an existing job. (To learn more about this perspective on organizational change, see Chapter 9 of Senge, 1990, and visit the Society for Organizational Learning at http://www.sol-ne.org.)

Practitioners who blame themselves for the contradictions that person-centered planning reveals between espoused values and current service performance are auditioning for martyrdom. Practitioners who want to mobilize action to resolve a contradiction begin by accepting responsibility for that contradiction as it affects the life of the person with whom they plan. Living up to that responsibility does not mean a single-handed, heroic effort to give the person whatever he wants; it means enlisting as many people as possible, beginning with the person himself and those who know and care about him, and supporting them to work together for positive change.

The group work that is particular to person-centered planning, the work that practitioners are responsible for skillfully facilitating, comprises four tasks and upholds an animating spirit. The first task is for a person and his or her allies to align around a common understanding of what is desirable for the person now and in the future. The second task is to generate creative actions that will immediately and over time realize more of what is desirable for the person. The third task is to support the person and his or her allies to negotiate for the accommodations, technology aids, services, supports, and funds required to realize more of what is desirable for him or her. The fourth task is to sustain focus on the person by supporting the person and his or her allies to deepen their understanding of what is desirable and to adapt their actions by reflecting on what they are doing. The spirit that animates effective person-centered planning calls on people to resist low expectations and social discrimination by imagining alternative ways that the person can express his or her particular capacities in the community.

A practitioner's skill in guiding people through the person-centered planning process influences his or her contribution to an organization's capacity to offer support consistent with its values. Yet, skill is not everything. A practitioner must decide that what matters to the focus person is important enough for the practitioner to accept responsibility for contradictions between service values and service capacity. There is one constructive way to decline responsibility for service contradictions: discovering a way that the person can realize at least some aspects of a desirable future outside of services. For example, person-centered planning allowed some people with developmental disabilities and their families to find jobs or leisure connections that fit their interests through their own social networks (Lyle O'Brien, Mount, O'Brien, & Rosen, in press).

There are many easy ways to resign from making a necessary change. Bandura and Barbaranelli (1996) inventoried mechanisms through which people disengage from moral responsibility. Thoughtful practitioners of person-centered planning will check themselves regularly for these five symptoms of ethical disengagement:

1. Disregarding consequences (e.g., "I have completed person-centered plans for my whole caseload but have not had time to discover the outcomes")

2. Making advantageous comparisons to worse practice (e.g., "Not much has happened for people, but the person-centered planning meetings we have now are much better than the individualized program planning meetings that we used to have")

3. Displacing responsibility (e.g., "The administration gave me a workload that makes it impossible for me to build relationships with the people I'm supposed to make plans for—what can you do?")

4. Diffusing responsibility (e.g., "I did my part—I facilitated the planning meeting and mailed out the minutes; implementation isn't in my job description")

5. Attributing blame (e.g., "Those parents make unrealistic demands—who would ever want to hire their daughter?")

Listening sufficiently to consider a person's desires reasonable and legitimate creates ethical conflicts when a service lacks the capacity to support the person's pursuit of those desires. It is understandable that disengagement will show up in people's thinking. Conducting person-centered planning requires noticing these maneuvers for what they are—a signal that something ethically important is at stake and at risk of being ignored—and then refocusing with the person to imagine and take a hopeful next step. Such steps only show themselves when practitioners of person-centered planning decide to work to discover them.

USES AND LIMITS OF NUMBERS

Numbers, as the products of well-designed studies or the tracks of a carefully designed schedule, may be beautiful and true. Nonetheless, they offer only limited guidance to a practitioner of person-centered planning who is deciding whether something is big enough to demand action or small enough to excuse absence. There is no adequate moral equation based on numerical inputs. The ethical decisions that determine whether person-centered planning keeps moving or stops are better understood in Taylor's terms:

> Much contemporary moral philosophy . . . has given such a narrow focus to morality that some critical connections are incomprehensible in its terms. This moral philosophy has tended to focus on what is right to do rather than on what it is good to be, on defining the content of obligation rather than the nature of good life; and has no conceptual place left for a notion of the good as the object of our love or allegiance or as the privileged focus of attention or will. (1989, p. 3)

Given the social and political realities in 2002, practitioners of person-centered planning should personally consider the following if they want inclusive communities where people with disabilities are free to exercise their human rights:

- The kind of people that it is good for them to strive to be
- The kind of relationships that they want to create
- The nature of the community that they want to foster

Although numbers do not help much with these ethical decisions, numbers are not unimportant. For those who choose to be influenced by them, numbers can indicate more or less fruitful ways to assist people. For example, Mank, Cioffi, and Yovanoff (2000) reported that people with severe disabilities in supported employment have higher wage levels and greater workplace integration when they experience typical employment conditions with the minimum necessary accommodation and assistance than they do when a supported employment program routinely creates special conditions in their hiring, job training, and workplace routines. This finding is important to practitioners who respond to people's desire for a particular real job. It is less salient to those who decide that the desire for a particular real job is a small thing that can be ignored. When the culture of a service supports their use, numbers can structure routines to ensure active support for people with disabilities to engage in everyday opportunities (see Chapter 11). Depending on the values that a service culture serves, however, numbers can also structure routines that promote staff behaviors with undesirable consequences. In the culture of habilitation described in Chapter 4, data collection, systematic scheduling, and a token economy created a setting in which people were denied control over many aspects of their lives and little regard was given to their values, preferences, and desires. The desire and skill to use numbers well can steer an intervention toward an important improvement in a person's life, as Holburn and Vietze described in their account of assisting Hal to stop hitting his mother (see Chapter 13). Numbers can also steer interventions that have little relevance to durable and meaningful life changes. Carr, Horner, and Turnbull (1999) reviewed a database of 109 published studies of positive behavioral support and found that

> Consumers . . . judge interventions in terms of their practicality and relevance and are concerned with how well intervention plans mesh with the realities of the complex social systems in which the consumers must function. The database [i.e., the 109 studies], more concerned with issues of rigor and demonstrations of experimental control, generally failed to focus on larger consumer goals. (p. 83)

Hal's story exemplifies a search for the relevance Carr and colleagues (1999) reported missing. Hal mattered as a person to the five members of his core team, who accompanied him on his 4-year journey from institutional to community life. They engaged more than 50 people in one or more of the 34 formal person-centered planning meetings they held to construct, remember, and revise a common understanding of Hal as a whole person and to make decisions in light of this understanding. They made the most of Hal's position—one of the last Willowbrook class members to move from an institution—to make more flexible a huge service system that was ill equipped for individualized supports. They learned with Hal by spending time doing new things alongside him, beginning with a risky walk around the block, and by offering him new opportunities, such as improved living conditions, stable connections to staff whom he liked, a routine that made sense to Hal, and support to experience his community. The team members used their personal contacts with system administrators and service providers to move services toward support for their vision of a desirable future for Hal. They made hard decisions, balancing the immediate availability of services that did not fit their shared understanding of Hal as a whole person against the time it took to develop better alternatives. Over and over, through difficulties and uncertainties, the team members continued to demonstrate fidelity to Hal. In this context, they deployed a systematic behavioral intervention that not only decreased Hal's hitting his mother but also shifted his parents' expectations of and for him. In this context, the team carried out person-centered planning.

Hal's story can be understood as an example of the systematic application of scientifically established laws of behavior (see Chapter 12). Environmental changes exposed Hal to fewer aversive events and provided him with ready access to reinforcers; thus, his challenging behavior decreased. Person-centered planning thereby provided an effective way to identify the aversive events and reinforcers. Yet, another reading of this situation is that people with the ability and willingness to act with Hal found a new way to see Hal's face. Then, they faithfully and persistently challenged what was assumed about Hal and his relationship to the system that served him until the settings and relationships that held Hal were transformed. The members of Hal's team were committed to changing things that others deemed impossible to change. Person-centered planning provided them with one way to focus and guide their efforts. Both of these readings risk reductionism, a bit like saying that *War and Peace* proves the folly of invading a big country during a difficult winter. Each may be true in some sense, but both offer too thin of an account to motivate and guide wise and positive action.

Resisting the temptation to oversimplify forms the foundation of understanding how person-centered planning contributes to better lives. Hal's father summarized a complex experience: "Person-centered planning is the Liquid-Plumr of DD [developmental disabilities]!" The meetings, graphic profiles, and vision statements that identify person-centered planning and are easily replicated would not have freed the service system's many clogs without the other elements of the story.

Holburn, Jacobson, Vietze, and Sersen (2000) developed a useful instrument as part of an ongoing research program to test the effects of person-centered planning on outcomes. The instrument enumerates 12 process factors believed to be associated with positive outcomes in person-centered planning, and it provides a way to count their presence or absence. It is instructive to map Hal's story onto an instrument that assesses such factors. However, any magic in person-centered planning is in people's relationships. Not even a carefully defined list captures the vitality of people working together out of commitment to a particular person to resolve the contradictions between a system's espoused values and its capacities. Process scales are more like a handbook of rhetorical devices than they are like Burton Blatt's "Family Secrets" (1977), the Presidential Address to the 100th anniversary convention of the American Association on Mental Deficiency. This powerful speech can be analyzed in rhetorical terms, but analysis cannot capture Blatt's passionate delivery or the speech's impact. As important as numbers may be, there is no adequate way to understand human action without story.

STORY AS A WAY OF KNOWING AND ORGANIZING

Brunner (1986) identified two distinct cognitive resources—complementary but not reducible to each other—that contribute to human knowing. The scientific mode of knowing proceeds logically to make empirical discoveries guided by reasoned hypotheses. The narrative mode of knowing seeks to disclose meaning in experience by creating and interpreting stories that trace the course of human purposes.

Some contributors to this book, perhaps because they define disability from a clinical perspective that suits their role in responding to difficult and dangerous behavior, seem to consider person-centered planning an instrument for scientific knowing and a fit object for scientific study. This legitimate way of knowing forms and tries to answer a question such as "Does offering people scheduled access to the preferred activities identified through person-centered planning decrease the incidence of problem behaviors?" (see Chapter 14) to contribute evidence to answer the question that interests the editors: "Does person-centered planning work?" Such questions classify person-centered planning as a form of clinical assessment or intervention and look for ways to isolate and test its effectiveness.

This structured and analytic form of inquiry sets aside some potentially important questions. As discussed in Chapter 14, Carl liked to vacuum his room, but offering him access to this activity actually increased problem behaviors. Did this empirical finding mean that Carl should no longer be allowed to vacuum his room? No, this finding led from science to story. It turned out that Carl got frustrated when he had difficulty operating the vacuum cleaner and when his teacher signaled him to stop. These facts indicated a need to review and revise the functional analysis of Carl's difficult behavior.

The reported story of Carl and his vacuum stops here. Yet, its incompleteness begs for resolution, so I speculatively provide it: Realizing that Carl hits or attempts property destruction more often when he is doing something that he prefers may open the way for systematically instructing Carl how to use the vacuum cleaner and how to judge when the task is finished. I supply this happy ending knowing that this agency gathers annually in the person's favorite restaurant to celebrate his accomplishments and to acknowledge his strengths before considering the possibilities generated by an assessment titled "And Here's What I Want." I also like that the authors call the commitments to action made at this meeting "promises." This is a great idea for guiding their organizational efforts to be accountable to the people whom they support.

For me and some other practitioners and students of person-centered planning, person-centered planning is best understood as an expression of the narrative mode. It is about composing and enacting good stories. These stories are not fictions; if invited, we could visit Hal at home. These stories are not "happily ever after"; it is reasonable to assume that Hal's life since establishing a stable community home has had its ups and downs. Yet, Hal's having a home matched to him had to be imagined as a story before it could be lived as a reality. The idea that a scientific instrument could predict the particular features that would make Hal comfortable and secure at home is as silly as the notion of a meter to measure his happiness.

Theorists of narrative (Tracy, 1986) draw attention to two features of stories like Hal's: they are 1) acts of resistance and 2) constructed through an interpretive process. The system that served Hal had no budget for a person to assist him in exploring and participating in his community, but Hal got an assistant because his person-centered planning team resisted the assumption that the system could not adapt to Hal. The team imagined and then negotiated payment for a community bridge builder, who was selected by Hal's parents and paid through a voucher signed by Hal's parents. Imagination can involve borrowing. The idea of community bridge builders did not originate with Hal's person-centered planning team; the team imagined that their enormous and complex system would make this highly individualized support available to Hal and his parents. The community bridge builder experience gave Hal's parents another reason to believe that Hal could be safe on their community's streets, which raised their expectations for Hal.

Like all good practitioners of person-centered planning, Hal's team members worked through many turns of an interpretive circle. Their thinking moved from a best attempt to express their understanding of Hal as a whole person to action to improve important particulars of his life and back again. Their vision of Hal as a participating community member, broad and somewhat tentative at first, provided a sufficient context to imagine and create a way for him to experience community. Their shared understanding of his responses to community life led them to a richer, better grounded picture of Hal as a whole person, which in turn helped them better understand the specifics of his life. The team members built a common understanding strong enough to create person-centered planning that could be described as "the Liquid-Plumr of DD."

REALIZING A DESIRABLE FUTURE

It is possible to listen appreciatively to a person's story and to think creatively about a desirable future with no other resource than a bit of quiet time. When services structure that person's life, the design and quality of the services determine how difficult it will be to move toward the desirable future revealed and enacted by careful listening, creative thinking, and courageous action.

Many pages of this book discuss efforts to change the culture, structure, and practices of service organizations. This emphasis makes me wonder if the book's central question—"Does person-centered planning work?"—might better be reformulated as "Under what conditions can a service honestly test the usefulness of person-centered planning?" The experience reflected in this book suggests three such conditions.

Organizational capacity to accommodate individual control: Because many service settings are organized to support groups of people with developmental disabilities, it can be so difficult to individualize supports that testing a person-centered planning team's ideas in action is impossible. Chapter 6 reports the positive effects of a large agency's revising its pattern of service to promote

- Staff continuity
- Decision making by people responsible for the service's responsiveness to the person's entire day
- Flexible transportation arrangements
- Personal space
- Individualized scheduling

This remarkable level of commitment to creating personalized supports—and, thus, creating the conditions for person-centered planning to make a real difference—exemplifies management taking responsibility for the contradiction between the organization's person-centered values and its actual capacities.

Microboards (see Chapter 7) emerged with the support of an agency that transformed itself from a provider of residential services to an organizer and supporter of people with developmental disabilities and their families. The microboards allowed people to both design and manage their own supports. This level of personalization would be very difficult without sufficient, flexible, and individualized government funding.

Organizational capacity to build staff teams able to keep and renew agreements that provide specific assistance: Even in small settings with stable staffing, simply following through on agreements to support continuing access to important opportunities can be difficult. Reaching toward new opportunities can be even more difficult. Chapter 5 identifies the importance of continued guidance, based on specific information about a person's everyday life, in increasing skilled staff's capacity to hold their focus on the person. This process, which included the creation and implementation of an Essential Team Plan to complement people's Essential Lifestyle Plans, supports the development of a stronger, more flexible team. Such a team is better able to respond to what it learns from person-centered planning.

Organizational capacity for learning: Person-centered planning helps an organization to test what it means when it says that its mission is to support inclusion, self-determination, or quality of life. Passing that test requires some organizations to change their culture, a process that calls for widespread learning about new skills and new reasons to do them. Chapter 4 describes an ongoing culture shift to make an institution as responsive as possible to its residents. Person-centered planning provided one element of a strategy for changing from a culture that successfully supported active treatment to a culture that offered residents greater respect and control. The managers took responsibility for their organization's change in functioning, which provided a reasonable context in which to test ideas that emerged from person-centered planning. Significant changes in the way things were done during the course of 10 years gave staff new conversation topics and shaped new roles with more direct responsibility. Everyone could track the effects of these changes in the following areas:

- Meals moved from the cafeteria to living units.
- Control of transportation and leisure activities shifted to living units.
- A functioning token economy was replaced by a procedure for negotiating with residents.
- Staff were encouraged to identify themselves as champions for individuals.

- Information was provided on increases in jobs.

- Information was given about decreases in use of emergency personal restraints.

- Information was provided regarding decreases in restrictive behavior reduction procedures.

- Information was given about use of medication for behavior management.

Responsible practitioners of person-centered planning will assist the people with whom they plan, as well as their allies, to assess these three capacities in the services that they use. When these conditions are present, participation in person-centered planning gives people a chance to develop more effective services while they pursue a desirable future. When these conditions are absent, progress will be difficult, and it will be especially important to build a strong person-centered planning group. This group will have to find ways that influence the service to increase its capacity to accommodate individual control, keep agreements about specific services, and learn new ways to provide support. If negotiations to improve organizational conditions fail, then the group will have to search for better quality alternative services or for other ways to realize a desirable future.

In 1965, Wolfensberger published the article "Diagnosis Diagnosed," in which he described a fallacy so appealing that it continues to entice people sincerely committed to improving service quality. In the 1960s, reformers talked of proper diagnosis. In the 1970s and 1980s, they talked of individualized program planning. In 2002, the "good guys" call for person-centered planning. Underneath the important differences among diagnosis, individual program planning, and person-centered planning lurks the same deception: Getting the plan right is the primary thing in helping someone to have a good life. This fallacy entices because it makes sense. Yet, it only makes sense to the degree that a capacity to respond exists that is at least as complex as the plan's requirements. As noted in Chapter 17, the thousands of hours of effort required in the late 1990s to produce grade-A, inspector-approved individual plans offered people little real improvement over the experiences of people whose diagnoses Wolfensberger analyzed 30 years before. What makes the difference to a person who relies on services is what the service itself offers every day, not what the plan says. If a system offers slots in boxes, then there is no need to decorate the interior walls of the boxes with colorful individual vision posters; its planning need not proceed beyond establishing eligibility and waiting list position. If an organization commits itself to the hard work of resolving the contradictions between its espoused values and its actual performance, then person-centered planning plays an important role. Responsible practitioners of person-centered planning will not get trapped hunting for the right words as if they were the key to a better life. They will encourage action for organizational change based on a common understanding of what is desirable for the person with whom they plan.

CONCLUSION: THE CENTRALITY OF DISCIPLINED IMAGINATION

At its best, person-centered planning lets disciplined imagination play in the lives of people who are profoundly vulnerable to low expectations and prejudices, which leave them on the sidelines of community life. It casts people with disabilities and their allies as the authors and enactors of positive stories about themselves as valued contributors to community life. As with any aesthetic activity, study, practice, and coaching build on natural ability to improve performance. Different media make different people come alive, so for some the activity will be more like playing basketball, piecing a quilt, composing a picture, or creating a dance than like telling a story. Poor stories are possible, so it is important to seek guidance and good examples.

Some people's ways of communicating leave the important people in their lives unable to hear their views about a life that would make sense. These other people have little choice but to create a story with a valued and central role for the person, whose preferences remain ambiguous. Then, these people make adjustments based on the person's responses to the real settings and experiences that resulted from their imagining (see Shafer, 1998, and O'Brien & Lyle O'Brien, 2000, for examples).

I like the idea, old as Aristotle, that the capacity to tell and respond to stories distinguishes zoe (biological life) from bios (human life). Shared narrative—whether communicated in drama, images, movement, or written words—is a source of the common understanding that makes possible community and compassion. Story is a foundation for phronesis, the practical wisdom necessary to make decisions that apply generally understood values in particular circumstances and draw a sensible balance among competing goods (e.g., freedom and safety). Story provides a channel for imagination to discover and broadcast the hopeful possibility that alternative realities are possible (Kearney, 2002). People with developmental disabilities come alive when careful attention is given to their stories. Person-centered planning can provide a social space for appreciating a person's story in a way that leads to meaningful new chapters. A decent community life begins with hearing and changing the stories of people who have been mindlessly excluded and controlled because of disability. Person-centered planning can provide a social space for shaping and learning from positive stories of community life for people with disabilities.

Because the people with developmental disabilities whom I know well face a long, tough struggle to claim and hold a valued place in community life, I like the idea that story, image, and dance help us—slowly and in our own time—to find meaning in disappointment, defeat, failure, tragic error, suffering, and death (Greene, 2001). People trapped in the box of segregation and socially sanctioned deprivation of opportunity need imagination almost as much as they need fresh air. Bringing disciplined imagination into people's lives is the privilege of those practitioners of person-centered planning who decide to honor people's concerns as worthy of attention.

REFERENCES

Auden, W.H. (1991). *Collected poems.* New York: Vintage Books.

Bandura, A., & Barbaranelli, C. (1996). Mechanisms of moral disengagement in the exercise of moral agency. *Journal of Personality and Social Psychology, 71*(2), 364–374.

Becker, H., Dumas, S., Houser, A., & Seay, P. (2000). How organizational factors contribute to innovations in service delivery. *Mental Retardation, 38*(5), 385–394.

Blatt, B. (1977). *The family papers.* Syracuse, NY: The Center on Human Policy.

Bruner, J. (1986). *Actual minds, possible worlds.* Cambridge, MA: Harvard University Press.

Carr, E., Horner, R., & Turnbull, A. (1999). *Positive behavior support for people with developmental disabilities: A research synthesis.* Washington, DC: American Association on Mental Retardation.

Greene, M. (2001). *Variations on a blue guitar: The Lincoln Center Institute lectures on aesthetic education.* New York: Teachers College Press.

Holburn, S., Jacobson, J., Vietze, P., & Sersen, E. (2000). Quantifying the process and outcomes of person-centered planning. *American Journal on Mental Retardation, 105*(5), 402–416.

Kearney, R. (2002). *On stories: Thinking in action.* New York: Routledge.

Lyle O'Brien, C., Mount, B., O'Brien, J., & Rosen, F. (in press). Pathfinders: Making a way from segregation to community life. In D. Fisher (Ed.), *Inclusive urban schools: Lessons learned in big city schools.* Baltimore: Paul H. Brookes Publishing Co.

Mank, D., Cioffi, A., & Yovanoff, P. (2000). Direct support in supported employment and its relation to job typicalness, co-worker involvement, and employment outcomes. *Mental Retardation, 38*(6), 506–516.

O'Brien, J., & Lyle O'Brien, C. (2000). *Walking toward freedom. One family's journey into self-determination.* Syracuse, NY: The Center on Human Policy.

Senge, P. (1990) *The fifth discipline: The art and practice of the learning organization.* New York: Doubleday.

Shafer, N. (1998). *Yes, she knows she's there!* Toronto: Inclusion Press.

Taylor, C. (1989). *Sources of the self: The making of the modern identity.* Cambridge, MA: Harvard University Press.

Tracy, D. (1986). *The analogical imagination.* New York: Crossroads.

Wolfensberger, W. (1965). Diagnosis diagnosed. *Journal of Mental Subnormality, 11*, 62–70.

Epilogue

In this book's preface we ask, "Does person-centered planning really work?" Now we ask, "Did we help answer that question?" We think so. In fact, we believe that this book sufficiently demonstrates that when people use person-centered principles as their true planning foundation, important life changes can and do occur. *Person-Centered Planning: Research, Practice, and Future Directions* illustrates an impressive range of changes that can occur, as well as the extent of those changes. It is not surprising that making more extensive changes takes more time and greater effort. Improvements in areas such as challenging behavior (Chapter 14), preference selection (Chapters 8 and 9), and team functioning (Chapter 15) occurred rather swiftly, but significant improvement in the more molar and often nebulous areas such as quality of life (Chapter 13), personal responsibility (Chapter 10), and organizational culture (Chapter 4) occurred only after person-centered planning had been underway for considerably longer periods of time.

Although the book focuses on research and evaluation, it also addresses historical and conceptual aspects of person-centered planning. When the philosophy and practice of person-centered planning are examined in the context of the history of services for people with disabilities, it is clear that person-centered planning is a young approach. Yet, its roots are old—many of which are fed by the normalization principle—whereas others are found in traditional group problem-solving techniques. More important, unlike theoretical frameworks such as the normalization principle and the new paradigm in developmental disabilities, person-centered planning offers a set of procedures designed to bring about the goals and aspirations espoused in these frameworks. One hundred years from now, this development might be regarded as an evolutionary leap in helping people with disabilities, but if the process is to survive and grow now, the method itself must make conceptual sense now. In other words, the improvements brought about from person-centered planning should be consistent with and should build on our current concepts of motivation, learning, culture, and disability. In this regard, as many of this book's authors contend, the principles and processes of person-centered planning indeed supplement and are compatible with what is already known about human behavior and society.

In presenting the effects of this long-term, multifaceted process, *Person-Centered Planning: Research, Practice, and Future Directions* can be viewed as an experiment in merging the philosophy of person-centered planning and the philosophy of science. The blending will be unsatisfying to the purist in either camp, yet it should pique the interests of both. The scientist may find new territory for social contribution, and the social advocate may discover new ways of informing the process of person-centered planning. Although one could argue that the research designs are quasi-experimental, many of the researchers who have contributed to this book have creatively and reliably measured outcomes considered by many investigators to be outside the realm of analysis. Conversely, although few examined the entire process of person-centered planning with all of its components, the contributors show how various principles and strategies of person-centered planning could be applied in innovative ways within service systems. There is a certain honesty in all of this, and there is no escaping the paradox that blending person-centered planning with scientific analysis dilutes but also strengthens both processes. We are convinced that the synergy of the two will advance the evolution of services and supports for people with disabilities.

Index

Page references followed by *f* and *t* indicate figures and tables, respectively